Bone Tumor Pathology

Editor

G. PETUR NIELSEN

SURGICAL PATHOLOGY CLINICS

www.surgpath.theclinics.com

Consulting Editor
JASON L. HORNICK

December 2021 • Volume 14 • Number 4

ELSEVIER

1600 John F. Kennedy Boulevard • Suite 1800 • Philadelphia, Pennsylvania, 19103-2899

http://www.theclinics.com

SURGICAL PATHOLOGY CLINICS Volume 14, Number 4
December 2021 ISSN 1875-9181, ISBN-13: 978-0-323-83562-6

Editor: Katerina Heidhausen
Developmental Editor: Diana Ang

Surgical Pathology Clinics (ISSN 1875-9181) is published quarterly by Elsevier Inc., 360 Park Avenue South, New York, NY 10010. Months of issue are March, June, September, and December. Business and Editorial Office: Elsevier Inc., 1600 John F. Kennedy Blvd., Ste. 1800, Philadelphia, PA 19103-2899. Accounting and Circulation Offices: Elsevier Inc., 3251 Riverport Lane, Maryland Heights, MO 63043. Periodicals postage paid at New York, NY and at additional mailing offices. Subscription prices are $228.00 per year (US individuals), $358.00 per year (US institutions), $100.00 per year (US students/residents), $283.00 per year (Canadian individuals), $383.00 per year (Canadian Institutions), $274.00 per year (foreign individuals), $383.00 per year (foreign institutions), and $120.00 per year (international students/residents), $100.00 per year (Canadian students/residents). Foreign air speed delivery is included in all *Clinics'* subscription prices. All prices are subject to change without notice. **POSTMASTER:** Send address changes to *Surgical Pathology Clinics*, Elsevier, 3251 Riverport Lane, Maryland Heights, MO 63043. **Customer Service: 1-800-654-2452 (US). From outside the United States, call 1-314-447-8871. Fax: 1-314-447-8029. E-mail:** JournalsCustomerServiceusa@elsevier.com **(for print support)** and JournalsOnlineSupport-usa@elsevier.com **(for online support)**.

Reprints. For copies of 100 or more, of articles in this publication, please contact the Commercial Reprints Department, Elsevier Inc., 360 Park Avenue South, New York, NY 10010-1710. Tel. 212-633-3874; Fax: 212-633-3820; E-mail: reprints@elsevier.com.

Surgical Pathology Clinics of North America is covered in *MEDLINE/PubMed (Index Medicus)*.

Contributors

CONSULTING EDITOR

JASON L. HORNICK, MD, PhD
Director of Surgical Pathology and
Immunohistochemistry, Brigham and Women's
Hospital, Professor of Pathology, Harvard
Medical School, Boston, Massachusetts, USA

EDITOR

G. PETUR NIELSEN, MD
Professor of Pathology, Harvard Medical
School, Pathologist, Department of Pathology,
Director of Bone and Soft Tissue Pathology,
Director of Electron Microscopy Unit,
Massachusetts General Hospital, Boston,
Massachusetts, USA

AUTHORS

FERNANDA AMARY, MD, PhD
Consultant Histopathologist, Histopathology
Department, Royal National Orthopaedic
Hospital, Stanmore, United Kingdom;
Honorary Associate Professor, Cancer
Institute, University College London, London,
United Kingdom

DANIEL BAUMHOER, MD
Bone Tumor Reference Center, Institute of
Medical Genetics and Pathology, University
Hospital Basel, University of Basel, Basel,
Switzerland

GIANLUCA BUSINELLO, MD
Department of Pathology, Azienda Ospedale-
Università Padova, Department of Medicine,
University of Padua School of Medicine,
Padua, Italy

CONNIE Y. CHANG, MD
Division of Musculoskeletal Imaging,
Department of Radiology, Radiologist,
Assistant Professor of Radiology, Harvard
Medical School, Massachusetts General
Hospital, Boston, Massachusetts, USA

IVAN CHEBIB, MD
James Homer Wright Pathology Laboratories,
Director of Immunohistochemistry Laboratory,
Assistant Professor of Pathology, Harvard
Medical School, Massachusetts General
Hospital, Boston, Massachusetts, USA

NICOLE A. CIPRIANI, MD
Department of Pathology, University of
Chicago Medical Center, Chicago, Illinois, USA

ANGELO P. DEI TOS, MD
Department of Pathology, Azienda Ospedale-
Università Padova, Department of Medicine,
University of Padua School of Medicine,
Padua, Italy

BRENDAN C. DICKSON, BA, BSc, MD, MSc, FRCPC
Staff Pathologist, Department of Pathology and
Laboratory Medicine, Mount Sinai Hospital,
Associate Professor, Department of
Laboratory Medicine and Pathobiology,
University of Toronto, Toronto, Ontario,
Canada

MATTEO FASSAN, MD
Department of Pathology, Azienda Ospedale-
Università Padova, Department of Medicine,
University of Padua School of Medicine,
Padua, Italy

ADRIENNE M. FLANAGAN, MD, PhD
Consultant Histopathologist, Histopathology
Department, Royal National Orthopaedic
Hospital, Stanmore, Middlesex, United
Kingdom; Professor of Pathology, UCL Cancer
Institute, University College London, London,
United Kingdom

MARCO GAMBAROTTI, MD
Unit of Surgical Pathology, Istituto Ortopedico
Rizzoli, Bologna, Italy

MEERA HAMEED, MD
Attending Pathologist and Member,
Department of Pathology, Memorial Sloan-
Kettering Cancer Center, New York, New York,
USA

DOROTHEE HARDER, MD
Department of Radiology, University Hospital
Basel, University of Basel, Basel, Switzerland

WOLFGANG HARTMANN, MD
Division of Translational Pathology, Gerhard-
Domagk-Institut of Pathology, University
Hospital Münster, Münster, Germany

YIN P. HUNG, MD, PhD
Assistant Pathologist, Assistant Professor,
Department of Pathology, Massachusetts
General Hospital, Harvard Medical School,
Boston, Massachusetts, USA

DARCY A. KERR, MD
Department of Pathology and Laboratory
Medicine, Dartmouth-Hitchcock Medical
Center, Lebanon, New Hampshire, USA;
Dartmouth Geisel School of Medicine,
Hanover, New Hampshire, USA

SCOTT E. KILPATRICK, MD
Director of Orthopedic Pathology, Staff
Pathologist, Department of Pathology,
Cleveland Clinic, Cleveland, Ohio, USA

SANTIAGO LOZANO-CALDERON, MD, PhD
Department of Orthopaedic Oncology,
Orthopedic Oncology Surgeon, Assistant
Professor of Orthopaedic Surgery, Harvard
Medical School, Massachusetts General
Hospital, Boston, Massachusetts, USA

ALESSANDRA F. NASCIMENTO, MD
Associate Professor, Department of Pathology,
Immunology and Laboratory Medicine,
University of Florida, Gainesville, Florida, USA

PAUL O'DONNELL, MD
Consultant Radiologist, Radiology
Department, Consultant, Department of
Histopathology, Royal National Orthopaedic
Hospital, Stanmore, United Kingdom;
Honorary Associate Professor, Cancer
Institute, University College London, London,
United Kingdom

JOHN D. REITH, MD
Staff Pathologist, Department of Pathology,
Cleveland Clinic, Cleveland, Ohio, USA

ALBERTO RIGHI, MD
Unit of Surgical Pathology, Istituto Ortopedico
Rizzoli, Bologna, Italy

MARTA SBARAGLIA, MD
Department of Pathology, Azienda Ospedale-
Università Padova, Department of Medicine,
University of Padua School of Medicine,
Padua, Italy

VAIYAPURI P. SUMATHI, MD, FRCPath
Consultant Histopathologist and Senior
Lecturer, Department of Musculoskeletal
Pathology, University Hospitals Birmingham,
The Royal Orthopaedic Hospital, Robert Aitken
Institute of Clinical Research, The Medical
School, University of Birmingham, Vincent
Drive, Birmingham, United Kingdom

ROBERTO TIRABOSCO
Consultant, Department of Histopathology,
Royal National Orthopaedic Hospital,
Stanmore, United Kingdom

AKIHIKO YOSHIDA, MD, PhD
Department of Diagnostic Pathology, National
Cancer Center Hospital, Tokyo, Japan

Contents

Benign bone-forming tumors comprise osteomas, osteoid osteomas, and osteoblastomas. Osteomas affect a wide age range and are usually discovered incidentally. They occur predominantly in the craniofacial skeleton and are classically composed of compact bone. Osteoid osteomas and osteoblastomas are painful lesions occurring in young patients. They are morphologically similar and characterized by FOS gene rearrangement and c-FOS expression at a protein level. Osteoid osteomas are usually smaller than 2 cm in maximum dimension with limited growth potential; osteoblastomas are larger than 2 cm and may be locally aggressive. Histologically both are composed of anastomosing trabeculae of woven bone.

Diagnosis of osteosarcoma can be challenging because of its diverse histological patterns and the lack of diagnostic biomarkers for most examples. This review summarizes the key pathologic findings of osteosarcoma subtypes (high-grade central, parosteal, low-grade central, periosteal, high-grade surface, and secondary) with an emphasis on describing and illustrating histological heterogeneity to help general pathologists. Differential diagnoses are listed for each entity, and histological subtype and distinguishing features, including molecular genetic findings (eg, *MDM2, IDH, H3F3A, FOS,* and *USP6*), are discussed. The review also covers recently established and emerging concepts and controversies regarding osteosarcoma.

Although uncommon in many pathology practices, cartilage-forming tumors represent some of the most frequent primary bone tumors. Diagnosis can be challenging given their variable histologic spectrum and the presence of overlapping morphologic, immunohistochemical, and genetic features between benign and malignant entities, particularly low-grade malignancies. Correlation with clinical findings and radiographic features is crucial for achieving an accurate diagnosis and appropriate clinical management, ranging from observation to excision. Tumors can be characterized broadly by their location in relation to the bone (surface or intramedullary). In specific instances, ancillary testing may help.

Chondrosarcomas are heterogeneous matrix-producing cartilaginous neoplasms with variable clinical behavior. Subtypes include conventional (75%), dedifferentiated (10%), clear cell (2%), mesenchymal (2%), and periosteal chondrosarcoma

(<1%). Tumor location and primary vs secondary also play a role. In conventional chondrosarcoma, histologic grading (I, II, and III) remains the gold standard for predicting recurrence and metastases. Due to the locally aggressive but overall nonmetastatic behavior, grade I chondrosarcomas (primary and secondary) of long and short tubular bones have been reclassified as atypical cartilaginous tumor. In this review, the pathologic features of malignant cartilage tumors are discussed with updates on recent genetic findings.

This review provides an overview of the spectrum of tumors showing notochordal differentiation. This spectrum encompasses benign entities that are mostly discovered incidentally on imaging, reported as benign notochordal cell tumor, usually not requiring surgical intervention; slowly growing and histologically low-grade tumors referred to as conventional chordoma but associated with a significant metastatic potential and mortality; and more aggressive disease represented by histologically higher-grade tumors including dedifferentiated chordoma, a high-grade biphasic tumor characterized by a conventional chordoma juxtaposed to a high-grade sarcoma, usually with a spindle or pleomorphic cell morphology, and associated with a poor prognosis and poorly differentiated chordoma.

Vascular tumors of bone can be diagnostically challenging because of their rarity and histologic overlap with diverse mimics. Vascular tumors of bone can be categorized as benign (hemangioma), intermediate-locally aggressive (epithelioid hemangioma), intermediate-rarely metastasizing (pseudomyogenic hemangioendothelioma), and malignant (epithelioid hemangioendothelioma and angiosarcoma). Recurrent genetic alterations have been described, such as FOSB rearrangements in pseudomyogenic hemangioendothelioma and a subset of epithelioid hemangiomas; CAMTA1 or TFE3 rearrangements in epithelioid hemangioendothelioma. This review discusses the clinical, histologic, and molecular features of vascular tumors of bone, along with diagnostic pitfalls and strategies for avoidance.

The intra-articular space is a relatively rare site of occurrence of neoplastic diseases. The 2 distinct groups of clinicopathologic entities that exhibit an almost exclusive tropism for the joints are represented by synovial chondromatosis and tenosynovial giant cell tumors (TGCT). Synovial chondromatosis is a locally aggressive chondrogenic neoplasm that very rarely can show malignant behavior. TGCT occur in 2 main variants, the localized variant and the more locally aggressive diffuse type. Malignant TCGT is exceedingly rare and is characterized by significant rates of both local recurrence and metastatic spread.

Undifferentiated small round cell sarcomas represent a heterogeneous group of mesenchymal neoplasms. While imprecise, this term nevertheless provides a useful framework for conceptualizing these tumors. This article highlights current trends in their classification based on morphology, immunohistochemistry, and advanced molecular techniques. As next-generation sequencing becomes commonplace in diagnostic laboratories pathologists can expect to differentiate these tumors with increasing confidence, and actively contribute to related discoveries. Ultimately, when synthesized with rigorous clinical outcome data and other investigative techniques, a more robust landscape for the molecular diagnosis and classification of undifferentiated small round cell sarcomas is expected to emerge in the future.

SURGICAL PATHOLOGY CLINICS

Preface
Bone Is Hard

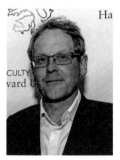

G. Petur Nielsen, MD
Editor

Bone is hard. Diagnosing bone tumors is a team approach that most importantly includes the pathologist and radiologist in conjunction with the orthopedic surgeon, along with the radiation and medical oncologist. It is imperative to emphasize that no bone tumor should ever be diagnosed without the pathologist studying the radiographic features, ideally with an experienced bone radiologist. Bone tumors are a diverse group of tumors, many of which are classified based on the matrix the neoplastic cells produce (ie, bone, cartilage). In recent years, there has been a lot of progress in understanding the genetics of bone tumors that in some instances can be diagnostically helpful (eg, *IDH1/2* mutation to distinguish high-grade chondrosarcoma from chondroblastic osteosarcoma, *USP6* translocation in an aneurysmal bone cyst, and immunohistochemical stains for H3K36M in chondroblastoma, and H3G34W in giant cell tumor of bone, to name a few).

The fifth edition of the World Health Organization (WHO) classification of bone tumors has recently been published. Compared with the previous edition,

1. Some tumors were moved between categories (eg, chondroblastoma was moved from intermediate rarely metastasizing to benign).

2. Some entities were deleted (such as liposarcoma, benign fibrous histiocytoma that is now considered a giant cell tumor of bone, and giant cell lesions of the small bones, which are now regarded as a solid aneurysmal bone cyst).

3. Some new entities were added (such as fibrocartilaginous mesenchymoma, hibernoma, and poorly differentiated chordoma).

One significant change in the WHO classification is the introduction of a separate "chapter" on undifferentiated small round cell sarcomas, where a number of these tumors are now classified based on the genetic alterations (such as *CIC* rearranged sarcoma and sarcoma with *BCOR* genetic alterations).

The concept of atypical cartilaginous tumor/chondrosarcoma grade 1 was first introduced in the fourth edition of the WHO classification in 2013. Few entities have caused as much confusion as the concept of atypical cartilaginous tumor. The most recent fifth edition of the WHO classification better defines atypical cartilaginous tumor and how that term should be used.

In this issue of *Surgical Pathology Clinics*, we have gathered renowned experts in bone pathology to discuss some of these most recent updates in selective tumors of bone and synovium,

Surgical Pathology 14 (2021) ix–x
https://doi.org/10.1016/j.path.2021.07.001
1875-9181/21/© 2021 Published by Elsevier Inc.

especially with regards to the current WHO classification and what changes have been made. This includes the discussion of new entities, updates on the molecular biology of bone tumors, and the application of immunohistochemistry in selected tumors. It is my hope that this selected review will be of diagnostic aid to the readers next time they encounter a tumor of the bone or the synovium.

G. Petur Nielsen, MD
Professor of Pathology, Harvard Medical School
Pathologist, Department of Pathology
Director of Bone and Soft Tissue Pathology
Director of Electron Microscopy Unit
Massachusetts General Hospital
55 Fruit Street
Boston, MA 02114, USA

E-mail address:
gnielsen@mgh.harvard.edu

Benign Bone-Forming Tumors

Fernanda Amary, MD, PhD[a,b,*], Adrienne M. Flanagan, MD, PhD[a,b], Paul O'Donnell, MD[b,c]

KEYWORDS

• Bone • Bone-forming • Benign • Osteoma • Osteoblastoma • Osteoma osteoid

Key points

- Osteomas occur in the craniofacial skeleton but on rare occasions they present as surface bone lesions in appendicular sites.
- Osteoid osteomas are small lesions, smaller than 2 cm in maximum dimension, usually intracortical and surrounded by dense sclerotic bone.
- Osteoblastomas are similar histologically to osteoid osteomas, usually larger than 2 cm in size, intramedullary, with a potential to grow. The most common site is the spine (neural arch).
- Osteoblastoma may display aggressive radiological features and needs to be differentiated from osteosarcoma.
- c-FOS expression and *FOS* gene rearrangement are present in most osteoid osteomas and osteoblastomas.

ABSTRACT

Benign bone-forming tumors comprise osteomas, osteoid osteomas, and osteoblastomas. Osteomas affect a wide age range and are usually discovered incidentally. They occur predominantly in the craniofacial skeleton and are classically composed of compact bone. Osteoid osteomas and osteoblastomas are painful lesions occurring in young patients. They are morphologically similar and characterized by *FOS* gene rearrangement and c-FOS expression at a protein level. Osteoid osteomas are usually smaller than 2 cm in maximum dimension with limited growth potential; osteoblastomas are larger than 2 cm and may be locally aggressive.

Histologically both are composed of anastomosing trabeculae of woven bone.

OSTEOMA

OVERVIEW

An osteoma is a benign bone-forming tumor arising on the surface of the bone, usually densely sclerotic, composed primarily of compact lamellar bone. Most occur in the craniofacial skeleton but on rare occasions they present in appendicular sites. Similar intramedullary lesions with characteristic imaging features are referred to as bone islands and are briefly discussed. Descriptive

[a] Histopathology Department, Royal National Orthopaedic Hospital, Brockley Hill, Stanmore, Greater London HA7 4LP, UK; [b] Cancer Institute, University College London, 72 Huntley Street, London WC1E 6DD, UK; [c] Radiology Department, Royal National Orthopaedic Hospital, Brockley Hill, Stanmore, Greater London HA7 4LP, UK
* Corresponding author. Histopathology Department, Royal National Orthopaedic Hospital, Brockley Hill, Stanmore, Greater London HA7 4LP, UK.
E-mail address: Fernanda.amary@nhs.net

Surgical Pathology 14 (2021) 549–565
https://doi.org/10.1016/j.path.2021.06.002
1875-9181/21/© 2021 Elsevier Inc. All rights reserved.

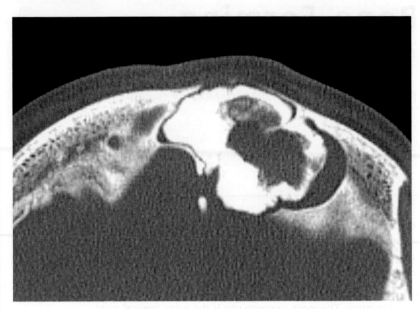

Fig. 1. Paranasal sinus osteoma. Axial CT shows a densely ossified mass in the frontal sinus containing eccentric lucency and causing marked erosion of the anterior and posterior cortex. Histology showed an osteoma with osteoblastoma-like features (see **Fig. 4**).

terms such as ivory exostosis (due to the density of paranasal sinus lesions), juxtacortical or parosteal osteoma (for lesions in the appendicular skeleton), and enostosis (bone island) are not recommended.[1]

Craniofacial osteomas are usually peripheral (surface) lesions but rarely may be central (intramedullary). They occur most frequently in the paranasal sinus, mandible, maxilla, or orbit,[2] but any craniofacial bone can be affected. Peripheral osteomas are considered to arise from the periosteum and, depending on their location, present as a mass: lesions on the mandibular condyle may prevent complete opening of the mouth.[3] Central osteomas arise from the endosteal surface[4] and may cause deformity if large: these are rare lesions unless associated with Gardner syndrome.[3] Osteomas occurring in the paranasal sinuses are slow growing and most are discovered incidentally: symptoms depend on location, size, and direction of growth. The frontal sinus is most frequently affected: headache, facial pain, sinus or nasal obstruction, exophthalmos, visual disturbance, and rarely symptoms from intracranial extension may result.[5–8] The earliest report of an osteoma dates from Ancient Egypt and was discovered in the frontal sinus of a mummy using computed tomography (CT).[9] As most lesions are discovered incidentally, the true incidence is unknown and ranges from 0.42% of 16,000 sinus radiographs to 6.4% of 1724 CT studies in patients with sinus disease.[10,11] Paranasal osteomas are usually detected in adults but affect a wide age range and there is a slight male predominance.[12]

Sporadic osteomas tend to be solitary. Multiple osteomas of the calvarium and mandible should raise the possibility of Gardner syndrome, a form of autosomal dominant familial adenomatous polyposis caused by mutations in the *APC* gene. Fifty percent to 80% of subjects with this condition have osteomas, with an average of 5.9 osteomas per person.[13] The frontal sinus is the most common location in Gardner syndrome, but a pedunculated osteoma at the angle of the mandible is also not uncommon and characteristic of the syndrome. Central osteomas may occur within the maxilla and mandible near the tooth roots, with additional multiple sclerotic lesions in flat and tubular bones.[14] Sporadic and syndromic osteomas occurring in the calvarium and sino-orbital areas are microscopically indistinguishable.

Osteomas of the appendicular skeleton are rare lesions that, in the largest series, accounted for only 0.035% of 40,000 bone lesions.[15] All were in long tubular bones, 86% in the lower limb. Patients, usually adults (21–66 years of age in the series of Bertoni and colleagues[15]) present with a slowly growing mass, occasional pain, and, rarely, restricted movement.

Bone islands are asymptomatic intramedullary sclerotic bone lesions consisting of compact bone, occurring in areas of the skeleton formed by endochondral ossification. The incidence of these lesions is approximately 1% on radiographs,[16] but they are frequent observations on cross-sectional imaging studies, occurring typically in the pelvis, femur, and spine: again, they may be found in any bone. Multiple bone islands occur in meta epiphyseal locations in osteopoikilosis.

RADIOLOGIC FEATURES

Paranasal sinus osteomas are usually peripheral lesions, arising from the bone surface and protruding into the lumen. They are typically smaller than 2 cm in diameter and when larger than 3 cm have been termed giant osteomas.[17] The imaging features are best shown by CT: they may be pedunculated, sessile, or appear as a small mass-like expansion of the thin bony septa that traverse the ethmoid air cells and the frontal sinus.[18] A homogeneously dense lobular mass is typically seen. Heterogeneous lesions, with central trabecular bone density or occasionally a "ground glass" appearance, and peripheral dense bone may be seen with cancellous/spongiose osteomas[19] and those containing osteoblastoma-like features.[20] MRI appearances reflect the homogeneous sclerotic bone of the compact osteoma (causing a signal "void" on all sequences) and marrow within a cancellous osteoma.[19] Large lesions expand the sinus, remodeling the surrounding cortical bone (**Fig. 1**), and are more likely to protrude into or erode the orbit, nasal cavity, and skull base.

Peripheral osteomas also occur on the inner and outer tables of the calvarium,[21] in the facial skeleton, and in the jaws. Again, they may be sessile or pedunculated and are often homogeneously dense. Sessile lesions show a lobular morphology when large and may be associated with remodeling or thickening of the adjacent cortex.[22]

Central craniofacial osteomas are well-defined intramedullary densities, which show somewhat nonspecific imaging appearances, overlapping with other inflammatory, traumatic, and neoplastic processes, including fibro-osseous lesions[3] and bone islands. Origin from the endosteal cortex, lobular morphology, and a well-defined border (not the brush border of a bone island, see later in this article) help to differentiate these similar lesions. Central osteomas usually grow slowly, causing expansile remodeling of the bone, tooth displacement, and occasionally tooth resorption.[23]

Appendicular osteomas are round or elongated ossified masses located on the bone surface (**Fig. 2**). They are homogeneous and show density similar to the cortex, with no significant internal lucency. The superficial surface is smooth or, in large lesions, lobular,[24] and the interface with adjacent soft tissue is usually well-defined, without invasion.[15,25] The cortex adjacent to the lesion may be thickened but a distinct periosteal reaction is almost invariably absent[15]; there is occasional

encroachment of dense tumor into the medulla.[15] Cortico-medullary continuity, the hallmark of an osteochondroma, is not identified and there is no lucent cleavage plane between the lesion and the cortex, which is a feature of parosteal osteosarcoma.[25] Radio-isotope bone scans are normal in the vascular and blood pool phases, but there is slightly increased activity on static images.[25] MRI shows a signal void similar to cortical bone, with no adjacent marrow edema or unossified component.[25]

Bone islands are intramedullary, homogeneous foci of dense bone. They are round or oval and when in a tubular bone, tend to be oriented along its long axis, parallel to cortex.[26] They usually measure smaller than 2 cm in diameter, but larger (giant) lesions are possible: bone islands may show slow growth or even become smaller.[27] The hallmark of a bone island is its nonaggressive, blended interface with surrounding trabecular bone: dense streaks radiate from the lesion, resulting in a feathered appearance/brush border (**Fig. 3**). It shows homogeneous low signal on

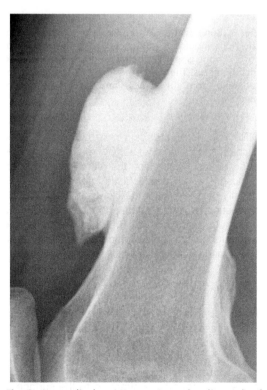

Fig. 2. Appendicular osteoma. Lateral radiograph of the distal femur showing an ossified, uniformly dense mass arising from the surface of the bone. It is well-defined but slightly lobulated superiorly and inferiorly. The cortex at the base of the lesion is thickened: there is no interposed lucent plane between the tumor and the femur.

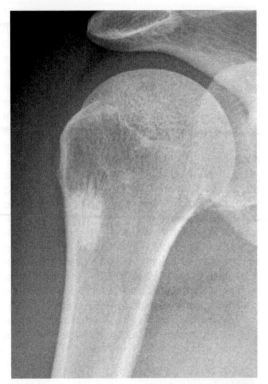

Fig. 3. Bone island. Anteroposterior radiograph of the right shoulder. A lesion showing the density of cortical bone is seen in the lateral aspect of the proximal humerus. There are fine linear bony projections radiating from the bone island into the adjacent medulla.

MRI, with no surrounding marrow edema. Bone islands show variable activity on radio-isotope bone scans, which are therefore unreliable for exclusion of an osteoblastic metastasis.[26] The density of the lesion on CT is useful to make this distinction: a mean attenuation of 885 HU and maximum attenuation of 1060 HU were reported as useful figures, below which a sclerotic metastasis was favored.[28]

GROSS FEATURES

Macroscopically, in the sino-orbital area, osteomas are densely ossific masses that usually do not exceed 2 cm in maximum dimension.

Osteomas that occur on the surface of long bones have macroscopic features of an ossified mass with broad base attached to the surface of the bone or the appearance of irregular cortical thickening (**Fig. 4A**).[15]

Bone islands consist of dense compact bone within the medullary cavity, with occasional slender attachment to the endosteal surface. They are ovoid areas with the long axis parallel

to the cortex, usually measuring up to 2 cm, most, however, being smaller than 1 cm in diameter.

MICROSCOPIC FEATURES

Classically osteomas are characterized by mature compact-type lamellar bone organized into Haversian canals and osteons. The periphery of the tumor is often composed predominantly of woven bone with osteoblastic rimming. However, osteomas may also show broad trabeculae of cancellous bone and fibrous stroma (**Fig. 5**). Osteoblastoma-like areas may be seen, particularly in sino-orbital osteomas, and are usually found where the tumor contacts or is attached to the host bone.[20] Another feature that may be observed is the presence of numerous cement lines giving it a Pagetoid appearance.

Osteomas of long bones also feature dense compact sclerotic lamellar bone with evident Haversian systems and cement lines, blending with host bone (**Fig. 4**). The pronounced cement lines usually give it a Pagetoid appearance. Invasion of the medullary canal is not seen.[15]

Bone islands are formed from compact lamellar bone and at the periphery, the thickened bone trabeculae merge with the surrounding lamellar bone in a spiculate pattern (**Fig. 6**).

MOLECULAR PATHOLOGY FEATURES

There are no specific molecular markers. Multiple osteomas are associated with Gardner syndrome (*APC* mutation). Multiple bone islands are seen in the setting of osteopoikilosis and *inactivating* mutations of the *LEMD3* gene.

DIFFERENTIAL DIAGNOSIS

Craniofacial osteomas may be misdiagnosed as osteoblastomas when osteoblastoma-like areas are present.[20] c-FOS immunohistochemistry can be useful in this differentiation.[29]

For osteomas of long bones, the differential diagnosis includes sessile osteochondromas and parosteal osteosarcoma.[24] In relation to the former, osteomas do not show continuity with the medullary bone or a cartilaginous cap usually seen in sessile osteochondromas. Parosteal osteosarcomas are expected to have lucent areas, with the periphery usually unmineralized. Chondroid areas, which are seen in a subset of parosteal osteosarcomas, are not present in osteomas. A spindle cell component is also not a feature of osteomas, nor is the presence of *MDM2* gene amplification, the molecular hallmark of parosteal osteosarcomas.

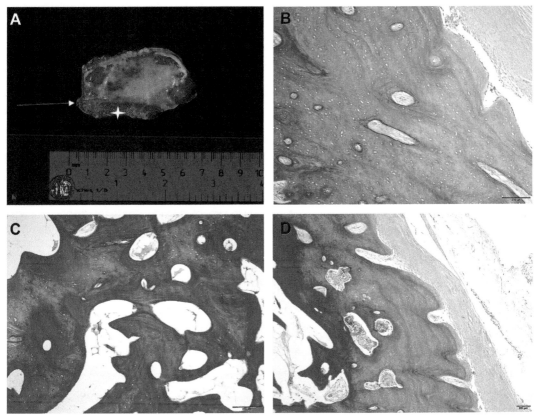

Fig. 4. Appendicular osteoma. (*A*) Macroscopic appearance of the resection specimen showing a surface sclerotic lesion with intact cortex (*arrow*) and uninvolved medullary canal (*star*). Microscopic features include compact lamellar bone showing prominent Haversian systems (*B*), cancellous and compact mixed woven and lamellar bone (*C*), and growing front covered by fibrous tissue (*D*).

Bone islands pose an important differential diagnosis with osteoblastic metastases.[28]

PROGNOSIS

The prognosis is excellent in most cases, and asymptomatic patients can be left untreated. Simple excision is usually curative.

- Pathologic Key Features of Osteoma
  - Compact/cortical lamellar (or mixed woven and lamellar) bone
  - Prominent Haversian systems
  - Broad trabeculae of woven bone and fibrous tissue at the growing front
- Differential Diagnosis and Pitfalls of Osteomas.
  - Osteoblastoma-like features may be seen in craniofacial osteomas.
  - Surface osteomas of the appendicular skeleton must be differentiated from:

- sessile osteochondromas (absence of continuity with medullary canal and no cartilaginous cap)
- parosteal osteosarcoma (absence of an intertrabecular spindle cell component and cartilaginous component. If in doubt, the absence of *MDM2* gene amplification should also help to confirm the diagnosis)
- Bone islands: careful differential diagnosis with osteosclerotic metastatic deposits.

OSTEOID OSTEOMA

OVERVIEW

An osteoid osteoma (OO) is defined by the World Health Organization (WHO) as "A benign bone-forming tumor characterized by small size (less than 2 cm) and limited growth potential."[30]

Most (75%) are intracortical, approximately 25% intramedullary and a small number subperiosteal or surface. Any bone can be affected, but the long bones of the lower limb are particularly

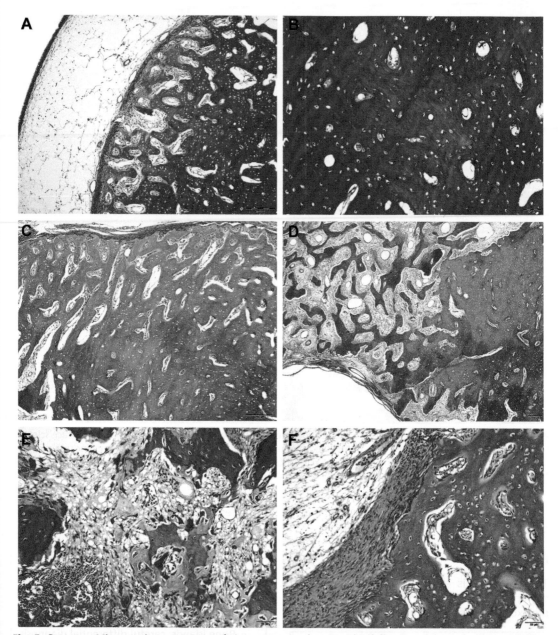

Fig. 5. Osteoma. Microscopic appearance of sinus osteoma showing the following: (*A*) respiratory epithelium overlying a lesion composed of compact bone; (*B*) compact predominantly woven bone with prominent Haversian system; (*C*) periphery of the lesion showing a looser cancellous pattern merging with fibrous tissue; (*D*) areas displaying a more trabecular pattern with intervening fibrous stroma and dilated blood vessels; (*E*) active bone remodeling with osteoblasts and areas of bone resorption (osteoclasts) giving an osteoblastoma-like appearance; and (*F*) growing front showing woven bone with osteoblastic rimming merging with a layer of cellular fibrous tissue.

common sites, accounting for approximately 50% of cases[31]: most femoral and tibial OOs are intra-cortical and diaphyseal. Other frequent locations include the spine, where OO occurs most frequently in the neural arch, and the small bones of the hands and feet.

Patients are usually young at the time of diagnosis (5–25 years) and male individuals are affected more commonly than female.[31] Most lesions present with pain, initially mild but becoming progressively more severe: night pain leading to disturbed sleep is common.[31] Nonsteroidal anti-

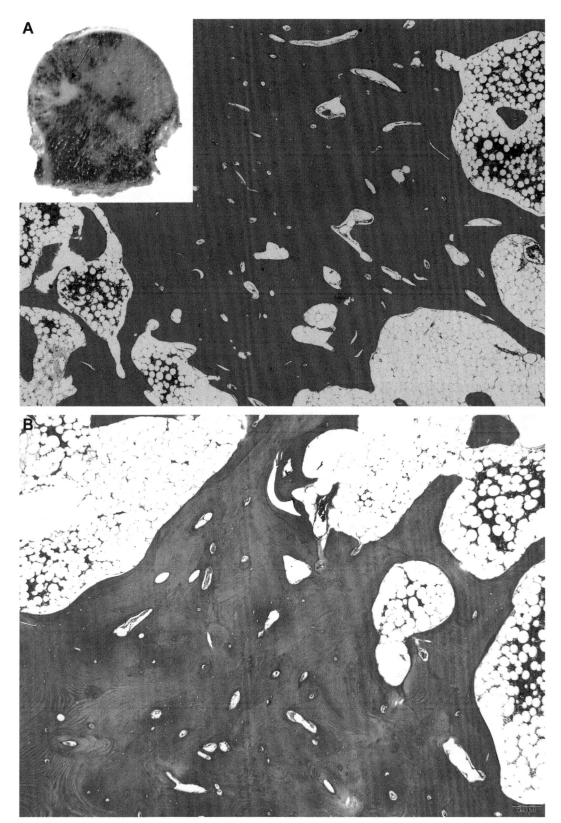

Fig. 6. Bone island. Photomicrograph showing a compact bone lesion merging with host lamellar bone trabeculae in a spiculated pattern (*A, B*). Inset (*top left corner*) showing the macroscopic appearance of a bone island formed by compact bone (*black arrow*) in a hip replacement specimen.

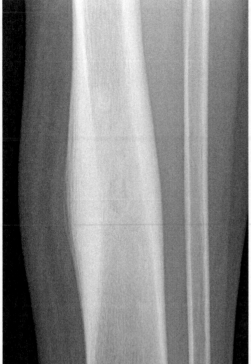

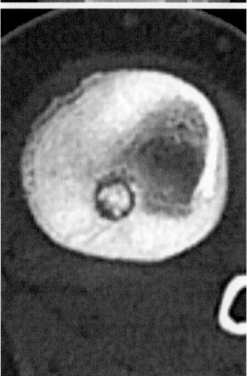

inflammatory medication relieves pain, at least temporarily.[32] Occasionally, OO is painless[33]: other presentations include a bony swelling (anterior tibial lesions), scoliosis, a limp (lesions within or near the hip) and a swollen, "drumstick," digit (OO in the phalanges).[34–37] Distal metaphyseal lesions adjacent to the open physis of a long bone may be associated with bone overgrowth and asymmetry.[38] Intra-articular lesions, accounting for approximately 10% of OO, present with relatively nonspecific features of an arthropathy and the diagnosis is often delayed.[39]

RADIOLOGIC FEATURES

Intracortical OO often shows characteristic imaging appearances.[40] The predominant feature is usually non-neoplastic new bone formation, causing fusiform, eccentric cortical thickening (**Fig. 7**A). Reactive new bone formation is also often seen in the medulla (endosteal sclerosis). The tumor ("nidus") is indicated by a round or ovoid lucency, often smaller than 10 mm in diameter (5–20 mm), surrounded by thickened cortex. The nidus is frequently occult on radiographs, requiring CT. CT also shows variable mineralization within the center of the nidus and there are often curvilinear lucent foci corresponding to vessels, extending from the periosteal surface of the bone toward the OO (vascular groove sign)[41] (**Fig. 7**B). The nidus is often seen on MRI, but small lesions may be occult.[42] It shows intermediate signal on T1-weighted images and intermediate to high signal on fluid-sensitive sequences (hyperintense to the surrounding thickened cortex on both sequences)[42]: lower signal is seen in the nidus in mineralized tumors. Hyperintensity in adjacent bone marrow and soft tissue, consistent with edema, is also typical. The nidus shows enhancement following contrast injection: using dynamic contrast enhanced scans, the nidus shows early arterial enhancement, typically within 6 seconds of the adjacent artery, and early partial wash-out, compared with the slower progressive enhancement of the adjacent marrow.[43,44]

Cancellous lesions cause medullary bone sclerosis and surrounding edema-like signal, but little by way of periosteal response or cortical thickening.[45] Heavily mineralized lesions resemble a bone island but usually lack the irregular margin: medullary sclerosis and marrow edema are also useful for differentiation (**Fig. 8**). Cancellous OOs are found most frequently in the spine, small bones of the hands and feet, and occasionally in long bones. Surface/subperiosteal lesions cause

Fig. 7. Intracortical OO. (*A*) Anteroposterior radiograph of the left tibia. There is eccentric cortical thickening, most marked medially, medullary sclerosis, and an oval lucency projected over the center of the bone (the nidus). (*B*) Axial CT of the left tibia. In cross-section, the nidus is round and located in the deep aspect of the thickened cortex. This lesion shows dense central ossification with a surrounding lucent halo. Faint linear lucencies extent from the cortical surface to the nidus, corresponding to vessels (the "vascular groove" sign).

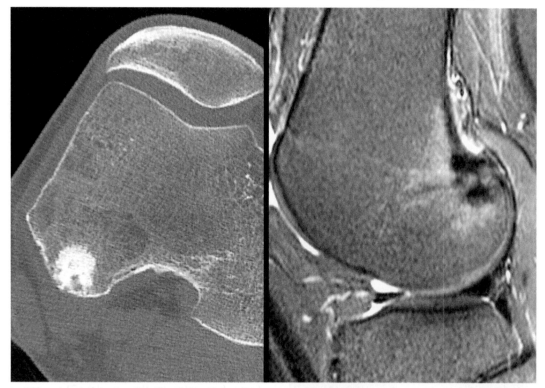

Fig. 8. Intramedullary OO. Axial CT through the right knee (*left*) shows a densely mineralized intramedullary tumor at the posterior aspect of the lateral femoral condyle, with an irregular edge, raising the possibility of a bone island. Sagittal STIR MRI (*right*) confirms that the lesion is surrounded by edema-like hyperintensity, which is not a feature of bone islands. A heavily calcified chondroblastoma could also show these appearances: OO was confirmed using CT-guided needle biopsy.

erosion of the outer cortex of the bone (**Fig. 9**), with no or only mild adjacent cortical thickening.[45] They are commonest at the medial aspect of the femoral neck and neck of the talus.[45,46]

Intra-articular OO (**Fig. 10**) shows distinct clinical and imaging features. More than 50% occur in the hip, with the OO typically intramedullary or on the bone surface.[47] Joint space may be reduced or widened, the latter reflecting synovial

Fig. 9. Surface (subperiosteal) OO. Axial CT of the left hip. The OO is eroding the surface of the bone, with adjacent medullary sclerosis but no significant cortical thickening.

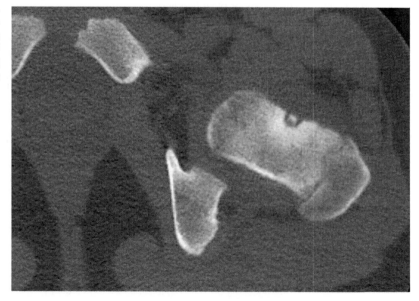

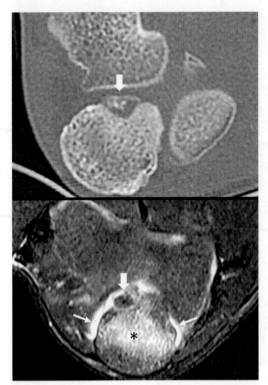

Fig. 10. Intra-articular OO. Axial CT (*upper image*) shows a mineralized nidus arising on the surface of the olecranon (*arrow*); the olecranon shows mild medullary sclerosis. Axial T2-weighted MRI with fat saturation (*lower image*) shows the hypointense nidus (*block arrow*), edema-like signal in adjacent marrow (*asterisk*) and high signal within the joint, consistent with synovitis/fluid (*arrows*).

proliferation.[48] Reactive cortical thickening may be seen at a distance from the lesion rather than in the joint; for example, inferior to the femoral neck or in the distal humerus: other plain film findings are osteopenia, thickening of the femoral neck, enlargement of the head (coxa magna) and osteophyte formation.[44,48] MRI usually shows a prominent effusion or synovitis and marrow edema-like signal, consistent with an arthropathy, and the nidus may be overlooked. On technetium isotope bone scans, which in appendicular sites usually show focal uptake in the nidus, diffuse activity may be seen.[49,50] The nidus is reliably localized by CT in intra-articular cases.

GROSS FEATURES

OOs are rarely excised, but historical cases show a central area of vascularized purplish to tan tissue (nidus), that is by definition smaller than 2 cm, but usually smaller than 1.5 cm in diameter. The nidus is surrounded by compact sclerotic bone in intracortical lesions.

MICROSCOPIC FEATURES

Histologically the tumor, referred to as the nidus, is composed of trabeculae of woven bone and osteoid lined by a single layer of osteoblasts (**Fig. 11**). There is intervening loose fibrovascular tissue, with dilated blood vessels and numerous scattered osteoblasts. This is surrounded, in most cases, by sclerotic/compact bone in different stages of maturation. The nidus also can have sclerotic areas, usually in the center, but the network of dilated blood vessels is usually still evident.

The osteoblastic cells usually show nuclear expression of c-FOS on immunohistochemistry.[29]

MOLECULAR PATHOLOGY FEATURES

OOs and osteoblastomas are associated with *FOS* or rarely *FOSB* gene rearrangement in the vast majority of cases.[29,51]

DIFFERENTIAL DIAGNOSIS

The main differential diagnosis is with osteoblastoma (see later in this article). They can be morphologically identical and arbitrarily separated by size, the latter larger than 2 cm and displaying a potential for continuous growth.[52,53] Reactive new bone formation is also in the differential diagnosis.

PROGNOSIS

OOs have limited growth and no aggressive features. Surgical or percutaneous image-guided treatments are usually curative.[54]

- Pathologic Key Features of Osteoid Osteoma
  - Interconnecting trabeculae of woven bone rimmed by plump osteoblasts.
  - Densely vascularized fibroblastic stroma with dilated capillary-type blood vessels.
  - Osteoclast-type giant cells.
  - Sclerotic lamellar bone surrounding the lesion (in intracortical tumors).
  - c-FOS nuclear expression in the osteoblastic component.

OSTEOBLASTOMA

OVERVIEW

Osteoblastomas are benign osteoblastic lesions, representing approximately 1% of primary bone

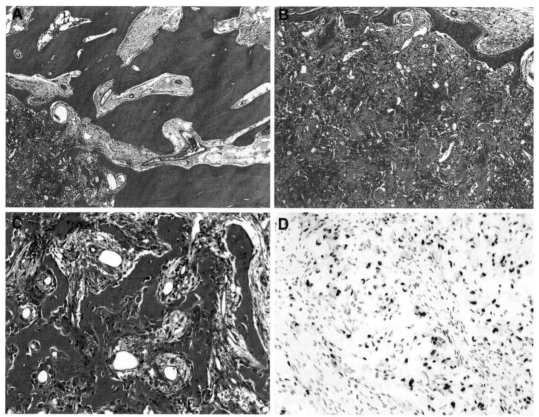

Fig. 11. OO. Photomicrograph of an OO showing (*A*) the nidus (*bottom left corner*) surrounded by sclerotic compact lamellar bone. (*B, C*) Woven bone trabeculae rimmed by plump osteoblasts in a richly vascularized fibroblastic stroma with dilated capillary-type blood vessels. (*D*) c-FOS nuclear expression limited to the osteoblastic component: the fibroblastic stroma is negative.

tumors[54] and therefore considerably rarer than OO. They can be indistinguishable from OOs on biopsies[55] and are differentiated by size, site, and radiological/macroscopic features. Osteoblastoma is defined by the WHO classification as a locally aggressive bone-forming tumor with potential for growth, generally measuring larger than 2 cm in diameter.[52]

Osteoblastomas are usually central intramedullary lesions with or without bone expansion,[55] but can occur on the surface of bone (intracortical and subperiosteal). They may arise in any bone,[53] but are most frequent in the spine, femur, tibia, mandible, and foot and ankle: rare cases have been reported in soft tissue and the skin.[56,57] A third of the cases present in the spine, the tumor usually located in the neural arch, but not infrequently extending to the vertebral body.[53,58] Like OO, osteoblastomas occur predominantly in the second and third decades, 70% in those younger than 31, and are twice as frequent in male individuals.[53,58]

Pain is the most common symptom, usually less responsive to nonsteroidal anti-inflammatories than OOs and not typically nocturnal.[53,54] Local swelling and tenderness at the site of the lesion, neurologic symptoms and deformity (scoliosis and torticollis) related to spinal osteoblastomas, and disuse atrophy and a limp due to lesions in the lower limb, are also common presenting symptoms.[59] Osteoblastomas also rarely present with systemic symptoms, including fever, anorexia, anemia, finger clubbing, and lymphadenopathy (so-called "toxic" osteoblastoma).[60]

IMAGING

Long bone tumors are usually located in the diaphysis or metadiaphysis. Typically, there is a well-demarcated, intramedullary lucent lesion. Ossification or occasionally punctate calcification resembling a cartilaginous matrix[61] is seen centrally, often surrounded by a lucent halo (**Fig. 12**) and expansile remodeling of the bone.[53] The

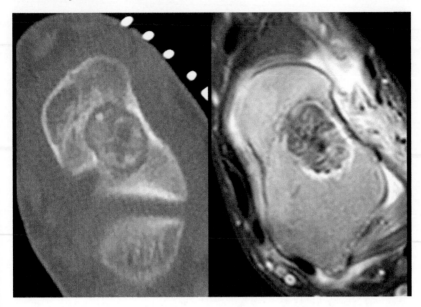

Fig. 12. Osteoblastoma of the left talus. Axial CT (*left*) at the time of biopsy shows a well-defined, ossified tumor. A lucent "halo" is seen peripherally and there is surrounding medullary and cortical sclerosis. Axial T2-weighted MRI with fat saturation (*right*) shows the mineralized tumor is hypointense, the halo hyperintense, and talar marrow diffusely edematous.

margin is usually sclerotic with adjacent medullary sclerosis. Cortical thickening, due in part to solid (nonaggressive) periosteal new bone formation is common. The features are usually nonaggressive and may resemble a large OO (**Fig. 13**); however, they may show aggressive features, including poor definition, lucency, cortical destruction, and a lamellated or spiculated periosteal response.[53] Toxic osteoblastomas (see previously) may be associated with periosteal new bone formation in other bones, either in the vicinity of the tumor or generalized, considered to be related to prostaglandin production,.[60,62] Subperiosteal osteoblastomas are mineralized masses protruding from the bone surface: they may show an ossified rim, lobular morphology, and mixed mineralized and lucent areas: occasionally they are predominantly lucent, with nonspecific imaging appearances.[61,63,64] The adjacent cortex may be thickened and the medulla sclerotic but otherwise intact.[63]

Vertebral osteoblastomas are typically expansile destructive tumors arising within the neural arch. They share many imaging features with long bone osteoblastomas. However, the cortex of the relatively small neural arch is often destroyed,[53] the lesion either surrounded by a shell of bone or partially devoid of an ossified

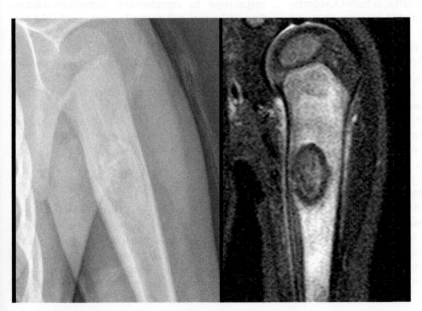

Fig. 13. Osteoblastoma of the left humerus. Anteroposterior radiograph (*left*) shows a mineralized medullary lesion resembling a large OO, with expansile remodeling and cortical thickening. The lesion is hypointense on short tau inversion recovery MRI (*right*), with extensive adjacent marrow edema-like signal.

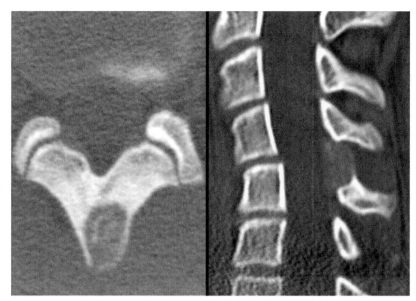

Fig. 14. Vertebral osteo-blastoma. Axial CT of the lumbar spine (*left*): mildly expansile lucent lesion in the spinous process of L3 with central ossification and adjacent medullary sclerosis. The cortex is thinned but largely intact. Sagittal CT reconstruction of the cervical spine (*right*) shows an osteoblastoma on the neural arch of C5, devoid of surrounding cortical bone and showing faint internal density.

margin. CT shows the extent of bone destruction, the type of matrix mineralization and adjacent cortical thickening (**Fig. 14**): features that are often poorly appreciated on radiographs.

Mineralized areas return low signal intensity on both T1-weighted and fluid-sensitive sequences. Nonmineralized tumor may show low, intermediate, or occasionally high signal on T1-weighted images, the latter due to the vascularized stroma[65]: these areas also tend to show hyperintensity on fluid-sensitive sequences.[34] MRI often shows hyperintensity in adjacent marrow and soft tissue, a feature shared with OO and called the "flare phenomenon," thought to represent prostaglandin-mediated inflammatory edema.[66] Fluid-fluid levels may be seen within medullary and periosteal osteoblastomas.[64,65,67] Radio-isotope bone scans show high uptake due to marked osteoblastic activity and vascularity.[65,68] Osteoblastomas show marked avidity for fluorodeoxyglucose on PET scans,[68] but these are rarely performed unless there is concern about malignancy.

GROSS FEATURES

Osteoblastomas are larger than OOs: on average 4 cm in maximum dimension. There is less pronounced sclerosis surrounding the lesion, but they are usually relatively well-defined. Bone expansion and cortical breach can be seen. When fresh, the rich vasculature gives a purplish/tan appearance to the tumor. Secondary aneurysmal bone cystlike changes may be present in the form of blood-filled spaces.

MICROSCOPIC FEATURES

Similar to OO, osteoblastomas are composed of anastomosing woven bone trabeculae rimmed by plump osteoblasts. The intervening fibrous stroma is richly vascularized with dilated capillary-type blood vessels, a feature that is usually easily appreciated at low power. Areas of sclerosis formed by confluent bone trabeculae may be seen within the tumor, occasionally forming a Pagetoid appearance.

In the absence of a nidus surrounded by sclerotic bone, a feature of OO, osteoblastomas and OO are histologically virtually identical.[55,69] Osteoblastomas are usually well-defined with peripheral maturation of the bone at the edge of the tumor[53] (**Fig. 15**), although osteoblastomas more frequently display large osteoblasts with bizarre nuclei (degenerative-type atypia).[53]

The so-called aggressive osteoblastoma is a controversial lesion, composed of large epithelioid osteoblasts that are usually more mitotically active.[54,70] Some tumors may be multinodular with a multifocal growth pattern that can mimic permeation.[53,70]

c-FOS nuclear expression is detected in most osteoblastomas (approximately 83%), limited to the osteoblastic component.[29] Although this is a useful diagnostic marker, focal expression may be present in up to 14% of osteosarcomas, requiring careful interpretation and clinical correlation.[29] Identification of *FOS* gene rearrangement using fluorescence in situ hybridization (FISH) is more specific in the setting of a bone-forming

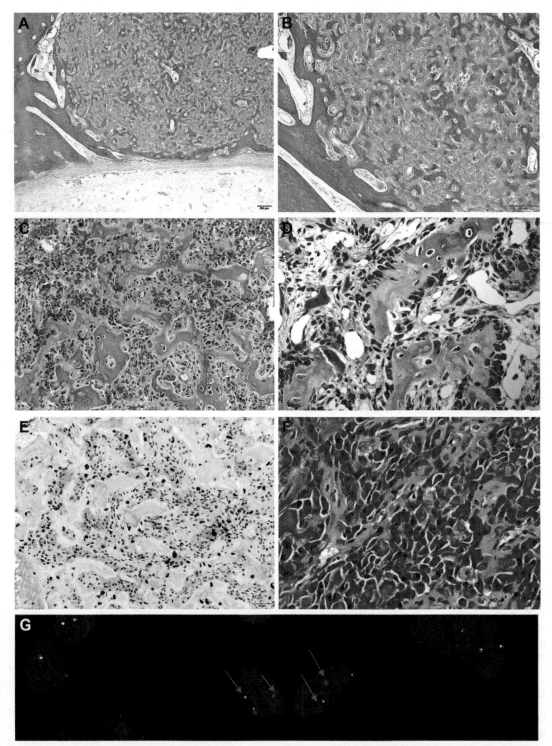

Fig. 15. Osteoblastoma showing well-defined borders (*A*) and peripheral maturation of the woven bone trabeculae merging with lamellar host bone (*B*). (*C*) Anastomosing woven bone trabeculae, osteoblasts, scattered osteoclasts, and dilated blood vessels. (*D*) Woven bone trabeculae in an osteoblastoma, rimmed by osteoblasts and scattered osteoclasts. Intervening loose fibrous stroma with dilated capillary-type blood vessels. (*E*) c-FOS nuclear expression highlighting plump osteoblastic cells. (*F*) Cellular epithelioid osteoblastoma. (*G*) Interphase FISH for c-*FOS* showing clear break-apart signals (arrows).

tumor.[29] Other markers of osteoblastic differentiation, such as SATB2, are also expressed by the osteoblastic component.[71]

MOLECULAR PATHOLOGY FEATURES

Both osteoblastomas and OOs are associated with rearrangement of *FOS* and rarely *FOSB* in the vast majority of cases, further supporting the association of these 2 tumors.[29,51] In addition, osteoblastomas are thought to have a "quiet" genome, with few somatic and copy number alterations, which may be helpful in excluding osteosarcoma in difficult cases.[51]

DIFFERENTIAL DIAGNOSIS

The main differential diagnosis when considering osteoblastoma is osteosarcoma, particularly the osteoblastoma-like variant that represents 1% of osteosarcomas.[72] This variant is frequently diagnosed as an osteoblastoma on needle core biopsies but they follow a more aggressive clinical course.[73] The most relevant morphologic features on which to make a diagnosis of osteosarcoma include infiltration of host bone (permeation), lack of maturation of bone at periphery of the tumor, and sheets of osteoblastic tumor cells without matrix production.[72]

PROGNOSIS

Osteoblastomas can be destructive locally aggressive lesions but by definition do not metastasize. They are usually managed surgically.[54,58]

- Pathologic Key Features of Osteoblastomas
  - Interconnecting trabeculae of woven bone rimmed by plump osteoblasts
  - Densely vascularized fibroblastic stroma with dilated capillary-type blood vessels.
  - Osteoclast-type giant cells.
  - Large polygonal osteoblasts with hyperchromatic nuclei may be seen.
  - The woven bone trabeculae tend to merge with the host bone at the periphery of the tumor.
  - c-FOS nuclear expression in the osteoblastic component.
- Differential Diagnosis and Pitfalls of Osteoid Osteomas and Osteoblastomas
  - OOs (smaller than 2 cm in size, showing limited growth) and osteoblastomas

---

(usually larger than 2 cm with growth potential).

- Osteoblastomas may display aggressive radiological features and the exclusion of osteosarcoma is paramount. Osteoblastomas should not permeate (entrap) host bone and are usually well-defined with peripheral maturation.
  - c-FOS expression is helpful but may be focally seen in up to 14% of osteosarcomas.
  - *FOS* gene rearrangement (detected by FISH) would strongly support the diagnosis of osteoblastoma over osteosarcoma.

DISCLOSURE

The authors have nothing to disclose.

REFERENCES

1. Baumhoer D, Bredella MA, Sumathi VP. Osteoma. In: WHO classification of tumours. Soft tissue and bone tumours. 5th edition. Lyon, France: IARC; 2020. p. 391–3.
2. Gundewar S, Kothari DS, Mokal NJ, et al. Osteomas of the craniofacial region: a case series and review of literature. Indian J Plast Surg 2013;46(3):479–85.
3. Kaplan I, Nicolaou Z, Hatuel D, et al. Solitary central osteoma of the jaws: a diagnostic dilemma. Oral Surg Oral Med Oral Pathol Oral Radiol Endod 2008;106(3):e22–9.
4. Larrea-Oyarbide N, Valmaseda-Castellon E, Berini-Aytes L, et al. Osteomas of the craniofacial region. Review of 106 cases. J Oral Pathol Med 2008; 37(1):38–42.
5. Boffano P, Roccia F, Campisi P, et al. Review of 43 osteomas of the craniomaxillofacial region. J Oral Maxillofac Surg 2012;70(5):1093–5.
6. Halawi AM, Maley JE, Robinson RA, et al. Craniofacial osteoma: clinical presentation and patterns of growth. Am J Rhinology Allergy 2013;27(2):128–33.
7. Koivunen P, Lopponen H, Fors AP, et al. The growth rate of osteomas of the paranasal sinuses. Clin Otolaryngol Allied Sci 1997;22(2):111–4.
8. Nah KS. Osteomas of the craniofacial region. Imaging Sci Dent 2011;41(3):107–13.
9. Seiler R, Ohrstrom LM, Eppenberger P, et al. The earliest known case of frontal sinus osteoma in man. Clin Anat 2019;32(1):105–9.
10. Eckel W, Palm D. [Statistical and roentgenological studies on some problems of osteoma of the paranasal sinuses]. Arch Ohren Nasen Kehlkopfheilkd 1959;174:440–57.
11. Lee DH, Jung SH, Yoon TM, et al. Characteristics of paranasal sinus osteoma and treatment outcomes. Acta Otolaryngol 2015;135(6):602–7.

12. Buyuklu F, Akdogan MV, Ozer C, et al. Growth characteristics and clinical manifestations of the paranasal sinus osteomas. Otolaryngol Head Neck Surg 2011;145(2):319–23.

13. Wesley RK, Cullen CL, Bloom WS. Gardner's syndrome with bilateral osteomas of coronoid process resulting in limited opening. Pediatr Dent 1987; 9(1):53–7.

14. Chang CH, Piatt ED, Thomas KE, et al. Bone abnormalities in Gardner's syndrome. Am J Roentgenol Radium Ther Nucl Med 1968;103(3): 645–52.

15. Bertoni F, Unni KK, Beabout JW, et al. Parosteal osteoma of bones other than of the skull and face. Cancer 1995;75(10):2466–73.

16. Kim SK, Barry WF Jr. Bone island. Am J Roentgenol Radium Ther Nucl Med 1964;92:1301–6.

17. Izci Y. Management of the large cranial osteoma: experience with 13 adult patients. Acta Neurochir (Wien) 2005;147(11):1151–5, [discussion: 1155].

18. Earwaker J. Paranasal sinus osteomas: a review of 46 cases. Skeletal Radiol 1993;22(6):417–23.

19. Becker M, Stefanelli S, Rougemont AL, et al. Nonodontogenic tumors of the facial bones in children and adolescents: role of multiparametric imaging. Neuroradiology 2017;59(4):327–42.

20. McHugh JB, Mukherji SK, Lucas DR. Sino-orbital osteoma: a clinicopathologic study of 45 surgically treated cases with emphasis on tumors with osteoblastoma-like features. Arch Pathol Lab Med 2009;133(10):1587–93.

21. Haddad FS, Haddad GF, Zaatari G. Cranial osteomas: their classification and management. Report on a giant osteoma and review of the literature. Surg Neurol 1997;48(2):143–7.

22. Tempaku A. Multiple skull osteomas in a 24-year-old woman. J Gen Fam Med 2017;18(6):468–9.

23. Bulut E, Ozan B, Gunhan O. Central osteoma associated with root resorption. J Craniofac Surg 2010; 21(2):419–21.

24. Sundaram M, Falbo S, McDonald D, et al. Surface osteomas of the appendicular skeleton. AJR Am J Roentgenol 1996;167(6):1529–33.

25. Lambiase RE, Levine SM, Terek RM, et al. Long bone surface osteomas: imaging features that may help avoid unnecessary biopsies. AJR Am J Roentgenol 1998;171(3):775–8.

26. Greenspan A. Bone island (enostosis): current concept–a review. Skeletal Radiol 1995;24(2):111–5.

27. Onitsuka H. Roentgenologic aspects of bone islands. Radiology 1977;123(3):607–12.

28. Ulano A, Bredella MA, Burke P, et al. Distinguishing untreated osteoblastic metastases from enostoses using CT attenuation measurements. AJR Am J Roentgenol 2016;207(2):362–8.

29. Amary F, Markert E, Berisha F, et al. FOS expression in osteoid osteoma and osteoblastoma: a valuable ancillary diagnostic tool. Am J Surg Pathol 2019; 43(12):1661–7.

30. Amary F, Bredella MA, Horvai AE, et al. Osteoid osteoma. In: WHO classification of tumours. Soft tissue and bone tumours. 5th Edition. Lyon, France: IARC; 2020. p. 394–6.

31. Kransdorf MJ, Stull MA, Gilkey FW, et al. Osteoid osteoma. Radiographics 1991;11(4):671–96.

32. Healey JH, Ghelman B. Osteoid osteoma and osteoblastoma. Current concepts and recent advances. Clin Orthop Relat Res 1986;204:76–85.

33. Basu S, Basu P, Dowell JK. Painless osteoid osteoma in a metacarpal. J Hand Surg Br 1999;24(1):133–4.

34. Kan P, Schmidt MH. Osteoid osteoma and osteoblastoma of the spine. Neurosurg Clin N Am 2008; 19(1):65–70.

35. Kiers L, Shield LK, Cole WG. Neurological manifestations of osteoid osteoma. Arch Dis Child 1990; 65(8):851–5.

36. Massei F, Laccetta G, Barrani M, et al. Osteoid osteoma mimicking monoarticular juvenile idiopathic arthritis in a girl. Pediatr Int 2016;58(8):791–4.

37. Soler JM, Piza G, Aliaga F. Special characteristics of osteoid osteoma in the proximal phalanx. J Hand Surg Br 1997;22(6):793–7.

38. Norman A, Dorfman HD. Osteoid-osteoma inducing pronounced overgrowth and deformity of bone. Clin Orthop Relat Res 1975;110:233–8.

39. Allen SD, Saifuddin A. Imaging of intra-articular osteoid osteoma. Clin Radiol 2003;58(11):845–52.

40. Chai JW, Hong SH, Choi JY, et al. Radiologic diagnosis of osteoid osteoma: from simple to challenging findings. Radiographics 2010;30(3):737–49.

41. Liu PT, Kujak JL, Roberts CC, et al. The vascular groove sign: a new CT finding associated with osteoid osteomas. AJR Am J Roentgenol 2011; 196(1):168–73.

42. Davies M, Cassar-Pullicino VN, Davies AM, et al. The diagnostic accuracy of MR imaging in osteoid osteoma. Skeletal Radiol 2002;31(10):559–69.

43. Liu PT, Chivers FS, Roberts CC, et al. Imaging of osteoid osteoma with dynamic gadolinium-enhanced MR imaging. Radiology 2003;227(3): 691–700.

44. Malghem J, Lecouvet F, Kirchgesner T, et al. Osteoid osteoma of the hip: imaging features. Skeletal Radiol 2020;49(11):1709–18.

45. Edeiken J, DePalma AF, Hodes PJ. Osteoid osteoma. (Roentgenographic emphasis). Clin Orthop Relat Res 1966;49:201–6.

46. Capanna R, Van Horn JR, Ayala A, et al. Osteoid osteoma and osteoblastoma of the talus. A report of 40 cases. Skeletal Radiol 1986;15(5):360–4.

47. Szendroi M, Kollo K, Antal I, et al. Intraarticular osteoid osteoma: clinical features, imaging results, and comparison with extraarticular localization. J Rheumatol 2004;31(5):957–64.

48. Cassar-Pullicino VN, McCall IW, Wan S. Intra-articular osteoid osteoma. Clin Radiol 1992;45(3):153–60.

49. Helms CA, Hattner RS, Vogler JB 3rd. Osteoid osteoma: radionuclide diagnosis. Radiology 1984;151(3):779–84.

50. Kattapuram SV, Kushner DC, Phillips WC, et al. Osteoid osteoma: an unusual cause of articular pain. Radiology 1983;147(2):383–7.

51. Fittall MW, Mifsud W, Pillay N, et al. Recurrent rearrangements of FOS and FOSB define osteoblastoma. Nat Commun 2018;9(1):2150.

52. Amary F, Bredella MA, Horvai AE, et al. Osteoblastoma. In: WHO classification of tumours. Soft tissue and bone tumours. 5th edition. Lyon, France: IARC; 2020. p. 397–9.

53. Lucas DR, Unni KK, McLeod RA, et al. Osteoblastoma: clinicopathologic study of 306 cases. Hum Pathol 1994;25(2):117–34.

54. Atesok KI, Alman BA, Schemitsch EH, et al. Osteoid osteoma and osteoblastoma. J Am Acad Orthop Surg 2011;19(11):678–89.

55. Barlow E, Davies AM, Cool WP, et al. Osteoid osteoma and osteoblastoma: novel histological and immunohistochemical observations as evidence for a single entity. J Clin Pathol 2013;66(9):768–74.

56. Deyrup AT, Monson DK, Dorfman HD. Aggressive (epithelioid) osteoblastoma arising in soft tissue. Int J Surg Pathol 2008;16(3):308–10.

57. Mohlman JS, Diaz KA, Schaber JD. Cutaneous epithelioid osteoblastoma. Am J Dermatopathol 2015;37(5):e61–3.

58. Berry M, Mankin H, Gebhardt M, et al. Osteoblastoma: a 30-year study of 99 cases. J Surg Oncol 2008;98(3):179–83.

59. McLeod RA, Dahlin DC, Beabout JW. The spectrum of osteoblastoma. AJR Am J Roentgenol 1976;126(2):321–5.

60. Mirra JM, Cove K, Theros E, et al. A case of osteoblastoma associated with severe systemic toxicity. Am J Surg Pathol 1979;3(5):463–71.

61. Bertoni F, Unni KK, Lucas DR, et al. Osteoblastoma with cartilaginous matrix. An unusual morphologic presentation in 18 cases. Am J Surg Pathol 1993;17(1):69–74.

62. Theologis T, Ostlere S, Gibbons CL, et al. Toxic osteoblastoma of the scapula. Skeletal Radiol 2007;36(3):253–7.

63. Mortazavi SM, Wenger D, Asadollahi S, et al. Periosteal osteoblastoma: report of a case with a rare histopathologic presentation and review of the literature. Skeletal Radiol 2007;36(3):259–64.

64. Biazzo A, Armiraglio E, Parafioriti A, et al. Periosteal osteoblastoma of the distal fibula with atypical radiological features: a case report. Acta Biomed 2018;89(2):269–73.

65. Wu M, Xu K, Xie Y, et al. Diagnostic and management options of osteoblastoma in the spine. Med Sci Monit 2019;25:1362–72.

66. Crim JR, Mirra JM, Eckardt JJ, et al. Widespread inflammatory response to osteoblastoma: the flare phenomenon. Radiology 1990;177(3):835–6.

67. Gutierrez LB, Link TM, Horvai AE, et al. Secondary aneurysmal bone cysts and associated primary lesions: imaging features of 49 cases. Clin Imaging 2020;62:23–32.

68. Huang Z, Fang T, Si Z, et al. Imaging algorithm and multimodality evaluation of spinal osteoblastoma. BMC Musculoskelet Disord 2020;21(1):240.

69. Byers PD. Solitary benign osteoblastic lesions of bone. Osteoid osteoma and benign osteoblastoma. Cancer 1968;22(1):43–57.

70. Zon Filippi R, Swee RG, Krishnan Unni K. Epithelioid multinodular osteoblastoma: a clinicopathologic analysis of 26 cases. Am J Surg Pathol 2007;31(8):1265–8.

71. Conner JR, Hornick JL. SATB2 is a novel marker of osteoblastic differentiation in bone and soft tissue tumours. Histopathology 2013;63(1):36–49.

72. Gambarotti M, Dei Tos AP, Vanel D, et al. Osteoblastoma-like osteosarcoma: high-grade or low-grade osteosarcoma? Histopathology 2019;74(3):494–503.

73. Ozger H, Alpan B, Soylemez MS, et al. Clinical management of a challenging malignancy, osteoblastoma-like osteosarcoma: a report of four cases and a review of the literature. Ther Clin Risk Manag 2016;12:1261–70.

Osteosarcoma
Old and New Challenges

Akihiko Yoshida, MD, PhD

KEYWORDS

• Bone • Osteoid • Neoplasm • Sarcoma • Osteosarcoma

Key points

- Osteosarcoma is a sarcoma that directly produces bone or osteoid.
- Osteosarcoma, particularly of the high-grade central type, displays a wide array of histologic patterns that can mimic other bone tumors, including benign lesions.
- The management of osteosarcoma is established, and accurate diagnosis is essential.
- Molecular genetic analysis may support the diagnosis of the rare low-grade subtype or exclude mimicking entities. Still, most osteosarcomas are diagnosed by closely correlating the clinical, radiological, and histologic features.

ABSTRACT

Diagnosis of osteosarcoma can be challenging because of its diverse histological patterns and the lack of diagnostic biomarkers for most examples. This review summarizes the key pathologic findings of osteosarcoma subtypes (high-grade central, parosteal, low-grade central, periosteal, high-grade surface, and secondary) with an emphasis on describing and illustrating histological heterogeneity to help general pathologists. Differential diagnoses are listed for each entity, and histological subtype and distinguishing features, including molecular genetic findings (eg, *MDM2*, *IDH*, *H3F3A*, *FOS*, and *USP6*), are discussed. The review also covers recently established and emerging concepts and controversies regarding osteosarcoma. with an emphasis on describing and illustrating histologic heterogeneity to help pathologists. Recent advances in classification and diagnostic methods are also addressed.

OVERVIEW

Osteosarcoma can be challenging to diagnose because of its highly diverse histologic patterns and the lack of diagnostic biomarkers for most examples. This review summarizes key pathologic findings of osteosarcoma subtypes and entities,

DEFINITION AND CLASSIFICATION

Osteosarcoma is defined as a malignant mesenchymal tumor of the bone that directly produces bone or osteoid. There is no minimum amount of tumor bone or osteoid required, and focal production is sufficient for the diagnosis.

The classification of osteosarcoma considers grade, location relative to the host bone, and histologic pattern. High-grade central and high-grade surface osteosarcomas are of high grade, whereas periosteal osteosarcoma is of intermediate grade, and parosteal and low-grade central osteosarcoma are of low grade. High-grade surface, periosteal, and parosteal osteosarcomas are surface tumors, whereas other variants arise in the medullary cavity. Pure intracortical osteosarcoma is exceptional. **Box 1** summarizes the classification of osteosarcoma. High-grade central osteosarcoma comprises greater than 90% of all osteosarcoma cases, whereas other entities are rarely

Department of Diagnostic Pathology, National Cancer Center Hospital, 5-1-1 Tsukiji, Chuo-ku, Tokyo 104-0045, Japan
E-mail address: akyoshid@ncc.go.jp

Surgical Pathology 14 (2021) 567–583
https://doi.org/10.1016/j.path.2021.06.003
1875-9181/21/© 2021 Elsevier Inc. All rights reserved.

Box 1
Classification of osteosarcoma

High-grade central osteosarcoma

  Common subtypes

    Osteoblastic

    Chondroblastic

    Fibroblastic

  Uncommon subtypes

    Osteoblastoma-like

    Chondroblastoma-like

    Sclerosing

    Epithelioid

    Small cell

    Chondromyxoid fibroma-like

    Undifferentiated pleomorphic sarcoma-like

    Giant cell rich

    Telangiectatic

Parosteal osteosarcoma

Low-grade central osteosarcoma

Periosteal osteosarcoma

High-grade surface osteosarcoma

Intracortical osteosarcoma

Secondary osteosarcoma

---

encountered. The "*conventional osteosarcoma*" terminology has been used widely for cases of high-grade central osteosarcoma; however, its exact definition varies among studies and textbooks. In the latest World Health Organization (WHO) classification,[1] conventional osteosarcoma seems to encompass all high-grade central osteosarcomas, except for small-cell predominant and telangiectatic-predominant tumors.

HIGH-GRADE CENTRAL OSTEOSARCOMA

CLINICAL FINDINGS

High-grade central osteosarcoma has a male predilection and the highest peak in the second decade. Any bone can be affected, but almost half occur around the knee (femur or tibia). Gnathic osteosarcomas tend to occur in older patients and may be associated with a more protracted course than extragnathic cases.[2] Osteosarcoma is usually diagnosed with biopsy and treated with neoadjuvant chemotherapy, followed by wide resection and adjuvant chemotherapy. Approximately 70% of patients with localized osteosarcoma of the extremities can survive. However, the 5-year survival rate is less than 30% for those who present with metastasis. The lung and bone are the most frequent metastatic sites. Skip metastasis is a characteristic form of spread with a rare (<5%) incidence in the contemporary literature. It is defined as metastasis present at the time of diagnosis in the same bone of the primary lesion or in the bone across a joint.[3] Major histologic response to neoadjuvant chemotherapy (<10% viable cells) is an important prognostic factor.

IMAGING

Radiologically, the tumor in long bones is often centered in the metaphysis, as an ill-defined and often eccentric lesion. The tumor shows a mixed lytic and sclerotic, "moth-eaten" appearance, but the findings range from purely lytic to highly sclerotic, depending on the amount of tumor bone (**Fig. 1**). The tumor characteristically shows fluffy internal mineralization, referred to as cotton or cloud, and represents tumor bone formation. There are frequent discontinuous periosteal reactions, such as Codman triangle. Spicula and

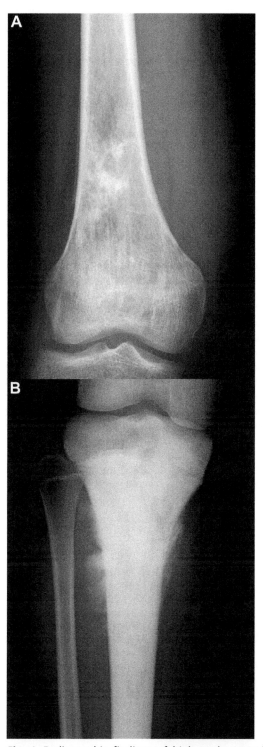

Fig. 1. Radiographic findings of high-grade central osteosarcoma. (*A*) This ill-defined mixed lytic and sclerotic tumor is eccentrically located in the metaphysis of the distal femur, associated with discontinuous periosteal reaction. (*B*) This highly sclerotic tumor is centered in the tibial metaphysis and displays extracortical extension and spiculated periosteal reaction.

onion-skin reactions may be observed. Chondroblastic osteosarcoma may show a ring and arc, stippled calcification. After neoadjuvant chemotherapy, the tumor often decreases in size with increased levels of sclerosis. However, some tumors may rapidly enlarge and demonstrate telangiectatic changes.

GROSS FINDINGS

The tumor typically displays an intramedullary, ill-defined tan fleshy tissue with gritty calcification, necrosis, and hemorrhage (**Fig. 2**). Extracortical extension with periosteal reaction is visible. The tumor tissue becomes fibroedematous with necrosis after chemotherapy.

MICROSCOPIC FINDINGS

Osteosarcoma is an infiltrating tumor, extending between host bone trabeculae. The tumor insinuates into the Haversian system and reaches the subperiosteal spaces and eventually the soft tissue (**Fig. 3**). Tumor cytology is variable, but in general, neoplastic cells show highly atypical and pleomorphic nuclei with hyperchromasia and nuclear membranous irregularity. Mitotic activity is often brisk, including atypical forms. Differentiating bone/osteoid from fibrosis/hyalinization can be challenging. There is no special stain or immunohistochemistry that is reliable for this purpose. Fibrosis tends to show a parallel fascicular arrangement of the collagen fibers, whereas osteoid shows more homogeneous multidirectional deposition. Osteoid has an intrinsic tendency to spontaneously calcify, and a bluish hue in lacelike osteoid is helpful for matrix typing in non-decalcified specimens.

HISTOLOGIC SUBTYPES

High-grade central osteosarcoma has been classically divided into osteoblastic, chondroblastic, and fibroblastic osteosarcomas, depending on the predominant pattern seen within the entire tumor, and each represents approximately 75%, 15%, and 10% of the cases, respectively. *Osteoblastic osteosarcoma* (**Fig. 4**) consists of osteoblast-like cells that produce delicate lacelike, trabecular, island, or sheetlike bone or osteoid. *Chondroblastic osteosarcoma* (**Fig. 5**) shows predominant neoplastic cartilage formation with a minor component of neoplastic bone. *Fibroblastic osteosarcoma* (**Fig. 6**) comprises fascicular to storiform growth of fibroblastic spindle cells, with only inconspicuous neoplastic bone formation.

However, osteosarcomas can display uncommon histologic patterns, for which several distinct

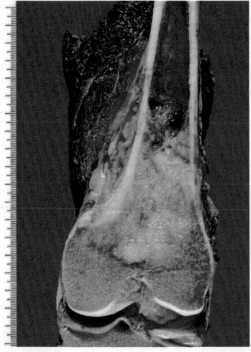

Fig. 2. Gross findings of high-grade central osteosarcoma. A poorly circumscribed tan fleshy tumor is present in the metaphyseal medullary cavity of the distal femur. Extracortical extension is associated with periosteal reaction.

names have been devised. When a tumor is predominated by such a pattern, it can be viewed as a subtype. *Osteoblastoma-like osteosarcoma* (**Fig.** 7A) shows uniform tumor osteoblasts that encircle trabecular tumor bone, often in a single layer, in association with edematous richly vascular stroma. *Chondroblastoma-like osteosarcoma* (**Fig.** 7B) features small uniform round cells with nuclear grooves that proliferate in sheets, occasionally producing islands of pink matrix. *Sclerosing osteosarcoma* (**Fig.** 7C) forms a highly sclerotic mass with scattered embedded tumor cells that often show only mild nuclear atypia (often referred to as "normalization"). *Epithelioid osteosarcoma* (**Fig.** 7D) mimics carcinoma metastasis because epithelioid tumor cells with ample cytoplasm grow in sheets or nests. *Small-cell osteosarcoma* (**Fig.** 8A) shows a relatively uniform small round cell morphology and mimics Ewing sarcoma. It is no longer considered an entity by the latest WHO classification,[1] because it has similar clinical features as osteosarcoma with other patterns. *Chondromyxoid fibroma-like osteosarcoma* (**Fig.** 8B) consists of lobulated tissue showing reticular proliferation of short spindle cells within the chondromyxoid matrix. *Undifferentiated pleomorphic sarcoma-like (malignant fibrous histiocytoma-like) osteosarcoma* (**Fig.** 8C) is characterized by fascicular and storiform growth of highly pleomorphic cells with only a minimal amount of tumor bone formation. *Giant cell–rich osteosarcoma* (**Fig.** 8D) is characterized by numerous osteoclast-like giant cells in addition to malignant mononuclear cells.

The most rigid definition of *telangiectatic osteosarcoma* requires a radiographically purely lytic lesion that grossly corresponds to hemorrhagic multilocular cysts with little solid component and

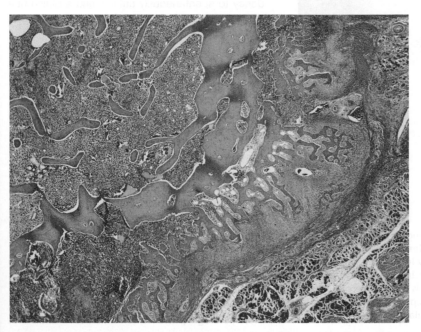

Fig. 3. Low-power view of high-grade central osteosarcoma. Osteosarcoma is an infiltrating disease, involving intertrabecular spaces, Haversian system, and extracortical tissues. Periosteal reaction is present (H&E, original magnification x20).

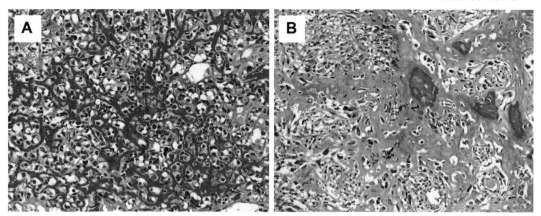

Fig. 4. Osteoblastic osteosarcoma. The tumor consists of highly atypical osteoblast-like cells that deposit neoplastic bone and osteoid. The matrix can be delicate and lacelike [hematoxylin-eosin stain, original magnification x100] (*A*) or in the form of broad trabeculae or sheets [hematoxylin-eosin stain, original magnification x100] (*B*).

no sclerosis[4] (**Fig. 9**A). Bone destruction is conspicuous, and fractures are common. Histologically, the tumor shows multiple blood-filled cysts with septa populated by highly atypical cells (**Fig. 9**B, C). Osteoclast-like giant cells are occasionally observed. Osteoid formation is scant and requires extensive searching. Telangiectatic osteosarcoma was previously considered a distinct entity.

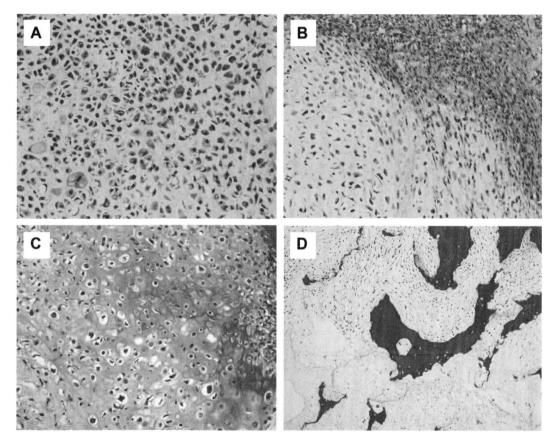

Fig. 5. Chondroblastic osteosarcoma. The cartilaginous component in most cases shows cellular proliferation of highly atypical cells, resembling grade 3 chondrosarcoma [hematoxylin-eosin stain, original magnification x200] (*A*). Noncartilaginous spindle cell proliferation often emerges at the periphery of the cartilage lobules [hematoxylin-eosin stain, original magnification x100] (*B*). The cartilaginous and osseous matrix often gradually merges to produce ambiguous stroma [hematoxylin-eosin stain, original magnification x200] (*C*). The tumor uncommonly harbors areas that resemble lower-grade chondrosarcoma [hematoxylin-eosin stain, original magnification x40] (*D*).

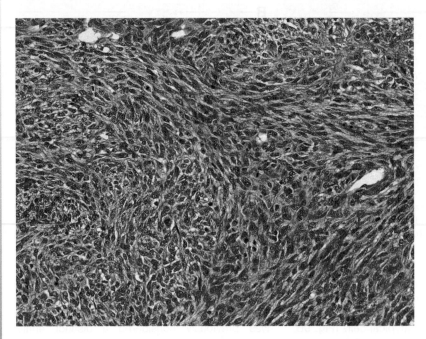

Fig. 6. Fibroblastic osteosarcoma. The tumor is predominated by fascicles of atypical spindle cells. A small amount of osteoid formation is present elsewhere (not shown) [hematoxylin-eosin stain, original magnification x200].

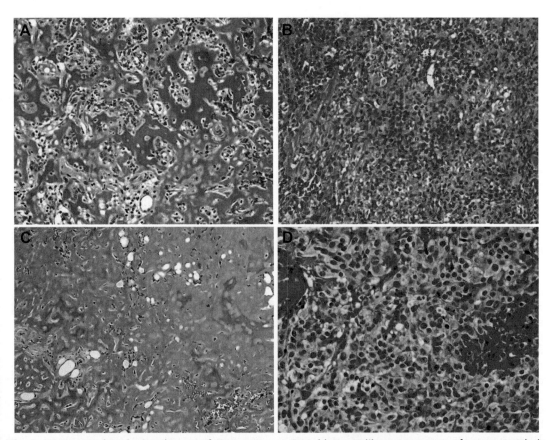

Fig. 7. Uncommon histologic subtypes of osteosarcoma. Osteoblastoma-like osteosarcoma features regularly deposited osteoid and intertrabecular hypervascular tissue [hematoxylin-eosin stain, original magnification x100] (*A*). Chondroblastoma-like osteosarcoma displays sheets of uniform cells with nuclear grooves within homogeneous eosinophilic matrix [hematoxylin-eosin stain, original magnification x200] (*B*). Sclerosing osteosarcoma is characterized by sheets of neoplastic bone, in which relatively bland tumor cells are embedded [hematoxylin-eosin stain, original magnification x100] (*C*). Epithelioid osteosarcoma mimics metastatic carcinoma [hematoxylin-eosin stain, original magnification x400] (*D*).

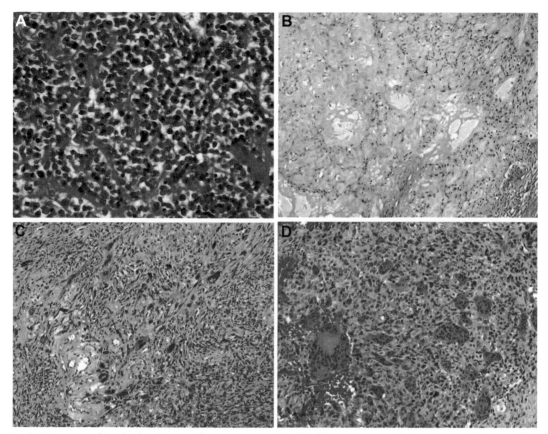

Fig. 8. Uncommon histologic subtypes of osteosarcoma. Small-cell osteosarcoma demonstrates diffuse proliferation of small round cells, reminiscent of Ewing sarcoma [hematoxylin-eosin stain, original magnification x400] (*A*). Chondromyxoid fibroma-like osteosarcoma shows lobulated growth of chondromyxoid tissue, in which tumor cells proliferate in a reticular pattern [hematoxylin-eosin stain, original magnification x40] (*B*). Undifferentiated pleomorphic sarcoma-like osteosarcoma is indistinguishable from undifferentiated pleomorphic sarcoma, except focal presence of bone/osteoid production (not shown, *C*) [hematoxylin-eosin stain, original magnification x100]. Giant cell–rich osteosarcoma features abundant osteoclast-like giant cells in addition to atypical mononuclear tumor cells [hematoxylin-eosin stain, original magnification x200] (*D*).

However, the rigid definition of radiologically/grossly purely lytic lesions without any sclerosis has not been uniformly applied in the literature, including the WHO classification,[1] and because otherwise typical high-grade osteosarcoma can show variable degrees of telangiectatic features, the distinction from such cases could be arbitrary. In addition, the epidemiology and prognosis of these tumors are not different from those of osteosarcoma with other patterns.

Although not a histologic subtype, *gnathic osteosarcoma* occasionally shows somewhat different histology from extragnathic osteosarcomas. These tumors can be chondroblastic, including the chondromyxoid fibroma-like pattern. Osteoblastic examples may show unusual maturation of tumor bone, and definitive diagnosis of malignancy can be challenging based on biopsy.

Osteosarcoma subtypes described above are considered to be of high grade according to the WHO classification, regardless of histologic pattern. However, a small number of osteosarcoma cases with apparently less aggressive clinical course have been reported in association with certain histologic patterns (eg, osteoblastoma-like, chondromyxoid fibroma-like).[5,6] Nevertheless, the significance of these associations remains difficult to determine because of the small number of cases and different criteria used, and the correlation between histology and behavior is overall unpredictable. The position held by the WHO classification is that all these tumors should be managed as high grade in order to avoid insufficient treatment, but future studies are required.

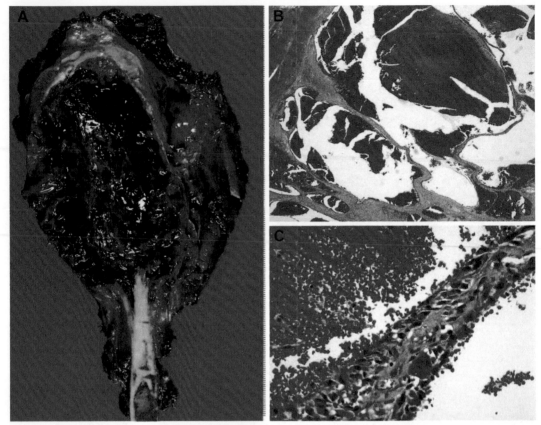

Fig. 9. Telangiectatic osteosarcoma. This classic example demonstrates a destructive hemorrhagic soft mass without any sclerotic component involving the fibular head (*A*). The tumor consists of multiple hemorrhagic cysts [hematoxylin-eosin stain, original magnification x20] (*B*), whose walls contained highly atypical spindle cells and a small number of osteoclast-like giant cells [hematoxylin-eosin stain, original magnification x400] (*C*) with minimal osteoid formation (not shown).

IMMUNOHISTOCHEMISTRY

The immunophenotype of osteosarcoma is variable, and in almost all cases, immunohistochemistry is not helpful for diagnosis. A subset of osteosarcoma is positive for cytokeratin, and if this happens in epithelioid osteosarcoma, differentiation from metastatic carcinoma can be challenging. SATB2 is diffusely positive in most osteoblastic osteosarcomas; however, the staining has low specificity.[7]

MOLECULAR GENETIC FINDINGS

High-grade central osteosarcoma has a highly complex genome with numerical and structural abnormalities, which may be derived from a single catastrophic event known as chromothripsis and chromoplexy. The most common mutation is that involving *TP53* including point mutation and gene rearrangement. Deletion of *RB1* or *CDKN2A* is also frequent. The region of recurrent amplification includes 6p (*RUNX2*, *VEGFA*), 8q (*MYC*), 4q

(*PDGFRA*, *KDR*, *KIT*), 12q (*MDM2*, *CDK4*), and 17p.[1,8] High-grade osteosarcoma with high-level *MDM2* amplification may represent a dedifferentiated low-grade osteosarcoma, because many such cases show at least focal low-grade component when carefully examined.[9] Genetic syndromes (and responsible mutant genes) that are associated with an increased incidence of osteosarcoma include Li-Fraumeni syndrome (*TP53*), bilateral retinoblastoma (*RB1*), Rothmund-Thomson syndrome (*RECQL4*), Bloom syndrome (*BLM*), and Werner syndrome (*WRN*).

DIFFERENTIAL DIAGNOSIS

Fracture callus (**Fig. 10**) may have histology similar to osteosarcoma in its early phase. Being aware of the underlying fracture is critical, particularly when the fracture line is inconspicuous in stress fracture. Stroma is often edematous and hypervascular. The proliferating cells harbor uniformly swollen normochromatic nuclei that lack pleomorphism. Fracture callus tissues extend through

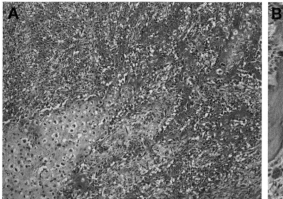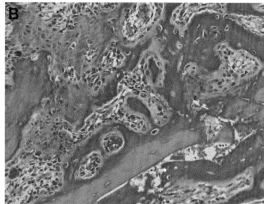

Fig. 10. Fracture callus. A jumbled admixture of osteoid, cartilage, and spindle cell proliferation characterizes an early phase of fracture callus [hematoxylin-eosin stain, original magnification x100] (*A*). The lesion involves intertrabecular tissues, mimicking infiltrating osteosarcoma [hematoxylin-eosin stain, original magnification x40] (*B*).

intertrabecular spaces, mimicking the invasive growth of osteosarcoma.

Osteoblastoma is radiologically well circumscribed, whereas osteoblastoma-like osteosarcoma is often ill defined. Osteoblastomas consist of regular deposition of trabecular bone lined by monolayered nonatypical osteoblasts, associated with hypervascular stroma, whereas in osteosarcoma, more mitotically active, atypical cells fill the intertrabecular spaces and often produce lacelike osteoid. However, in a rare variant, epithelioid osteoblastoma, the tumor cells can be large and mildly atypical, and intertrabecular spaces can be filled by sheets of tumor cells. The most reliable differentiating criterion is the invasive growth of osteosarcoma.[6] Osteoblastoma often harbors *FOS* (or rarely, *FOSB*) gene fusion, which is a specific finding not observed in osteosarcoma.[10] The presence of *FOS* fusion is translated to diffuse strong c-FOS immunoreactivity in osteoblastomas, and this finding can be helpful in difficult cases. However, a small subset of osteoblastomas lack *FOS* rearrangement, and some osteosarcomas express c-FOS despite the lack of *FOS* rearrangement, requiring care.[11,12]

Chondroblastoma typically manifests as a well-circumscribed lytic lesion with a sclerotic rim in the epiphysis, and these findings are distinct from those of chondroblastoma-like osteosarcoma. Osteosarcoma shows nuclear atypia and permeating intertrabecular growth. More than 95% of chondroblastomas harbor a specific H3.3 K36M mutation (*H3F3B* > *H3F3A*), and its detection using a specific monoclonal antibody can be helpful. Although chondroblastoma is considered benign, exceptional examples, particularly in older patients, show infiltrative growth, metastasize, or even become fatal. Recently, 1 study[13] described

a small number of H3.3K36M-positive bone tumors that were clinically and/or histologically malignant, among cases that were originally diagnosed as chondroblastoma-like osteosarcoma, suggesting that a subset of them may represent a malignant chondroblastoma.

Sclerosing osteosarcoma may resemble *bone island* or *reactive bone sclerosis* based solely on histology. Radiologically, osteosarcoma is a large, ill-defined tumor. The key to osteosarcoma diagnosis is an invasive growth, which can be represented by an entrapped native lamellar bone within the neoplastic woven bone, which is best seen under polarized light (**Fig. 11**). Sclerosing osteosarcoma may show inconspicuous nuclear atypia and mitotic activity, but close examination often reveals hyperchromasia or mild nuclear membrane irregularity.

Unlike *Ewing sarcoma*, small-cell osteosarcoma usually at least focally exhibits some degree of nuclear pleomorphism when searched, and identifying neoplastic bone/osteoid is the key for differentiation. Notably, Ewing sarcoma may be associated with reactive bone formation, and a small subset may even manifest as a radiologically sclerotic mass. Intercellular fibrin deposition in Ewing sarcoma is another pitfall, particularly during intraoperative consultation. Diffuse strong membranous CD99 expression, as classically seen in Ewing sarcoma, is not a feature of most osteosarcoma. Small-cell osteosarcoma is negative for NKX2.2 and positive for SATB2, an opposite phenotype of Ewing sarcoma.[14,15] Although not necessary in most cases, demonstrating a specific *EWSR1-FLI1* fusion could help with the diagnosis of Ewing sarcoma.

A small number of sarcomas originally diagnosed as osteosarcoma were reported to harbor

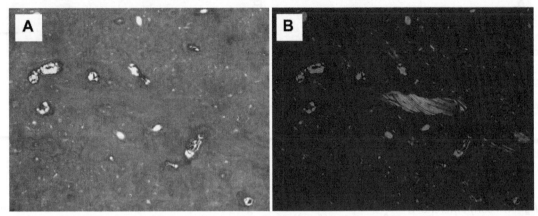

Fig. 11. The use of polarizing light in osteosarcoma diagnosis. Sclerosing osteosarcoma such as this may be confused with benign bone sclerosis [hematoxylin-eosin stain, original magnification x100] (*A*). However, examination under polarized light highlights a preexisting lamellar bone trabecula amid tumor-woven bone, evidencing infiltrating growth of sarcoma [hematoxylin-eosin stain under polarized light, x100] (*B*).

EWSR1-CREB3L1 or related fusion transcripts, and they are increasingly considered a variant of *sclerosing epithelioid fibrosarcoma of bone*.[16–18] These tumors often show well-circumscribed expansile lytic lesions with or without a sclerotic rim and consist of MUC4-positive uniform round cells embedded in hyalinizing tissue. A subset of cases harbors a minor component of bone formation.

Chondrosarcoma can be confused with chondroblastic osteosarcoma. Osteosarcoma should be favored in pediatric patients. Conventional chondrosarcomas are virtually nonexistent in jaw bones, where chondroblastic osteosarcoma or mesenchymal chondrosarcoma should be considered. Radiologically, aggressive periosteal reactions, such as a Codman triangle and spicula, are not expected in chondrosarcoma unless dedifferentiated. Histologically, the cartilage in chondroblastic osteosarcoma shows highly cellular tissues with severe nuclear atypia and mitoses, which would correspond to grade 3 if they were chondrosarcomas (see **Fig. 5**A). Lobulation is less well developed than chondrosarcoma, and nonchondrogenic highly atypical spindle cells often emerge in the periphery of lobulation (see **Fig. 5**B). The neoplastic matrix often shows areas of ambiguous quality between the bone and cartilage (see **Fig. 5**C). Osteosarcoma mimicking grade 1 to 2 chondrosarcomas is uncommon (see **Fig. 5**D). Direct bone formation by malignant cells can be scant and may not be present in the biopsy. Chondrosarcoma can have cellular fibrous interlobular septa and enchondral ossification, which should not be mistaken as evidence of tumor bone. The dedifferentiated component of dedifferentiated chondrosarcoma may sometimes take the form of osteosarcoma (which can be chondroblastic). Immunohistochemistry is not useful for distinguishing between osteosarcoma and chondrosarcoma. *IDH1/2* mutation testing can be helpful because chondrosarcoma harbors this mutation in about half of the cases, whereas it is not present in osteosarcoma.[19] However, the testing suggests chondrosarcoma diagnosis only when *IDH* is mutated, and it is noncontributory when the mutation is absent.

Differentiating osteosarcoma from *undifferentiated pleomorphic sarcoma* primarily depends on the identification of neoplastic bone/osteoid, and the distinction is often impossible on biopsy. Radiological evidence of mineralization may be suggestive of osteosarcoma, and the significance of the findings should be discussed with clinicians and radiologists. In pediatric patients, bone sarcoma with an undifferentiated pleomorphic histology on biopsy may be treated similarly to osteosarcoma.

Differentiation of telangiectatic osteosarcoma from *aneurysmal bone cyst* is critical, and radiological findings may be similar. Atypical spindle cells with frequent mitoses, including abnormal forms, suggest osteosarcoma diagnosis. *USP6* rearrangement, as seen in most primary aneurysmal bone cysts, is lacking in telangiectatic osteosarcoma.

Giant cell tumor of bone generally presents as a purely lytic well-circumscribed lesion in an epiphysis to metaepiphysis of a skeletally mature patient, which is unusual for osteosarcoma. Giant cell–rich osteosarcoma often shows nuclear atypia and pleomorphism in the mononuclear cells (see **Fig. 8**D). Mitotic activity tends to be high (>20/ 10 high-power field) in osteosarcoma, including atypical forms, and giant cells are typically smaller than giant cell tumors. However, rare osteosarcoma may show bland cytologic features, indistinguishable from giant cell tumors. The bone in a giant cell tumor is often trabecular along incipient fibrous septa, surrounded by monolayered osteoblasts. Giant cell tumors principally lack intratumoral lamellar bone trabeculae, whereas osteosarcoma diffusely entraps native cancellous bone as a reflection of its invasive growth. Giant cell tumor harbors *H3F3A* G34 mutation in greater than 95% of cases, and most frequent mutations can be detected using mutation-specific immunohistochemistry. However, this same mutation can be present in malignant giant cell tumors and rare osteosarcomas that lack history or histology of giant cell tumor. Because the latter tumors are usually located in the epiphysis in young adults, suggesting a relationship with giant cell tumor, there is a proposal to expand the definition of a primary malignant giant cell tumor on the basis of *H3F3A* G34 mutation.[20] Of note, although many sarcomas with *H3F3A* G34 mutations are rich in giant cells, only a small subset of giant cell–rich osteosarcoma harbors this mutation.[21]

PAROSTEAL OSTEOSARCOMA AND LOW-GRADE CENTRAL OSTEOSARCOMA

CLINICAL FINDINGS

Parosteal osteosarcoma and low-grade central osteosarcoma are low-grade osteosarcomas that are distinguished based on their location relative to the native bone. These tumors account for 5% of all osteosarcomas. There is a mild female predilection, and the peak incidence is in the third decade of life, a decade later than that for high-grade central osteosarcomas. Parosteal osteosarcomas develop on the surface of the bone as a sclerotic broad-based mass, most commonly involving the distal femur or proximal tibia. Low-grade central osteosarcomas arise within the medullary cavity, often of long bones, such as the femur and tibia. The preoperative period of these tumors is often longer than that of conventional osteosarcoma, which can be greater than 10 years. Low-grade osteosarcoma grows slowly and has almost no intrinsic capacity for metastasis. When widely resected, the 10-year overall survival rate is greater than 80%. Approximately 15% of low-grade osteosarcoma cases shows high-grade progression (referred to as "dedifferentiation," although many examples show a rather gradual transition and high-grade components often retain osteoblastic differentiation), either at presentation or at recurrence. The presence of dedifferentiation confers a worse prognosis with a high metastatic rate and requires treatment with standard chemotherapy. There seems to be no significant survival difference between dedifferentiated osteosarcoma and de novo high-grade osteosarcoma, but the former is associated with less chemotherapy effect.[22]

IMAGING

Parosteal osteosarcoma forms a well-circumscribed, highly sclerotic mass plastered on the cortex of the host bone (**Fig. 12**). Low-grade central osteosarcoma commonly manifests as a large lytic and sclerotic lesion in the metaphysis or metadiaphysis with a trabeculated appearance, often with a relatively well-circumscribed border and expanded adjacent cortex (**Fig. 13**). Active periosteal reaction is uncommon unless progression to high-grade sarcoma occurs.

MICROSCOPIC FINDINGS

Both parosteal and low-grade central osteosarcomas have a similar appearance and are composed of fascicles of mildly atypical long spindle cell proliferation and well-formed trabeculae of neoplastic bone (**Fig. 14**B). Thick bone is typically

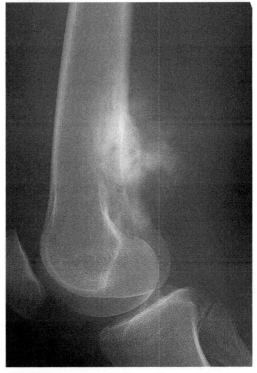

Fig. 12. Radiographic findings of parosteal osteosarcoma. A sclerotic mass is attached on the surface of the posterior cortex of the distal femur.

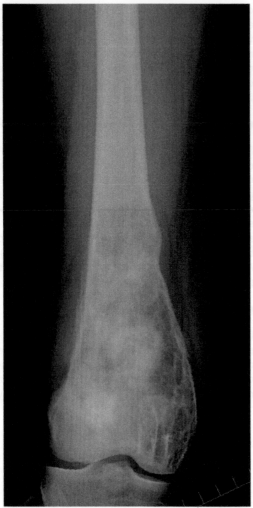

Fig. 13. Radiographic findings of low-grade central osteosarcoma. A relatively well-circumscribed mixed lytic and sclerotic lesion is present in the distal femur, associated with mild cortical expansion and trabeculated appearance.

disposed in a parallel distribution (**Fig. 14**A), but it can be thinner and more irregular (**Fig. 14**C). The marrow component in parosteal osteosarcoma, if present, is fatty. Pagetoid bone with irregular cement lines may be observed. Soft tissue invasion and/or permeation between host bone trabeculae are present. Mitotic activity is low. Some tumors are predominated by fibrosclerotic tissues without matrix production (**Fig. 14**D). Cartilage formation may be focally present, which may form a cap at the periphery of parosteal osteosarcoma (**Fig. 14**E). Dedifferentiation often takes the form of high-grade osteosarcoma, with a sharp or gradual border (**Fig. 14**F). Because of their significant clinical impact, detecting dedifferentiated

foci is critical in the evaluation of low-grade osteosarcomas. Some tumors present with predominantly high-grade osteosarcoma with only an inconspicuous low-grade precursor component.

MOLECULAR GENETIC FINDINGS

Parosteal and low-grade central osteosarcomas commonly harbor high-level amplification of 12q13-15 involving *MDM2* and *CDK4*. *MDM2* amplification is maintained in the dedifferentiated component. Although most parosteal osteosarcomas harbor *MDM2* amplification, it is lacking in a significant minority of low-grade central osteosarcoma, and the genetic background of such cases remains unknown.

DIFFERENTIAL DIAGNOSIS

In general, high-level *MDM2* amplification (**Fig. 15**A), detectable by fluorescence in situ hybridization (FISH) or other methods, is helpful for differentiating low-grade osteosarcoma from mimics. When genetic analysis is unavailable, immunohistochemical reactivity of MDM2 and/or CDK4 (**Fig. 15**B) in low-grade osteosarcoma can be useful.[23,24]

Fibrous dysplasia is a well-demarcated lesion that lacks intertrabecular or soft tissue invasion. Vaguely storiform growth of typically oval bland cells in fibrous dysplasia contrasts with fascicles of long spindle cells with hyperchromatic nuclei in low-grade osteosarcoma. Mitotic figures are usually not detectable in fibrous dysplasia, in contrast to low-grade osteosarcoma. Most cases of fibrous dysplasia harbor *GNAS* activating mutation, which is lacking in low-grade osteosarcoma.[25]

Myositis ossificans adjacent to the cortex may be confused with parosteal osteosarcoma. Myositis ossificans typically shows zoning architecture with an immature center and maturing bone at the periphery and is characterized by regularly connected bone trabeculae and hypervascular intertrabecular spaces. The findings contrast with parallel seams of bone trabeculae and sclerotic stroma in parosteal osteosarcoma. A subset of myositis ossificans harbors *USP6* rearrangement, unlike osteosarcoma.

Osteochondroma may look similar to parosteal osteosarcoma with peripheral cartilaginous differentiation. On imaging, osteochondroma shows medullary continuity to the host bone, whereas parosteal osteosarcoma is attached to the intact cortex. The stalk of osteochondroma is fatty and devoid of fibrous tissue and spindle cells, unless complicated by fracture.

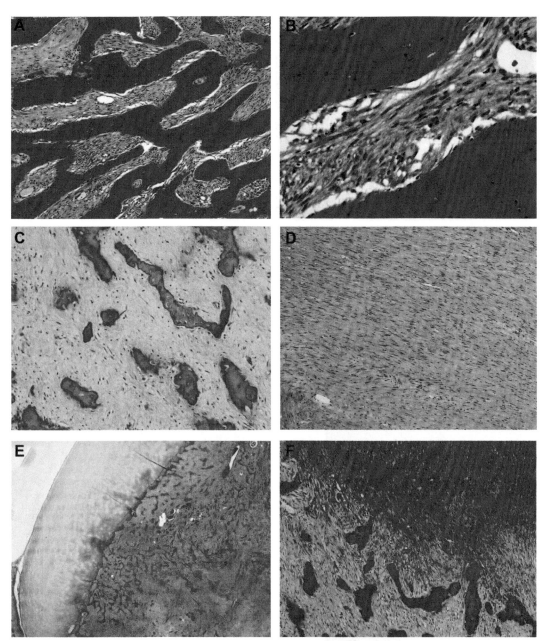

Fig. 14. Histologic findings of low-grade osteosarcoma. The tumor consists of fibrous tissue and well-formed bone trabeculae, often arranged in parallel arrays [hematoxylin-eosin stain, original magnification x40] (*A*). The fibrous tissue is populated by mild to moderately cellular fascicles of spindle cells with mild nuclear atypia [hematoxylin-eosin stain, original magnification x400] (*B*). Some examples show more irregularly shaped bone within fibroedematous stroma, mimicking fibrous dysplasia [hematoxylin-eosin stain, original magnification x40] (*C*). Uncommonly, the tumor can be focally devoid of bone formation, mimicking desmoplastic fibroma [hematoxylin-eosin stain, original magnification x100] (*D*). Cartilaginous differentiation is present in a subset, and when it occurs at the periphery of parosteal osteosarcoma, the tumor resembles osteochondroma [hematoxylin-eosin stain, original magnification x20] (*E*). Low-grade osteosarcoma can progress to high-grade sarcoma, a phenomenon known as "dedifferentiation" [hematoxylin-eosin stain, original magnification x40] (*F*, high-grade component is in the right upper half).

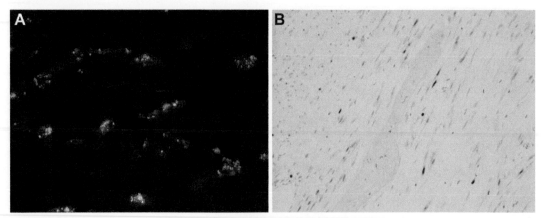

Fig. 15. MDM2 analysis of low-grade osteosarcoma. Most low-grade osteosarcomas harbor high-level *MDM2* amplification (*A, MDM2* FISH; green signals indicate *MDM2*). Positive MDM2 immunohistochemical reactivity is a surrogate of *MDM2* amplification [hematoxylin-eosin stain, original magnification x200] (*B*).

Giant cell tumor of bone post denosumab therapy often consists of fascicles of spindle cells associated with trabecular bone formation, which can mimic low-grade central osteosarcoma. Knowing the history of drug administration is key. Giant cell tumor involves epiphysis, is well defined, and lacks intertrabecular infiltration and nuclear atypia.

When low-grade central osteosarcoma is predominated by fibrous tissue without matrix, the

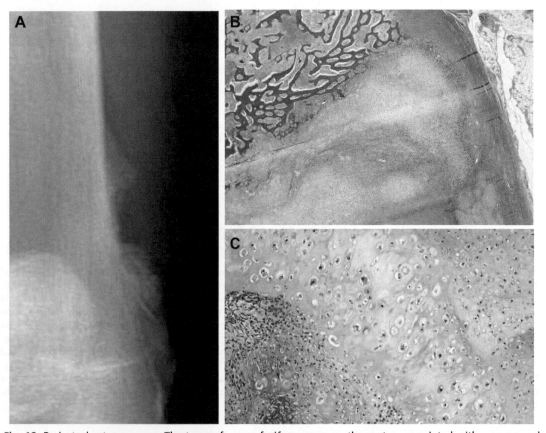

Fig. 16. Periosteal osteosarcoma. The tumor forms a fusiform mass on the cortex, associated with pronounced periosteal reaction (*A*). Histologically, the tumor is located beneath the elevated periosteum [hematoxylin-eosin stain, original magnification x20] (*B*) and consists of lobulated growth of malignant cartilage that is septated by atypical, bone-producing spindle cells [hematoxylin-eosin stain, original magnification x100] (*C*).

histology is indistinguishable from that of *desmoplastic fibroma* or *low-grade fibrosarcoma*. *MDM2* analysis is required for diagnosing the latter diseases, which are rarer than low-grade osteosarcoma.

High-grade osteosarcoma arising from precursor low-grade osteosarcoma can be difficult to distinguish from *conventional osteosarcoma*. Older age, longer preoperative period, unusual imaging (eg, cortical expansion or better circumscription), and history of previous treatment of "benign" bone tumor at the same site should raise suspicion, and identification of a low-grade component in the present or previous specimens settles the diagnosis. This differentiation can be aided by analyzing *MDM2* amplification or immunohistochemical coexpression of MDM2 and CDK4.[9]

PERIOSTEAL OSTEOSARCOMA

Periosteal osteosarcoma is an intermediate-grade chondroblastic osteosarcoma on the bone surface, accounting for 1% of osteosarcoma cases. The tumor has a peak incidence in the second decade with a mild female predilection. The tumor most commonly involves the diaphysis or metadiaphysis of the femur and tibia. On imaging, the tumor forms a fusiform mass on the cortex beneath the periosteum, associated with a pronounced periosteal reaction (**Fig. 16**A). Histologically, periosteal osteosarcoma consists of lobulated growth of atypical cartilage septated by atypical spindle cells with neoplastic bone formation (**Fig. 16**B, C). Minimal medullary invasion is accepted.[1] *MDM2* amplification and *IDH* mutation are not present in contrast to parosteal osteosarcoma and periosteal chondroma/chondrosarcoma, respectively.[26] Additional differential diagnoses include florid periosteal reaction and high-grade surface osteosarcoma. Wide resection with chemotherapy is often used for treatment, but the chemotherapy treatment effect is not predictive of survival. Periosteal osteosarcoma has a better prognosis than conventional osteosarcoma, with a 5-year survival rate of 89%.[27]

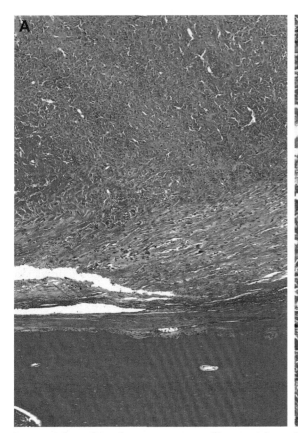
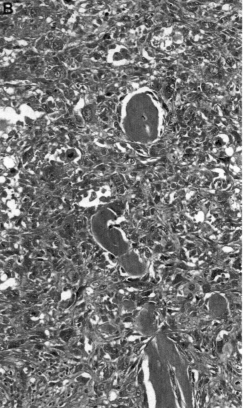

Fig. 17. High-grade surface osteosarcoma. The tumor is on the surface of the cortex (*A*, [hematoxylin-eosin stain, original magnification x20] cortex is in the lower half). The histology is of high-grade osteoblastic osteosarcoma in most cases [hematoxylin-eosin stain, original magnification x200] (*B*).

HIGH-GRADE SURFACE OSTEOSARCOMA

High-grade surface osteosarcoma is an extremely rare (<1% of osteosarcoma) entity, arising on the surface of the bone. It has a similar age and sex distribution as conventional osteosarcoma and typically involves the diaphysis or metadiaphysis of the femur, tibia, or humerus. Radiologically, an ill-defined mass with fluffy calcification lies on the bone surface. The tumor shows histology comparable to that of conventional osteosarcoma, with most examples being osteoblastic (**Fig. 17**). Medullary invasion should be absent or minimal.[28] Differential diagnoses include fracture callus, conventional osteosarcoma with predominant surface component, periosteal osteosarcoma, dedifferentiated parosteal osteosarcoma, and extraskeletal osteosarcoma. The presence of *MDM2* amplification should suggest the diagnosis of dedifferentiated parosteal osteosarcoma. High-grade surface osteosarcoma behaves similarly to conventional osteosarcoma.

SECONDARY OSTEOSARCOMA

Secondary osteosarcoma is an osteosarcoma that occurs in abnormal bone or secondary to extrinsic causes. The suggested cause includes Paget disease of the bone, bone infarct, radiation therapy, and prosthesis. The histologic findings of the tumors are indistinguishable from those of conventional osteosarcoma. The clinical management is also the same, but the prognosis is often worse than in cases with primary osteosarcomas.

SUMMARY

Recent advancements in molecular genetics have provided some support for the diagnosis of osteosarcoma, but mostly in the setting of a rare low-grade variant (*MDM2*) or for the exclusion of mimicking entities (*IDH*, *H3F3A*, *FOS*, and *UPS6*). A large wilderness of high-grade central or "conventional" osteosarcoma is still diagnosed by conventional morphologic methods, in close correlation with clinical and radiological findings.

DISCLOSURE

The author has nothing to disclose.

REFERENCES

1. WHO classification of tumours editorial board. WHO classification of tumours 5th edition, soft tissue and bone tumours. Lyon: IARC; 2020.
2. Baumhoer D, Brunner P, Eppenberger-Castori S, et al. Osteosarcomas of the jaws differ from their peripheral counterparts and require a distinct treatment approach. Experiences from the DOESAK Registry. Oral Oncol 2014;50:147–53.
3. Kager L, Zoubek A, Kastner U, et al. Skip metastases in osteosarcoma: experience of the Cooperative Osteosarcoma Study Group. J Clin Oncol 2006;24:1535–41.
4. Matsuno T, Unni KK, McLeod RA, et al. Telangiectatic osteogenic sarcoma. Cancer 1976;38:2538–47.
5. Chow LT, Lin J, Yip KM, et al. Chondromyxoid fibroma-like osteosarcoma: a distinct variant of low-grade osteosarcoma. Histopathology 1996;29:429–36.
6. Gambarotti M, Dei Tos AP, Vanel D, et al. Osteoblastoma-like osteosarcoma: high-grade or low-grade osteosarcoma? Histopathology 2019;74:494–503.
7. Davis JL, Horvai AE. Special AT-rich sequence-binding protein 2 (SATB2) expression is sensitive but may not be specific for osteosarcoma as compared with other high-grade primary bone sarcomas. Histopathology 2016;69:84–90.
8. Suehara Y, Alex D, Bowman A, et al. Clinical genomic sequencing of pediatric and adult osteosarcoma reveals distinct molecular subsets with potentially targetable alterations. Clin Cancer Res 2019;25:6346–56.
9. Yoshida A, Ushiku T, Motoi T, et al. MDM2 and CDK4 immunohistochemical coexpression in high-grade osteosarcoma: correlation with a dedifferentiated subtype. Am J Surg Pathol 2012;36:423–31.
10. Fittall MW, Mifsud W, Pillay N, et al. Recurrent rearrangements of FOS and FOSB define osteoblastoma. Nat Commun 2018;9:2150.
11. Lam SW, Cleven AHG, Kroon HM, et al. Utility of FOS as diagnostic marker for osteoid osteoma and osteoblastoma. Virchows Arch 2020;476:455–63.
12. Amary F, Markert E, Berisha F, et al. FOS expression in osteoid osteoma and osteoblastoma: a valuable ancillary diagnostic tool. Am J Surg Pathol 2019;43:1661–7.
13. Papke DJ, Hung YP, Schaefer IM, et al. Clinicopathologic characterization of malignant chondroblastoma: a neoplasm with locally aggressive behavior and metastatic potential that closely mimics chondroblastoma-like osteosarcoma. Mod Pathol 2020;33:2295–306.
14. Machado I, Navarro S, Picci P, et al. The utility of SATB2 immunohistochemical expression in distinguishing between osteosarcomas and their malignant bone tumor mimickers, such as Ewing sarcomas and chondrosarcomas. Pathol Res Pract 2016;212:811–6.
15. Yoshida A, Sekine S, Tsuta K, et al. NKX2.2 is a useful immunohistochemical marker for Ewing sarcoma. Am J Surg Pathol 2012;36:993–9.

16. Debelenko LV, McGregor LM, Shivakumar BR, et al. A novel EWSR1-CREB3L1 fusion transcript in a case of small cell osteosarcoma. Genes Chromosomes Cancer 2011;50:1054–62.

17. Wojcik JB, Bellizzi AM, Dal Cin P, et al. Primary sclerosing epithelioid fibrosarcoma of bone: analysis of a series. Am J Surg Pathol 2014;38:1538–44.

18. Tsuda Y, Dickson BC, Dry SM, et al. Clinical and molecular characterization of primary sclerosing epithelioid fibrosarcoma of bone and review of the literature. Genes Chromosomes Cancer 2020;59:217–24.

19. Kerr DA, Lopez HU, Deshpande V, et al. Molecular distinction of chondrosarcoma from chondroblastic osteosarcoma through IDH1/2 mutations. Am J Surg Pathol 2013;37:787–95.

20. Amary F, Berisha F, Ye H, et al. H3F3A (histone 3.3) G34W immunohistochemistry: a reliable marker defining benign and malignant giant cell tumor of bone. Am J Surg Pathol 2017;41:1059–68.

21. Yoshida KI, Nakano Y, Honda-Kitahara M, et al. Absence of H3F3A mutation in a subset of malignant giant cell tumor of bone. Mod Pathol 2019;32:1751–61.

22. Toki S, Kobayashi E, Yoshida A, et al. A clinical comparison between dedifferentiated low-grade osteosarcoma and conventional osteosarcoma. Bone Joint J 2019;101-B:745–52.

23. Dujardin F, Binh MB, Bouvier C, et al. MDM2 and CDK4 immunohistochemistry is a valuable tool in the differential diagnosis of low-grade osteosarcomas and other primary fibro-osseous lesions of the bone. Mod Pathol 2011;24:624–37.

24. Yoshida A, Ushiku T, Motoi T, et al. Immunohistochemical analysis of MDM2 and CDK4 distinguishes low-grade osteosarcoma from benign mimics. Mod Pathol 2010;23:1279–88.

25. Salinas-Souza C, De Andrea C, Bihl M, et al. GNAS mutations are not detected in parosteal and low-grade central osteosarcomas. Mod Pathol 2015;28:1336–42.

26. Righi A, Gambarotti M, Benini S, et al. MDM2 and CDK4 expression in periosteal osteosarcoma. Hum Pathol 2015;46:549–53.

27. Grimer RJ, Bielack S, Flege S, et al. Periosteal osteosarcoma–a European review of outcome. Eur J Cancer 2005;41:2806–11.

28. Wold LE, Unni KK, Beabout JW, et al. High-grade surface osteosarcomas. Am J Surg Pathol 1984;8:181–6.

Benign Cartilage-forming Tumors

Darcy A. Kerr, MD[a,b,*], Nicole A. Cipriani, MD[c]

KEYWORDS

• Cartilage • Benign • Neoplasm • Chondroid • Chondroma • Chondroblastoma

---

Key Points

- Cartilage-forming tumors are among the most commonly encountered primary bone neoplasms, and benign neoplasms vastly outnumber their malignant counterparts.
- Significant morphologic, genetic, and radiographic overlap exists between benign and low-grade malignant cartilaginous neoplasms, potentially creating diagnostic challenges.
- Careful morphologic assessment with clinical and radiographic correlation is essential for accurate diagnosis and optimal patient management.

ABSTRACT

Although uncommon in many pathology practices, cartilage-forming tumors represent some of the most frequent primary bone tumors. Diagnosis can be challenging given their variable histologic spectrum and the presence of overlapping morphologic, immunohistochemical, and genetic features between benign and malignant entities, particularly low-grade malignancies. Correlation with clinical findings and radiographic features is crucial for achieving an accurate diagnosis and appropriate clinical management, ranging from observation to excision. Tumors can be characterized broadly by their location in relation to the bone (surface or intramedullary). In specific instances, ancillary testing may help.

OVERVIEW

Cartilage-forming tumors are common primary bone neoplasms, but they are often asymptomatic and clinically undetected, making their overall incidence likely underestimated.[1] The use of more sensitive imaging modalities over the last decade has increased the detection of benign and low-grade malignant cartilaginous neoplasms.[2]

Histologically, the formation of a cartilaginous matrix characterizes this group of neoplasms. The matrix is usually of hyaline type with a smooth, basophilic to amphophilic quality. Individual chondrocytes reside in lacunae. Radiographically, the cartilaginous matrix demonstrates mineralization in the form of rings and arcs or popcorn calcifications; endochondral ossification around the periphery of cartilage lobules is the microscopic correlate.[3]

Biopsy frequently guides management toward observation or surgical intervention. Although lesions on the extremes of the biological spectrum are straightforward to diagnose, the distinction between benign and low-grade malignant can be problematic, particularly in limited biopsy specimens and radiographically equivocal cases. There is significant interobserver variability in the diagnosis of well-differentiated tumors, even among orthopedic pathologists.[4,5] Fortunately, treatment paradigms largely overlap for these tumors: for instance, aggressive curettage is the treatment of choice for enchondroma as well as atypical cartilaginous tumor/chondrosarcoma, grade 1 (ACT/

---

[a] Department of Pathology and Laboratory Medicine, Dartmouth-Hitchcock Medical Center, One Medical Center Drive, Lebanon, NH 03756, USA; [b] Geisel School of Medicine at Dartmouth, Hanover, NH, USA; [c] Department of Pathology, University of Chicago Medical Center, 5841 South Maryland Avenue, Chicago, IL 60637, USA
* Corresponding author.
E-mail address: Darcy.A.Kerr@hitchcock.org
Twitter: @darcykerrMD (D.A.K.); @nicolecipriani (N.A.C.)

Surgical Pathology 14 (2021) 585–603
https://doi.org/10.1016/j.path.2021.06.004

CSA1) in the appendicular skeleton. The term ACT was recently defined in the fifth edition (2020) of the World Health Organization tumor classification to better reflect the indolent biologic behavior of such lesions in the appendicular skeleton compared with the axial skeleton (still termed CSA1).[1] Distinguishing benign or low-grade from high-grade cartilaginous neoplasms is more clinically relevant and reliable, both histologically and radiographically.

As with other primary bone tumors, correlation with radiographic findings is essential. Plain radiographs serve as a barometer for a neoplasm's biologic potential. Computed tomography scans and MRI help to assess mineralization patterns, cortical integrity, and associated soft tissue components. MRI with gadolinium enhancement, PET, and bone scan can help to further biologically stratify lesions, were absent to low enhancement, low maximum standardized uptake values, and less avid technetium uptake, respectively, portend a benign diagnosis.[3]

This review examines the commonly encountered benign cartilage-producing neoplasms, emphasizing the clinical and radiographic context, molecular pathogenesis, and relevant genetic syndromes, while highlighting when to consider the possibility of malignancy. Two of these lesions, chondromyxoid fibroma and chondroblastoma, were recently reclassified as benign by the World Health Organization, after historically being categorized as intermediate (locally aggressive/rarely metastasizing) neoplasms.[1] Differential diagnoses are also presented in tables (**Table 1** [surface tumors] and **Table 2** [intramedullary tumors]) and syndromes in boxes.

SURFACE TUMORS

OSTEOCHONDROMA

Osteochondroma is an exophytic cartilaginous neoplasm arising on the bone surface with a bony stalk. It is the most common benign cartilage tumor (35%), representing 8% of all bone tumors. The metaphysis of the distal femur, proximal tibia, and proximal humerus are the most common sites, although osteochondromas can affect any bone formed by endochondral ossification (therefore, they are uncommon in the craniofacial skeleton or clavicles). Patients are typically adolescents and young adults, with a peak incidence in the second decade of life. Osteochondromas often are discovered incidentally on imaging or noted as firm, long-standing, slow-growing masses. They are generally painless, except in the presence of complications (local compression, bursitis,

or stalk fracture). Most (approximately 85%) are solitary. Multiple lesions occur in patients with the autosomal-dominant disorder, multiple osteochondromas (multiple hereditary exostoses).[6]

Radiographically, osteochondroma is an exophytic, pedunculated, occasionally sessile bony excrescence capped by cartilage (**Fig. 1**). A hallmark feature is the contiguity of the lesional cortex and medulla with that of the underlying bone. MRI is helpful to assess the thickness of the cartilage cap.[7]

On gross examination, osteochondroma demonstrates a thin (1–2 cm) cartilage cap with a bony stalk (**Fig. 2**A). The cap thickness is a factor used in the assessment of potential malignant transformation and should be documented. The configuration of the cartilage cap varies, ranging from a single dome or mushroom-shaped cap to numerous bosselated excrescences.

Histologically, osteochondromas are composed of a thin outer fibrous layer, followed by the cartilaginous cap that recapitulates a growth plate (**Fig. 2**B–D). Superficial chondrocytes may be haphazardly distributed, but they have a columnar arrangement in the ossification zone. Nuclear atypia is absent. In the growing skeleton, lesions may be cellular with prominent primary spongiosa-like areas. The base undergoes endochondral ossification and shows a transition to lamellar cancellous bone with fatty or hematopoietic marrow. Older lesions may be composed principally of bone owing to pronounced ossification.

Osteochondromas are caused by loss of function mutations in tumor-suppressor genes exostosin 1 or 2 (*EXT1* or *EXT2*).[8,9] The heparan sulfate structure is thereby modified, affecting chondrocyte proliferation, differentiation, and organization in the growth plate.[8] These genes are also implicated in the hereditary syndrome multiple osteochondromas (**Box 1**, **Fig. 3**).

Surgical excision of sporadic osteochondroma is usually curative. Recurrence is possible with incomplete excision.[10]

Malignant Transformation in Osteochondroma

The incidence of malignant transformation in sporadic osteochondroma is low, at approximately 0.4% to 2.0%. Clinically, the rapid growth of a preexisting osteochondroma and/or the presence of pain in an older patient raise concern for malignancy, particularly in the proximal skeleton.[10] Radiographically, a thick cartilaginous cap (>2 cm) in a skeletally mature individual, inhomogeneous mineralization, an irregular margin, and an associated soft tissue mass are features

Table 1
Benign/low-grade[a] surface cartilage tumors: Differential diagnosis and useful distinguishing features

	Surface Cartilaginous Lesions					Surface Osteosarcomas	
	BPOP	Osteochondroma	Secondary Peripheral Chondrosarcoma	Periosteal Chondroma	Periosteal Chondrosarcoma	Periosteal osteosarcoma[a]	Parosteal Osteosarcoma
Demographics	Adults, 3rd–4th decades M = F	Adolescents, 2nd decade M>F (2:1)	Older than benign osteochondroma Risk increased in MO	Children, young adults, 2nd–3rd decades M>F (1.5:1)	Young adults, 3rd decade M>F	Adolescents, 2nd decade M = F	Young adults, 3rd decade M<F (1:1.3)
Clinical presentation	Painless swelling Rapid growth possible	Asymptomatic Pain with bursitis, stalk fracture	Growth of known osteochondroma Pain	Asymptomatic	Painful swelling Impaired range of motion	Short duration Painful swelling Firm, fixed mass	Long duration Occasionally painful Impaired range of motion
Size	0.5–3.0 cm	3–6 cm; can be larger	>10 cm; can be smaller	<5 cm (1–3 cm)	>5 cm	10 cm	9 cm
Site	Hands and feet (75%)	Long bones Metaphysis	Proximal skeleton	Hands and feet Proximal humerus Metaphysis	Long bones (distal femur and humerus) Metaphysis	Long bones (femur and tibia) Diaphysis	Long bones (tibia and humerus) Posterior distal tibial metaphysis (70%)
Imaging	Well-circumscribed Mineralized Lacks continuity with underlying bone	Cartilage cap 1–2 cm Continuity with underlying bone	Consider when cartilage cap >2 cm Irregular mineralization Soft tissue component	Well-demarcated Radiolucent Cortical sclerosis and lateral buttressing Lacks continuity with underlying bone	Lobulated Coarse calcification with or without a shell Cortex thick or thin Lacks continuity with underlying bone	Fusiform with broad-based surface attachment Radiolucent with intratumoral linear bone radiating from base Cortical thickening and scalloping, infrequent invasion Cartilaginous component bright on T2-weighted MRI	Lobular, surface based Densely mineralized Well-delineated with no or little periosteal reaction Cortical invasion in 50%

(continued on next page)

Table 1
(continued)

	Surface Cartilaginous Lesions					Surface Osteosarcomas	
	BPOP	Osteochondroma	Secondary Peripheral Chondrosarcoma	Periosteal Chondroma	Periosteal Chondrosarcoma	Periosteal osteosarcoma[a]	Parosteal Osteosarcoma
Morphology	Triphasic: variably cellular fibrous tissue, cartilage, (blue) bone With or without hypercellularity, chondrocyte enlargement	Resembles growth plate Thin overlying perichondrium Ossifies with age No infiltration	Permeative growth involving bone or soft tissue Myxoid/cystic change of matrix Wide fibrous bands Disordered chondrocytes Hypercellularity Mitotic activity or pleomorphism (uncommon)	Lobulated Low to moderately cellular hyaline cartilage Impingement of medullary cavity but not true invasion	Lobulated Moderately cellular hyaline cartilage Permeative growth of underlying cortex Marrow usually not involved	Predominantly chondroblastic Intermediate grade Neoplastic bone/ osteoid often in center of cartilage lobules With or without Fascicles of spindle cells Rare high-grade dedifferentiated component	Predominantly osteoblastic Low grade Long seams of well-formed woven bone, with or without cement lines Atypical spindle cells Cartilaginous cap with mildly atypical chondrocytes Rare high-grade dedifferentiated component
Genetics	t(1;17) or variant inv(7) or inv(6)	*EXT1* and *EXT2* mutations	*EXT1* and *EXT2* mutations	*IDH1/2* mutations	*IDH1* mutations Wnt/β-catenin alterations Lacks *MDM2* and *TP53* alterations	No consistent genetic signature (with or without *TP53* mutations) Lacks *IDH1/2* and *MDM2* alterations	Overexpression of MDM2 and CDK4 by IHC and amplification of *MDM2* by FISH

Abbreviations: BPOP, bizarre parosteal osteochondromatous proliferation; MO, multiple osteochondromas; IHC, immunohistochemistry; FISH, fluorescence in situ hybridization.
 [a] Surface osteosarcomas can be biologically low grade (parosteal osteosarcoma) or high grade (periosteal osteosarcoma or high-grade surface osteosarcoma). Although not technically low grade, periosteal osteosarcoma is included as a differential diagnosis in this table given the potential morphologic overlap with other surface-based cartilaginous tumors.

Benign/low-grade malignant intramedullary cartilage tumors: Differential diagnosis and useful distinguishing features

	Enchondroma	Atypical Cartilaginous Tumor/ Chondrosarcoma Grade 1	Chondroblastoma	Malignant Chondroblastoma	Chondroblastoma-like Osteosarcoma	Clear Cell Chondrosarcoma	Chondromyxoid Fibroma	Chondromyxoid Fibroma-like Osteosarcoma
Demographics	Adults, 3rd–4th decades M = F	Adults, 5th–7th decades M>F	Skeletally immature, 2nd–3rd decades M>F (2:1)	Skeletally mature, 5th decade M>F (6:1)	Adults, 3rd–4th decades M > F (2:1)	Adults, 3rd–5th decades M>F (3:1)	Adolescents, young adults, 2nd–3rd decades M>F (1.5:1)	Adults, 3rd–5th decades M = F
Clinical presentation	Asymptomatic Pain with pathologic fracture	Painful enlarging mass, can be of long duration	Pain, swelling Stiffness Limp	Limited information available	Limited information available	Pain, often of long duration	Pain, can be of long duration Swelling especially in hands and feet	Mass, with or without pain
Size	<3 cm, but up to 5 cm	>10 cm; can be smaller	<5 cm	6.4 cm	6.5 cm	5–10 cm	3–4 cm; can be smaller or larger	Not well-described; often <5 cm
Site	Hands and feet Long bones Diaphysis	Pelvis > long bones	Long bones (femur, tibia, humerus) Epiphysis > apophysis	Ribs, scapula, talus, radius Epiphysis or epiphyseal equivalent	<50% in long bones (humerus) Ribs, scapula, vertebra Epiphysis or epiphyseal equivalent	Femoral or humeral head (wide anatomic distribution) Epiphysis	Long bones > flat bones Metaphysis	Long bones (femur); wide anatomic distribution (including craniofacial) Variable location within bone
Imaging	Lobulated Nonsclerotic margin Matrix mineralization (rings and arcs) With or without cortical scalloping or thinning, bone expansion Less avid technetium uptake on bone scan, low SUV on PET/CT	Matrix mineralization (rings and arcs) Lytic areas with geographic destruction Permeation of cortex, soft tissue more often in high-grade CSA More avid technetium uptake on bone scan, higher SUV on PET/CT	Well-demarcated Central or eccentric Lytic with sclerotic rim With or without punctate calcifications	Expansile, lytic Thin sclerotic margins Internal trabeculations With or without cortical breakthrough Increased SUV on PET/CT scan	Expansile, lytic Internal trabeculations Cortical breakthrough	Lytic, well-demarcated Sclerotic rim With or without radiodensities (cartilage matrix) Overlap with chondroblastoma	Well-demarcated Lobulated, lytic Often eccentric, can be central	Variable, ranging from lytic to sclerotic Often infiltrative With or without cortical destruction

(continued on next page)

Table 2
(continued)

	Enchondroma	Atypical Cartilaginous Tumor/ Chondrosarcoma Grade 1	Chondroblastoma	Malignant Chondroblastoma	Chondroblastoma-like Osteosarcoma	Clear Cell Chondrosarcoma	Chondromyxoid Fibroma	Chondromyxoid Fibroma-like Osteosarcoma
Morph-ology	Mature hyaline cartilage Low cellularity Cytologic atypia, myxoid stromal change, moderate cellularity especially in small bones or in enchon-dromatosis Endochondral ossification at periphery No invasion or mitoses	Infiltrative Mature hyaline to myxoid cartilage Low to moderate cellularity Rare mitoses	Mononuclear cells with nuclear grooves Osteoclast-type giant cells Pink "fibroch-ondroid" islands "Chicken-wire" calcifications With or without secondary ABC-like changes	Resembles chondroblastoma but with cytologic atypia and infiltration With or without sheets of cells or tenosynovial giant cell tumor-like morphology With or without lymphovascular invasion or necrosis	Some resemblance to chondroblastoma, but with significant cytologic atypia (more than in malignant chondroblastoma) Tumor cells produce neoplastic bone matrix Infiltration Necrosis	Lobules of cell with abundant clear to lightly eosinophilic cytoplasm and well-defined cell borders Woven bone with osteoclast-type giant cells Foci of conventional low-grade chondrosarcoma in approximately 50%	Lobular growth Oval-stellate cells in chondroid-myxoid matrix Peripheral hypercellularity with osteoclast-type giant cells and "staghorn-like" vasculature Coarse purple calcifications With or without secondary ABC-like changes	Some resemblance to chondromyxoid fibroma, but infiltrative and with cytologic atypia Tumor cells produce neoplastic bone matrix Mitoses
Genetics	*IDH1/2* mutations (IHC not helpful)	*IDH1/2* mutations (IHC not helpful)	Histone *H3F3B* or *H3F3A* gene mutations (H3K36M IHC; DOG1 IHC)	H3K36M IHC Not well-described (with or without copy number alterations)	Lacks histone mutations	Retinoblastoma pathway implicated Rare *TP53*, *CDKN2A*, or *H3F3B* K36M mutations	Possible GRM1 overexpression	Not well-described

Abbreviations: ABC, aneurysmal bone cyst; CSA, chondrosarcoma; CT, computed tomography; IHC, immunohistochemistry; SUV, standardized uptake value.

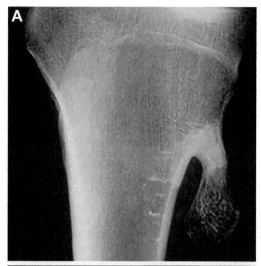

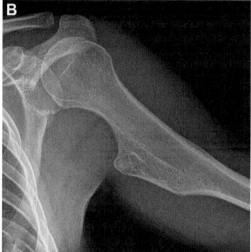

Fig. 1. (*A*) A pedunculated osteochondroma of the proximal tibia on a conventional radiograph. (*B*) Some osteochondromas show broad-based bony attachment, including characteristic contiguity between the cortex and marrow of the lesion and that of the underlying bone.

associated with malignancy.[7] Histologically, nodular cartilage with wide fibrous septae, infiltration of preexisting bone, and mitotic activity or nuclear pleomorphism support malignant transformation (see **Fig. 3**C). The diagnosis can be difficult, and the final determination is best made in a multidisciplinary setting.[5]

BIZARRE PAROSTEAL OSTEOCHONDROMATOUS PROLIFERATION

Bizarre parosteal osteochondromatous proliferation or a Nora lesion is an uncommon surface proliferation of bone and cartilage. It typically affects the small bones of the hands and feet (75%) but may involve long bones. Bizarre parosteal osteochondromatous proliferation generally affects adults in the third to fourth decades of life. Clinically, patients present with a localized, usually painless, swelling that may demonstrate rapid growth.[11] Subungual exostosis shares similar morphologic features but is now known to be a distinct entity with a different underlying genetic change.

Radiographic studies show intact cortex with a surface-based, well-demarcated, mineralized mass. Gross specimens demonstrate a 0.5 to 3.0 cm lobulated, cartilaginous mass with a bony stalk (**Fig. 4**A). Microscopically, a disorganized proliferation of fibrous tissue, cartilage, and bone characterizes bizarre parosteal osteochondromatous proliferation. The surface fibrous tissue ranges in cellularity, with hypercellularity possible. The cartilaginous component demonstrates endochondral ossification that may show distinctive basophilic mineralization (*blue bone*), noted to persist even after decalcification (**Fig. 4**B, C).[12] The cartilage may be hypercellular with enlarged and binucleated chondrocytes (*bizarre*), without atypical mitoses or pleomorphism.

Ancillary studies are usually not used. Most cases demonstrate a t(1;17) or variant thereof. A subset demonstrates inv(7) or inv(6).[12,13]

Treatment is simple surgical excision, although asymptomatic lesions can be observed. About one-half of cases recur, sometimes multiply, likely owing to incomplete excision. No metastases have been reported.

PERIOSTEAL CHONDROMA

Periosteal (surface or juxtacortical) chondroma is an uncommon benign cartilage tumor involving the surface of bone and frequently eroding the underlying cortex. It typically affects the small bones of the hands and feet or the long bones of the appendicular skeleton, in particular the proximal humerus. All age groups are affected, with a peak in the second and third decades of life. Tumors are usually asymptomatic, solitary, and found incidentally on imaging. Presentation with a painful, palpable mass is also possible.[14]

Radiographically, periosteal chondromas are small (1–3 cm), well-demarcated, and radiolucent, with or without internal mineralization. They are attached to the cortex and demonstrate superficial cortical erosion, underlying sclerosis, and occasionally peripheral periosteal calcification. MRI shows a T2-bright signal (**Fig. 5**).

Gross examination shows firm, pale blue, translucent cartilage nodules with a sharp cortical

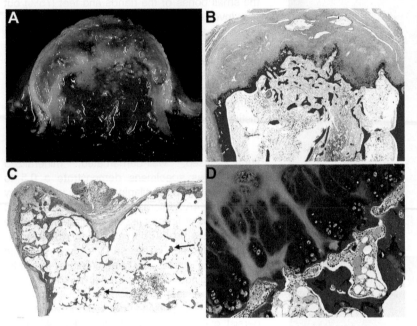

Fig. 2. (*A*) On resection, osteochondroma shows an exophytic mass with a thin, glistening, grey–blue cartilage cap overlying bone. (*B*) It is surfaced by fibrous perichondrium and undergoes endochondral ossification at the base (hematoxylin-eosin, original magnification x6). (*C*) The cartilaginous cap undergoes progressive endochondral ossification with time such that long-standing lesions may be composed predominantly of bone. Scattered residual cores of cartilage (*arrows*) are visible within the medullary cavity (hematoxylin-eosin, original magnification x5). (*D*) Osteochondroma recapitulates growth plate architecture, demonstrating a columnar arrangement of chondrocytes (hematoxylin-eosin, original magnification x20).

interface. A zone of sclerotic bone can frequently be appreciated (**Fig. 6**A). Medullary cavity impingement is possible by reactive endosteal bone, but it is not invaded by the tumor.

Microscopically, periosteal chondroma consists of lobules of low to moderately cellular hyaline cartilage. The interface with the underlying bone is sharp, and permeation of the Haversian canals

---

Box 1
Multiple osteochondromas (multiple hereditary exostoses)

- Autosomal dominant; germline alterations in *EXT1* (at 8q24.11) or *EXT2* (11p11.2) in more than 90% of patients

- Estimated prevalence of at least 1 in 50,000

- Seventy-five percent of patients have a family history (incomplete penetrance and variable expressivity)

- Rarely a manifestation of separate continuous deletion syndromes:
  ○ Lenger–Giedion syndrome (*EXT1* and *TRPS1*)
  ○ Potocki–Schaffer syndrome (*EXT2* and *ALX4*)

- Clinical presentation within the first 2 decades of life; tumor growth until skeletal maturity

- Pain and decreased quality of life in the majority (>80%) of patients; occasionally asymptomatic

- Sequelae include bone deformities requiring multiple surgeries, arthritis, impingement, and bursa formation

- Rate of malignant transformation estimated at 0.5% to 5.0% (slightly higher than sporadic lesions) (see **Fig. 3**)
  ○ Mostly to ACT/CSA1 (90%)
  ○ Occasionally to high-grade chondrosarcoma

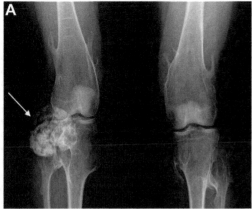

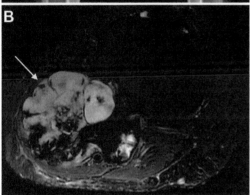

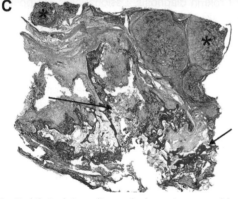

Fig. 3. (*A*) A plain radiograph shows innumerable osteochondromas of the femur, tibia, and fibula bilaterally in a patient with multiple osteochondromas. The cartilage caps are oriented away from the joint. A dominant osteochondroma arising from the posterior proximal tibia demonstrates irregular mineralization and showed growth over several years, raising suspicion for chondrosarcomatous transformation (*arrow*). (*B*) Corresponding T2-weighted MRI demonstrates a large hyperintense cartilaginous cap (*arrow*). (*C*) Histologically, the residual underlying mineralized osteochondroma (*arrows*) transitions into a multinodular mass of hyaline cartilage with fibrous bands, increased cellularity, and pushing growth into soft tissue (*), indicative of transformation to atypical cartilaginous tumor/low-grade chondrosarcoma (hematoxylin-eosin , original magnification x5).

or medulla is absent. Chondrocytes are bland, with at most mild to moderate atypia (**Fig. 6**B, C). Binucleated chondrocytes and chondrocyte drop can occur. Rare tumors have focal myxoid matrix or hypercellularity.

Immunohistochemistry is not useful for diagnosis. Genetically, many periosteal chondromas harbor mutations in *IDH1*.[15]

Treatment is surgical removal by curettage or simple excision, and recurrence is uncommon.[16] Malignant transformation is exceedingly rare. Clinical and morphologic overlap make distinguishing periosteal chondroma from periosteal chondrosarcoma challenging. Periosteal chondrosarcomas are typically large (>5 cm), with increased cellularity and atypia; cortical invasion is diagnostic (see **Table 1**).[17]

INTRAMEDULLARY TUMORS

ENCHONDROMA

Enchondroma is a benign intramedullary tumor of hyaline cartilage. It is the second most common benign cartilage neoplasm and represents 12% to 24% of primary bone tumors.[18] Although its true incidence is unknown because it is frequently discovered incidentally, enchondromas have been identified in 2% to 3% of patients undergoing routine knee or shoulder MRIs.[3]

The distal appendicular skeleton is most frequently involved, with approximately 60% occurring in the phalanges. Other sites include the long tubular bones (femur, tibia, humerus, and fibula). Enchondromas are rare in the pelvis (<3%), but can involve any bone derived from endochondral ossification. The age range is wide, with most patients in the third to fourth decades of life.

Clinically, enchondromas are painless except in cases of pathologic fracture; a painful intraosseous cartilaginous lesion raises concern for chondrosarcoma. Approximately 10% of patients with enchondroma will have multiple tumors. These patients are usually young and may possess 1 of 3 clinical syndromes: enchondromatosis (Maffucci syndrome or Ollier disease) or, rarely, metachondromatosis (multiple enchondromas and osteochondromas) (**Box 2**).[18]

Imaging studies show a centrally located intramedullary lesion with variable mineralization. Plain films often demonstrate ring and arc or popcorn calcifications. By computed tomography scans, enchondromas are well-circumscribed and mineralized. They are T2-bright by MRI (**Fig. 7**). Expansile growth with an intact cortex and sclerotic rim is common, and endosteal scalloping can be

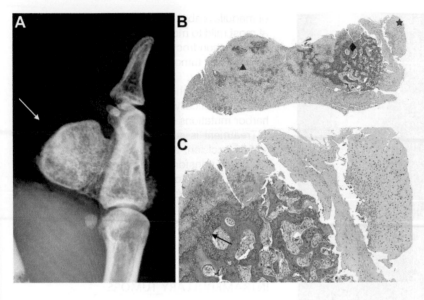

Fig. 4. (*A*) Conventional radiograph of bizarre parosteal osteochondromatous proliferation (BPOP) shows a well-demarcated, exophytic, mineralized mass arising on the surface of the first proximal phalanx with intact underlying cortex and an associated soft tissue swelling (*arrow*). (*B*) Histologically, the lesion demonstrates a triphasic morphology including cartilage (*star*), bone (*diamond*), and fibroblasts (*triangle*) [hematoxylin-eosin , original magnification x10]. (*C*) Cartilaginous areas contain enlarged, occasionally binucleated chondrocytes. Areas of ossification may contain characteristic "blue bone" (*arrow*) [hematoxylin-eosin , original magnification x40].

present in active lesions. Periosteal reaction is absent unless there is a pathologic fracture.

Grossly, most specimens represent curettages, consisting of coalescing pale to translucent hyaline cartilage nodules. Admixed gritty white–tan hard bone may be present. Resection specimens show a well-demarcated tumor with a rim of sclerotic bone (**Fig. 8**A).

Histologic sections demonstrate coalescing nodules of pale blue hyaline cartilage within the medullary cavity. There is a sharp interface between the cartilage and bone, with peripheral endochondral ossification of cartilage lobules (**Fig. 8**B). There is no permeation of preexisting bony trabeculae or invasion within Haversian canals. Chondrocytes are distributed evenly throughout and lack a columnar orientation. Nuclei are round, small, and dark (**Fig. 8**C). Mitotic activity is absent. Enchondromas in small bones of the hands and feet, in children, and in enchondromatosis syndromes can show increased cellularity, mild cytologic atypia, and myxoid matrix change (**Fig. 8**D).[8,19]

Molecularly, more than 50% of solitary enchondromas and approximately 90% of enchondromas in the setting of Ollier disease or Maffucci syndrome harbor gain-of-function mutations involving arginase residues in the genes encoding isocitrate dehydrogenase, *IDH1* (R132) or *IDH2* (R140 and R172).[15,20] IDH gains neomorphic activity and converts alpha-ketoglutarate into the oncometabolite D-2-hydroxyglutarate, affecting DNA hypermethylation at CpG sites and other metabolic activities.[8] These genes are also implicated in enchondromatosis (**Fig. 9**).

Immunohistochemistry does not play a significant role in diagnosis. Lesional cells are positive for S-100 protein, similar to other cartilaginous tumors. Both ACT/CSA1 and enchondroma may express ERG, limiting its discriminative usefulness.[18,21] The available IDH1 antibodies used in glial tumors cover less than 30% of the mutations in central and peripheral cartilaginous and are therefore of limited diagnostic usefulness.[8,15]

Asymptomatic enchondromas can be followed clinically and radiographically. Symptomatic lesions or those with questionable radiographic features should be biopsied or curetted. Sizable lesions (>5 cm) or those in expendable bones may be excised. Recurrence is uncommon and may be due to incomplete curettage, but should raise concern for chondrosarcoma. Malignant transformation to conventional or dedifferentiated chondrosarcoma occurs in a small percentage of cases (<1% in a nonsyndromic setting) although it is not uncommon to see areas resembling enchondroma in association with central chondrosarcoma.[8]

Clinically, new-onset pain may be a harbinger of malignant transformation. Salient radiographic features include permeative growth, changing radiographic margins with areas of lucency, periosteal reaction, cortical thickening or disruption, and soft tissue extension.[3]

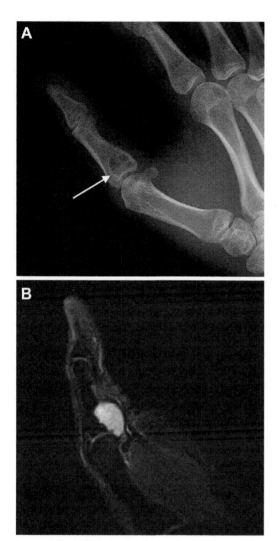

Fig. 5. (A) A plain radiograph of periosteal chondroma demonstrates a 2-cm mass involving the proximal phalanx of the thumb that is lobulated with a sclerotic border (*arrow*). (B) The corresponding MRI more clearly demonstrates its surface-based location. It is heterogeneously bright on T2-weighted sequences with cortical erosion.

Histologically, the threshold for diagnosing ACT/CSA1 is somewhat variable depending on site, clinical context, and age. A combination of 5 features (hypercellularity, open chromatin, age >45 years, bone invasion, and ≥20% myxoid matrix) has been proposed, with the last 2 being the most discriminatory for ACT/CSA1.[4] In the small bones of the hands and feet as well as in enchondromatosis syndromes, the diagnosis of ACT/CSA1 usually hinges on unequivocal invasion. Specific location is also helpful to inform pretest probability: well-differentiated cartilaginous tumors of the phalanges are usually enchondromas

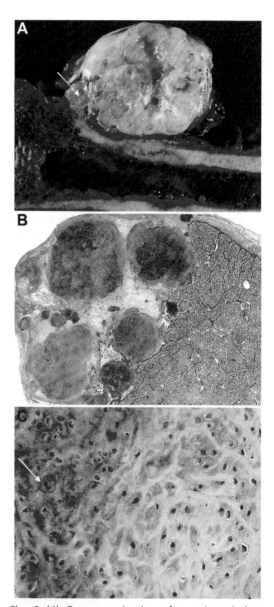

Fig. 6. (A) Gross examination of a periosteal chondroma demonstrates a surface lobular proliferation of glistening hyaline cartilage, partially surrounded by a sclerotic rim of bone (*arrow*). (B) Histologically, nodules of hyaline cartilage coalesce into a multinodular tumor covered by periosteum, with a well-demarcated, pushing border (hematoxylin-eosin , original magnification x5). (C) Cellularity is low to moderate with small chondrocytes lacking nuclear atypia. Binucleated chondrocytes (*arrow*) may be present, and some cases may exhibit a higher degree of cellularity and atypia compared with an enchondroma (hematoxylin-eosin , original magnification x200).

whereas in the axial skeleton they generally represent CSA1.

Molecular analysis is of limited usefulness in separating enchondroma from ACT/CSA1. *IDH1/*

Box 2
Multiple enchondromas

- Enchondromatosis (Maffucci syndrome or Ollier disease) (see **Fig. 9**)
  - ○ Noninherited; postzygotic mosaic mutations in *IDH1* and *IHD2*
  - ○ Multiple enchondromas of the metaphyseal regions of tubular, and, less commonly, flat bones
  - ○ Associated with other nonskeletal malignancies
  - ○ Maffucci syndrome also manifests soft tissue hemangiomas, often spindle cell hemangioma
  - ○ The lifetime risk of malignant transformation approximately 40% (higher than sporadic lesions), highest in pelvic enchondromas
  - ○ Patients need careful radiographic surveillance and clinical management
- Metachondromatosis (multiple enchondromas and osteochondromas)
  - ○ Autosomal dominant; *PTPN11* loss-of-function mutations
  - ○ No apparent increased risk of malignant transformation

---

2 mutations are an early oncogenic event in cartilaginous tumors (including conventional and dedifferentiated chondrosarcoma) and cannot be used to separate these entities.[15,22] Similarly, alterations in the *COL2A1* gene, important for type II collagen fiber formation, are seen in both enchondroma and chondrosarcoma.[8] Chondrosarcoma shows additional numerical and structural karyotypic aberrations, increasing with histologic grade; p53, Rb, and Hedgehog pathways are implicated.[8]

CHONDROBLASTOMA

Chondroblastoma is a benign tumor composed of chondroblastic cells and matrix, typically involving the epiphysis. It is rare (<1% of primary bone tumors). Chondroblastoma preferentially involves skeletally immature individuals (adolescents and young adults) and is rare in older adults.[23,24]

Pain is the most common symptom, often several months to years in duration.[24] Gait abnormality, joint effusion, swelling, muscle atrophy, or decreased mobility can be seen. Most chondroblastomas involve epiphyses of long bones; however, a range of sites can be affected, in particular the phalanges and flat bones in adults.[23]

Radiographically, chondroblastoma is nearly always unifocal and sharply marginated, predominantly lytic, and rimmed by sclerotic bone. Tumors are centered in the epiphysis, but may cross the physis into the metaphysis. Approximately 25% of cases are apophyseal. Matrix calcification is seen in 25% to 33%.[24] Periosteal reaction is uncommon, but MRI often demonstrates tumor-associated reactive marrow changes (**Fig. 10**).

Gross examination of curetted material shows firm, pink–gray tissue, occasionally with gritty

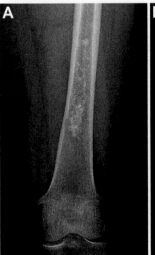
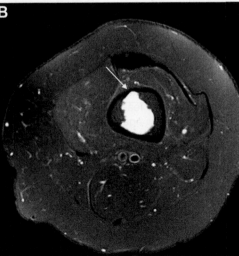

Fig. 7. (*A*) A plain film of an enchondroma demonstrates stippled intramedullary calcifications indicative of chondroid matrix with associated calcification. (*B*) On MRI, the cartilaginous matrix is bright on T2-weighted sequences, and this case shows minor endosteal cortical scalloping (*arrow*).

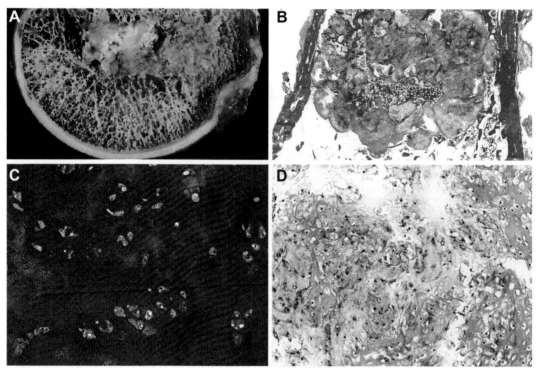

Fig. 8. (*A*) Gross examination of a resected enchondroma demonstrates multiple coalescing intramedullary nodules of pearly white–blue cartilage with central gritty white ossification. (*B*) At low power, enchondroma is composed of coalescing nodules of hyaline cartilage, some surrounded by a rim of bone, with a well-demarcated peripheral border (lower portion of image) [hematoxylin-eosin , original magnification x6]. (*C*) Higher magnification shows well-formed hyaline cartilage with basophilic matrix, low cellularity, and chondrocytes with small, round, dark nuclei (hematoxylin-eosin , original magnification x130). (*D*) Enchondromas of small bones can show somewhat increased cellularity and may demonstrate foci of myxoid matrix (hematoxylin-eosin , original magnification x120).

calcifications, hemorrhage, and cystic change. Resection demonstrates a well-demarcated, round to oval mass generally less than 5 cm, surrounded by a thin rim of sclerotic bone.

Histologically, chondroblastoma is characterized by sheets of ovoid mononuclear chondroblasts, irregularly distributed osteoclast-type giant cells, and islands of pink cartilage. The chondroblasts have pale eosinophilic cytoplasm, relatively well-defined cytoplasmic membranes, and eccentric nuclei with lobulated contours and grooves (**Fig. 11**A, B). Distinguishing features include eosinophilic fibrochondroid matrix and pericellular delicate, stippled chicken wire calcifications (present in 35% of cases). Denser calcifications may be seen.[23] Well-developed hyaline cartilage is almost never identified. Mitotic activity is present but low. Secondary aneurysmal bone cyst change is not uncommon.

Molecularly, the majority (approximately 90%) of chondroblastomas harbor driver mutations in *H3F3B* or, less commonly, *H3F3A*, genes encoding histone H3.3 protein, leading to epigenetic alterations and a highly altered transcriptome.[25] A specific antibody for H3K36M, the most common mutation, serves as a useful diagnostic adjunct (**Fig. 11**C).[26] The mutation-specific antibody for giant cell tumor of bone, H3G34W, is negative.[26] DOG1 expression may also serve as a diagnostic marker, albeit with less sensitivity and specificity. The chondroblasts are typically positive for S-100 protein (may be focal) and SOX9, and they may express cytokeratin and p63.[27,28] A recent study demonstrated increased expression of receptor activator of nuclear factor-κB ligand (RANKL) by in situ hybridization.[29]

Most cases are successfully treated by curettage. Recurrence rates range from 5%[30] to 14%[31] and vary by anatomic site: lower in long bones and higher in flat and craniofacial bones. Histologically benign chondroblastoma can exceptionally produce lung metastasis (<1%), usually related to multiple prior recurrences or pathologic fracture. The recent demonstration of increased RANKL expression raises the possibility of denosumab as a potential therapeutic avenue.[29]

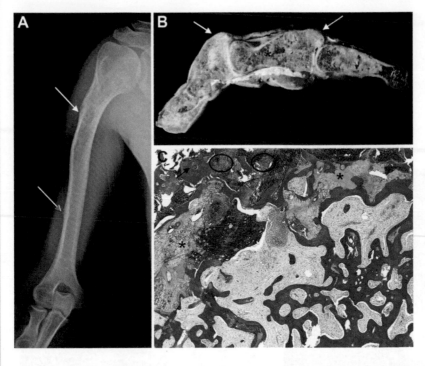

Fig. 9. (*A*) In a patient with enchondromatosis (Ollier disease), a plain radiograph shows a bowing deformity with multifocal mixed radiolucent and radiodense lesions throughout the humerus, including a dominant well-defined lucent lesion with cortical thinning (*white arrow*). Although most lesions are intramedullary, patients with enchondromatosis frequently also have periosteal and cortical tumors (*yellow arrow*). (*B*) Gross examination of a resected finger in a patient with Ollier disease shows multiple intramedullary enchondromas (***) with foci of chondrosarcomatous transformation evidenced by multifocal cortical transgression with soft tissue extension (*arrows*). (*C*) Histologically, an underlying mineralized enchondroma is present (***) with areas of chondrosarcomatous transformation with frank infiltrative growth, circumferentially encasing preexisting bony trabeculae (*circles*) and permeating Haversian systems (*arrow*) [hematoxylin-eosin , original magnification x10].

Malignant chondroblastoma is exceedingly rare. It is defined as chondroblastoma with cytologic atypia and permeative growth.[32] The identification of the molecular driver of chondroblastoma has facilitated understanding of this disease. Some previously reported chondroblastoma-like osteosarcoma cases might represent malignant chondroblastoma.[32,33]

CHONDROMYXOID FIBROMA

Chondromyxoid fibroma is a benign cartilaginous and myofibroblastic neoplasm with distinctive lobulated, zonal architecture. It is rare (<1% of primary bone tumors). This tumor is most frequent in long bones (proximal tibia and distal femur), but can occur in any osseous site including the pelvis, skull, and phalanges. Age range at presentation is wide, with a peak in the second and third decades of life. Chondromyxoid fibroma is usually intramedullary, but juxtacortical tumors are possible, particularly in a slightly older age group.[34]

Pain is a common presenting symptom, but is usually mild and of long duration.[35] Swelling and tenderness are usually restricted to lesions of the small bones of the distal extremities.

On imaging, chondromyxoid fibroma is eccentric, metaphyseal, lucent, and multilobated with internal septations (**Fig. 12**). Sclerotic margins with scalloping and matrix calcifications are occasionally present. It characteristically causes a fusiform expansion of the involved bone along its longest axis. Cortical erosion with soft tissue extension may be present, but the periosteum is intact.[35] On MRI, chondromyxoid fibroma shows high intensity on T2-weighted images and low-to-intermediate intensity on T1-weighted sequences.

Most gross specimens are curettage samples showing rubbery to firm, tan-white glistening tissue with gritty areas. Resected tumors are well-demarcated and lobulated with a sclerotic rim. The average tumor size is 3 cm (range, 1–10 cm).

Histologically, the low-power lobular and zonal architecture with peripheral hypercellularity is characteristic. The matrix is composed of poorly formed hyaline cartilage with focal well-formed hyaline cartilage in a minority of cases (20%). The neoplastic cells are spindled to stellate, with interconnecting cytoplasmic processes. In the chondroid areas, the lesional cells are rounded and occupy lacunae. Osteoclast-like giant cells and chondroblast-like cells are present in the

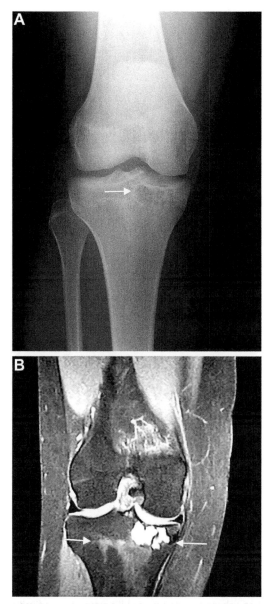

Fig. 10. (*A*) Chondroblastoma of the proximal tibial epiphysis shows a well-defined, radiolucent mass with lobu-lated margins and a thin sclerotic rim (*arrow*) on radiographs. (*B*) On MRI, this T2-weighted sequence shows a well-defined, lobulated lesion extending inferiorly across the physis (*arrows*).

periphery. Delicate, branching vasculature is not uncommon and is unique among the low-grade cartilage tumors. Approximately 25% of cases harbor coarse, globular calcifications, and 10% demonstrate secondary aneurysmal bone cyst-like changes (**Fig. 13**). Pseudomalignant change (enlarged, hyperchromatic nuclei with smudgy, degenerative-type atypia) is well-documented. Necrosis and mitotic activity are uncommon.

Immunohistochemically, SOX9 and S-100 pro-tein are expressed in the chondrogenic areas of chondromyxoid fibroma. Myofibroblastic differen-tiation is evident in the spindle cells, with the expression of HHF35 and smooth muscle actin.[36]

Clonal rearrangements of chromosome 6 have been described as the sole or as 1 of multiple karyotypic abnormalities. Recurrent *GRM1* gene fusions have also been implicated in the

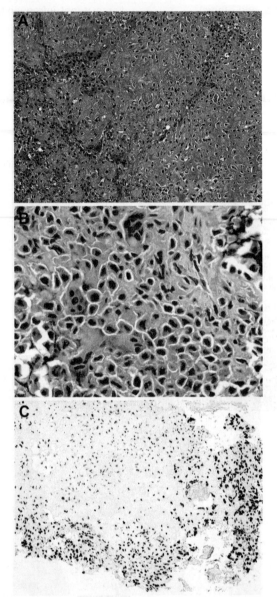

Fig. 11. (*A*) Chondroblastoma has a characteristic eosinophilic matrix that is fibrillary to dense (hematoxylin-eosin , original magnification x100). (*B*) The neoplastic mononuclear cells have eosinophilic cytoplasm, well-defined cell borders, and folded, grooved nuclei. The matrix shows calcification in a "chicken-wire" distribution (*top right*) [hematoxylin-eosin , original magnification x400]. (*C*) Immunohistochemistry with the mutation-specific anti-body, H3K36M, highlights the neoplastic mononuclear cells (hematoxylin-eosin , original magnification x100).

pathogenesis of chondromyxoid fibroma and are believed to be the driving event.[37]

Most cases of chondromyxoid fibroma are treated by curettage or, less commonly, conservative en bloc resection. Recurrence occurs in up to 15% of cases.[38] Metastasis has not been documented. Malignant transformation is exceptionally rare. Chondromyxoid fibroma-like osteosarcoma occasionally enters the differential diagnosis (see **Table 2**).[39]

Fig. 12. (*A*) Chondromyx-oid fibroma eccentrically located along the posterior aspect of the distal tibia on conventional radiograph, centered in the metaphysis. (*B*) Characteristically, its long axis is parallel to the long bone, and it has lobulated borders with internal septations. Thinning of the posterior cortex is seen (*arrow*).

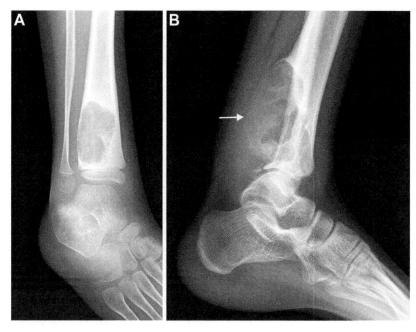

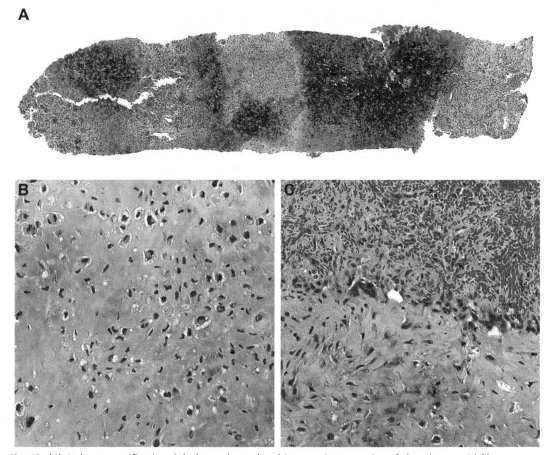

Fig. 13. (*A*) At low magnification, lobular and zonal architecture is suggestive of chondromyxoid fibroma, even on core biopsy (hematoxylin-eosin , original magnification x6). Matrix-rich, hypocellular regions transition to hypercellular zones containing tumor cells admixed with osteoclast-type giant cells. (*B*) The lesional cells are oval to polyhedral and reside within lacunae or are stellate in shape, suspended in myxoid matrix (hematoxylin-eosin , original magnification x200). (*C*) Secondary aneurysmal bone cyst-like changes can be seen (hematoxylin-eosin, original magnification x150).

SUMMARY

Benign cartilage-forming tumors can represent diagnostic challenges owing to overlap with low-grade malignant cartilage-forming tumors. However, careful histologic assessment, correlation with clinical and radiographic features, and selective use of ancillary testing will lead to appropriate diagnosis and treatment in most instances. A multidisciplinary team approach is an invaluable aspect of this diagnostic process.

CLINICS CARE POINTS

- Radiographically, cartilage-forming tumors usually demonstrate characteristic matrix mineralization, and correlation with imaging findings is essential in establishing a diagnosis.

- In low-grade cartilaginous tumors, the diagnostic threshold for malignancy is influenced by patient age, tumor location, and the presence of an underlying genetic syndrome.

- Invasion of preexisting bone or adjacent soft tissue is generally incompatible with a benign diagnosis.

- The separation of benign and low-grade malignant tumors remains challenging in some instances; however, these categories of tumors are frequently treated clinically in a similar fashion.

SOURCE OF FUNDING

None.

DISCLOSURE

The authors have no conflicts of interest to declare.

REFERENCES

1. WHO Classification of Tumours Editorial Board. Soft tissue and bone tumours. International Agency for Research on Cancer; 2020.
2. van Praag Veroniek VM, Rueten-Budde AJ, Ho V, et al. Incidence, outcomes and prognostic factors during 25 years of treatment of chondrosarcomas. Surg Oncol 2018;27:402–8.
3. Afonso PD, Isaac A, Villagrán JM. Chondroid tumors as incidental findings and differential diagnosis between enchondromas and low-grade chondrosarcomas. Semin Musculoskelet Radiol 2019;23:3–18.
4. Eefting D, Schrage YM, Geirnaerdt MJA, et al. Assessment of interobserver variability and histologic parameters to improve reliability in classification and grading of central cartilaginous tumors. Am J Surg Pathol 2009;33:50–7.
5. de Andrea CE, Kroon HM, Wolterbeek R, et al. Interobserver reliability in the histopathological diagnosis of cartilaginous tumors in patients with multiple osteochondromas. Mod Pathol 2012;25:1275–83.
6. Bovée JVMG. Multiple osteochondromas. Orphanet J Rare Dis 2008;3:3.
7. Bernard SA, Murphey MD, Flemming DJ, et al. Improved differentiation of benign osteochondromas from secondary chondrosarcomas with standardized measurement of cartilage cap at CT and MR imaging. Radiology 2010;255:857–65.
8. de Andrea CE, San-Julian M, Bovée JVMG. Integrating morphology and genetics in the diagnosis of cartilage tumors. Surg Pathol Clin 2017;10: 537–52.
9. Hameetman L, Szuhai K, Yavas A, et al. The role of EXT1 in nonhereditary osteochondroma: identification of homozygous deletions. J Natl Cancer Inst 2007;99:396–406.
10. Florez B, Mönckeberg J, Castillo G, et al. Solitary osteochondroma long-term follow-up. J Pediatr Orthop B 2008;17:91–4.
11. Nora FE, Dahlin DC, Beabout JW. Bizarre parosteal osteochondromatous proliferations of the hands and feet. Am J Surg Pathol 1983;7:245–50.
12. Cocks M, Helmke E, Meyers CA, et al. Bizarre parosteal osteochondromatous proliferation: 16 Cases with a focus on histologic variability. J Orthop 2018;15:138–42.
13. Nilsson M, Domanski HA, Mertens F, et al. Molecular cytogenetic characterization of recurrent translocation breakpoints in bizarre parosteal osteochondromatous proliferation (Nora's lesion). Hum Pathol 2004;35:1063–9.
14. Bauer TW, Dorfman HD, Latham JT Jr. Periosteal chondroma. A clinicopathologic study of 23 cases. Am J Surg Pathol 1982;6:631–7.
15. Amary MF, Bacsi K, Maggiani F, et al. IDH1 and IDH2 mutations are frequent events in central chondrosarcoma and central and periosteal chondromas but not in other mesenchymal tumours. J Pathol 2011;224:334–43.
16. Lewis MM, Kenan S, Yabut SM, et al. Periosteal chondroma. A report of ten cases and review of the literature. Clin Orthop Relat Res 1990;185–92.
17. Cleven AHG, Zwartkruis E, Hogendoorn PCW, et al. Periosteal chondrosarcoma: a histopathological and

molecular analysis of a rare chondrosarcoma subtype. Histopathology 2015;67:483–90.

18. Suster D, Hung YP, Nielsen GP. Differential diagnosis of cartilaginous lesions of bone. Arch Pathol Lab Med 2020;144:71–82.

19. Bierry G, Kerr DA, Nielsen GP, et al. Enchondromas in children: imaging appearance with pathological correlation. Skeletal Radiol 2012;41:1223–9.

20. Pansuriya TC, van Eijk R, d'Adamo P, et al. Somatic mosaic IDH1 and IDH2 mutations are associated with enchondroma and spindle cell hemangioma in Ollier disease and Maffucci syndrome. NatGenet 2011;43:1256–61.

21. Shon W, Folpe AL, Fritchie KJ. ERG expression in chondrogenic bone and soft tissue tumours. J Clin Pathol 2015;68:125–9.

22. Kerr DA, Lopez HU, Deshpande V, et al. Molecular distinction of chondrosarcoma from chondroblastic osteosarcoma through IDH1/2 mutations. Am J Surg Pathol 2013;37:787.

23. John I, Inwards CY, Wenger DE, et al. Chondroblastomas presenting in adulthood: a study of 39 patients with emphasis on histological features and skeletal distribution. Histopathology 2020;76:308–17.

24. Bloem JL, Mulder JD. Chondroblastoma: a clinical and radiological study of 104 cases. Skeletal Radiol 1985;14:1–9.

25. Behjati S, Tarpey PS, Presneau N, et al. Distinct H3F3A and H3F3B driver mutations define chondroblastoma and giant cell tumor of bone. Nat Genet 2013;45:1479–82.

26. Schaefer IM, Fletcher JA, Nielsen GP, et al. Immunohistochemistry for histone H3G34W and H3K36M is highly specific for giant cell tumor of bone and chondroblastoma, respectively, in FNA and core needle biopsy. Cancer Cytopathol 2018;126:552–66.

27. Akpalo H, Lange C, Zustin J. Discovered on gastrointestinal stromal tumour 1 (DOG1): a useful immunohistochemical marker for diagnosing chondroblastoma. Histopathology 2012;60:1099–106.

28. Cleven AHG, Briaire-de Bruijn I, Szuhai K, et al. DOG1 expression in giant-cell-containing bone tumours. Histopathology 2016;68:942–5.

29. Suster DI, Kurzawa P, Neyaz A, et al. Chondroblastoma expresses RANKL by RNA in situ hybridization and may respond to denosumab therapy. Am J Surg Pathol 2020;44:1581–90.

30. Ebeid WA, Hasan BZ, Badr IT, et al. Functional and oncological outcome after treatment of chondroblastoma with intralesional curettage. J Pediatr Orthop 2019;39:e312–7.

31. Laitinen MK, Stevenson JD, Evans S, et al. Chondroblastoma in pelvis and extremities- a single centre study of 177 cases. J Bone Oncol 2019;17:100248.

32. Papke DJ, Hung YP, Schaefer I-M, et al. Clinicopathologic characterization of malignant chondroblastoma: a neoplasm with locally aggressive behavior and metastatic potential that closely mimics chondroblastoma-like osteosarcoma. Mod Pathol 2020;33:2295–306.

33. Hmada YA, Bernieh A, Morris RW, et al. Chondroblastoma-like Osteosarcoma. Arch Pathol Lab Med 2020;144:15–7.

34. Baker AC, Rezeanu L, O'Laughlin S, et al. Juxtacortical chondromyxoid fibroma of bone: a unique variant: a case study of 20 patients. Am J Surg Pathol 2007;31:1662–8.

35. Wu CT, Inwards CY, O'Laughlin S, et al. Chondromyxoid fibroma of bone: a clinicopathologic review of 278 cases. Hum Pathol 1998;29:438–46.

36. Nielsen GP, Keel SB, Dickersin GR, et al. Chondromyxoid fibroma: a tumor showing myofibroblastic, myochondroblastic, and chondrocytic differentiation. Mod Pathol 1999;12:514–7.

37. Baumhoer D, Amary F, Flanagan AM. An update of molecular pathology of bone tumors. Lessons learned from investigating samples by next generation sequencing. Genes Chromosomes Cancer 2019;58(2):88–99.

38. Bhamra JS, Al-Khateeb H, Dhinsa BS, et al. Chondromyxoid fibroma management: a single institution experience of 22 cases. World J Surg Oncol 2014;12:283.

39. Zhong J, Si L, Geng J, et al. Chondromyxoid fibroma-like osteosarcoma: a case series and literature review. BMC Musculoskelet Disord 2020;21:53.

Malignant Cartilage-Forming Tumors

Meera Hameed, MD

KEYWORDS

- Conventional • Dedifferentiated • Secondary • Periosteal • Clear cell • Mesenchymal • *IDH1/2 mutations* • *Hey1-NCOA2 rearrangement*

Key points

- Chondrosarcoma is classified into central and peripheral types
- Secondary chondrosarcoma is associated with benign preexisting lesion such as osteochondroma
- IDH1/2 mutations are seen in about 50% cases of central chondrosarcoma
- Hey1-NCOA2 fusion is diagnostic for mesenchymal chondrosarcoma

ABSTRACT

Chondrosarcomas are heterogeneous matrix-producing cartilaginous neoplasms with variable clinical behavior. Subtypes include conventional (75%), dedifferentiated (10%), clear cell (2%), mesenchymal (2%), and periosteal chondrosarcoma (<1%). Tumor location and primary vs secondary also play a role. In conventional chondrosarcoma, histologic grading (I, II, and III) remains the gold standard for predicting recurrence and metastases. Due to the locally aggressive but overall nonmetastatic behavior, grade I chondrosarcomas (primary and secondary) of long and short tubular bones have been reclassified as atypical cartilaginous tumor. In this review, the pathologic features of malignant cartilage tumors are discussed with updates on recent genetic findings.

CONVENTIONAL CHONDROSARCOMA

INTRODUCTION

Chondrosarcomas (CSs) comprise about 20% of primary osseous malignancies with an estimated incidence of 1:20,000.[1,2] Of these central type predominates (about 75%) and peripheral CSs account for 10%, both defined by the production of neoplastic hyaline cartilage by tumor cells whose pathologic grade and location affect therapeutic outcome.[3–6] Tumors occur in adults between third and sixth decades of life with pelvis, femur, humerus, and rib being common locations.[4] Pathologic grading into atypical cartilaginous tumor (ACT) and grade 1 CS (long tubular bones and axial skeleton, respectively) and grades II and III CS influence 10-year survival.[7–9] Clinically, pain is a common symptom often waking the patient at night, and radiopathological correlation is essential for histologic diagnosis of CS especially in ACT/grade I CS. Surgery is the mainstay of treatment with extended curettage with adjuvant therapies for low-grade intramedullary tumors in long tubular bones and en bloc resection for grades II and III CS.[10] Low-grade tumors relapse as high grade in about 13% of the cases.[6] At present, radiation and chemotherapy are of limited benefit in relapsed and metastatic disease.[10] About 50% of central conventional CSs possess hotspot mutations in isocitrate dehydrogenase 1 and 2 (*IDH1/2*) leading to gain of function of oncometabolite D-2-hydroxyglutarate, resulting in epigenetic changes of a hypermethylated phenotype.[11,12] There are ongoing clinical trials exploring mutant IDH1 inhibitors in patients with CS.[13]

Department of Pathology, Memorial Sloan-Kettering Cancer Center, 1275 York Avenue, New York, NY 10065, USA

E-mail address: hameedm@mskcc.org

Surgical Pathology 14 (2021) 605–617
https://doi.org/10.1016/j.path.2021.06.005

surgpath.theclinics.com

IMAGING FEATURES

CSs commonly affect metaphyseal regions (50%) of long bones followed by diaphyseal (36%) and epiphyseal regions (16%).[2] Radiographs typically show lytic and sclerotic lesion showing chondroid-type matrix mineralization with "rings and arcs," endosteal scalloping (**Fig. 1A and B**), cortical expansion, and cortical penetration and soft tissue mass in some cases. Deep endosteal scalloping (more than two-thirds of the depth of cortex) is considered a sensitive indicator to distinguish central CS from enchondroma.[14] MRI shows a lobular growth pattern with low to intermediate T1-weighted signal and high T2-weighted signal due to high water content[14] (**Fig. 1C and D**).

GROSS AND MICROSCOPIC FEATURES

ACT/CS I is generally treated by curettage and grossly shows bluish gray fragments with admixed bone marrow and bone. Resected specimens (most often CS II and III) show a lobulated bluish gray/white tumor with glistening surface (**Fig. 1E**). Myxoid and cystic changes are apparent as is cortical destruction and penetration. Microscopically, the tumor is composed of lobules of hyaline cartilage composed of chondrocytes sitting in lacunar spaces with uni or binucleated nuclei. The diagnosis is established by the presence of entrapped preexisting viable bony trabeculae within lobules of cartilage or cortical erosion by tumor cells. In grade II CS, cellularity is higher than ACT/CS I; additionally, myxoid changes with chondrocytes arranged in cords without lacunar spaces may be present. The nuclei are condensed or more open with nucleoli, and mitoses may be seen. In grade III CSs, nuclei are larger and more hyperchromatic, have more easily identifiable mitoses, and spindling of cells at the periphery and myxoid changes can be seen (**Fig. 1F–I**). Necrosis can be seen regardless of the grade of tumor. In small bones of hands and feet, increased cellularity or myxoid changes by itself is not sufficient

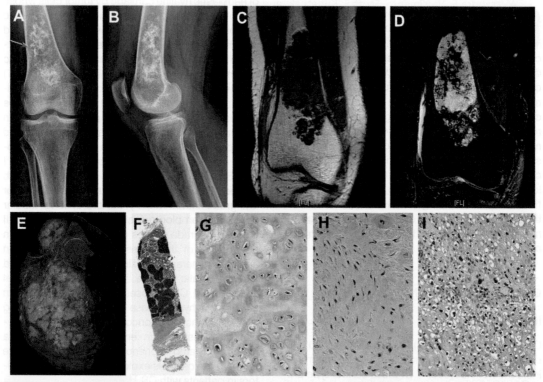

Fig. 1. (*A, B*) Atypical cartilaginous tumor/low-grade chondrosarcoma: anteroposterior (AP) and lateral views of distal femoral metadiaphyseal lesion show ring and arc-type calcifications and endosteal scalloping (*arrow*). (*C, D*) Coronal T1-weighted and fat-suppressed T2-weighted MRI showing lobulated chondroid lesion, with hyperintense signal on T2. (*E*) Gross photograph of a pelvic chondrosarcoma with destruction of acetabular roof. The tumor is composed of lobules of glistening cartilage with calcifications. (*F*) Photomicrograph of chondrosarcoma grade 1 of pubis with cortical invasion (low power, ×10). [Photomicrograph ((*G–I*) Photomicrographs of chondrosarcoma grades I, II, and III showing increasing cellularity with increasing grade of chondrocytes [Photomicrograph (hematoxylin-eosin stain)]. Myxoid changes with loss of lacunar spaces are seen in grade II CS (*H*). Photomicrograph (hematoxylin-eosin, original magnification×200).

and cortical destruction and soft tissue extension is needed to establish malignancy.

MOLECULAR PATHOLOGY

It is well established that about 50% of conventional CSs harbor heterozygous missense mutations in *IDH1* R132 and *IDH2* R172.[11] *IDH1* R132 is the most common variant, and of the various substitutions, R132C is seen in ~40% of the *IDH* mutated tumors. Gain of function of the oncometabolite D-2-hydroxyglutarate is the direct consequence of *IDH1/2* mutations resulting in inhibition of demethylation enzyme Tet methylcytosine dioxygenase 2 (TET2) ultimately leading to a hypermethylation phenotype altering various transcriptional pathways.[12,15] About 37% of CSs have mutations in *COL2A1*, a major cartilage collagen gene, in the form of insertions, deletions, or rearrangements. Disruption of collagen maturation and matrix deposition has been proposed as the mechanism of promoting oncogenesis.[16] Additional genomic alterations include alterations in *TP53* (20%), *RB1* pathway (33%), Hedgehog pathway (18%), *CDKN2A/B* (30%), and *TERT/ATRX* (20%–26%).[16–19] Recently a multiomics classification has been proposed based on 3 molecular features in cartilage tumor progression, which include *IDH1/2* mutations leading to broad hypermethylation, loss of expression of 14q32 locus, specifically miRNA cluster at this locus, and a transcriptome with increased mitotic potential, together showing superior prognostic value when compared with traditional grading methods.[20]

DIFFERENTIAL DIAGNOSIS

The major differential diagnosis for ACT/CS 1 is enchondroma, which can have overlapping histologic and imaging characteristics. The difficulties in distinguishing these 2 entities have been emphasized in a few studies where interobserver variabilities have been highlighted in both imaging and histologic features[21,22]; this underscores the importance of a multidisciplinary approach, which takes into account clinical, imaging, and pathologic findings. Histologically difficulties are also related to fragmentation of tissue in curettings, which precludes accurate assessment of architectural patterns. Nevertheless, entrapment of preexisting viable lamellar bone within cartilage lobules and erosion or invasion of cortex are pathologic signs of malignancy. In high-grade CSs, the aggressive nature is often evident on imaging with permeative cortical destruction and/or soft tissue extension. In biopsy samples, a chondroblastic osteosarcoma can be difficult to distinguish

if neoplastic osteoid is not present, and additional studies such as *IDH1/2* mutation analysis may be necessary. In skull-based lesions a chondroid chordoma can mimic a CS and will stain for brachyury and keratin, which would aid their distinction.

PROGNOSIS

Pathologic grading remains the major prognostic indicator, and the corresponding 10-year survival for ACT/CS I, CS II, and CS III ranges from 79% to 100%, 53% to 90%, and 29% to 55%, respectively.[7–9] Metastatic rates of 10% to 30% and 32% to 71% are reported for grade II and grade III CSs, respectively.[3,6,8,9] Tumors at axial location have a worse outcome than those at extremities.[23,24] Chen and colleagues[25] have reported a nomogram based on sex, pathologic grade, tumor size, stage, and surgery to predict overall survival in pelvic CSs. The role of *IDH* mutations in overall survival is not clear now.[19,26–28]

DEDIFFERENTIATED CHONDROSARCOMA

INTRODUCTION

Dedifferentiated chondrosarcoma (DDCS) is the most aggressive subtype representing about 11% of all CSs and is defined by biphasic morphology with a low-grade cartilaginous component juxtaposed with a high-grade noncartilaginous sarcomatous component.[29,30] DDCS is a tumor of older adults (59–66 years) with equal sex distribution, commonly affecting the femur (55%), pelvis (23%), and humerus (10%), but other bones such as the scapula, ribs, tibia, and fibula can also be affected.[31] Although most tumors arise centrally as components of a conventional CS, rare tumors develop from peripheral tumors (transformation in osteochondroma).[32] About 20% present with metastatic disease,[31] and the 5-year survival is about 18%.[33] Surgery with wide margins is considered the optimal treatment of choice, and any adjuvant therapy is currently investigational.[30,33–35]

IMAGING FEATURES

Radiological features show features of high-grade CS with chondroid-type matrix mineralization in most cases adjacent to a lytic area associated with cortical destruction and soft tissue extension (Fig. 2A). Pathologic fracture can be present in one-third of the cases. MRI shows the bimorphic pattern with chondroid and nonchondroid components.[14]

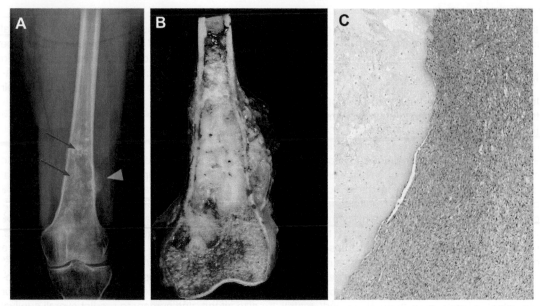

Fig. 2. (*A*) Dedifferentiated chondrosarcoma: AP view of a distal femur shows a metadiaphyseal lesion with rings and arc-like chondroid matrix calcification (*arrows*) with destructive lytic areas and periosteal reaction (*arrowhead*). (*B*) Gross photograph of dedifferentiated chondrosarcoma showing an intramedullary cartilage lesion with white glistening lobules of cartilage associated with soft tissue extension with gray fleshy appearance representing the dedifferentiated component. (*C*) Photomicrograph showing a biphasic histology of a well-differentiated chondrosarcoma juxtaposed to a noncartilaginous high-grade spindle cell sarcoma Photomicrograph (hematoxylin-eosin, original magnification×100).

GROSS AND MICROSCOPIC FEATURES

The 2 components are usually clearly visible with bluish lobulated cartilage within medullary cavity juxtaposed with a fleshy tan yellow/brown non-chondroid component often extending into the soft tissue (**Fig. 2**B). Microscopically, the tumor is composed of 2 components, a well-differentiated cartilage component with features ranging from enchondroma to CS grade I or II with abrupt transition to a high-grade noncartilaginous component composed of a sarcoma with features of undifferentiated pleomorphic sarcoma, osteosarcoma, spindle cell sarcoma not otherwise specified (NOS), and other rare types such as angiosarcoma and rhabdomyosarcoma (**Fig. 2**C).[36] Rarely the dedifferentiated component is made up of squamous, epithelial, or adamantinomalike areas.[37–39] The dedifferentiated component is variable and can be as little as 2% or as high as 98% in any individual tumor.[40]

MOLECULAR PATHOLOGY

Similar to conventional CS, *IDH1/2* and *COL2A1* are frequently mutated in DDCS and show additional genetic changes in the dedifferentiated component, such as *TP53* alterations.[11,16,41] In a recent study, next-generation sequencing of matched chondroid and dedifferentiated components of DDCS has shown identical *IDH1/2*, *COL2A1*, and *TERT* promoter mutations suggesting a monoclonal origin with divergence into 2 lineages, and these mutations are likely early events in tumorigenesis.[42] Rare metachronous tumors have been reported suggesting a time-dependent progression whose molecular characteristics are unknown.[43,44] Loss of histone-H3k27me3 by immunohistochemistry has been reported in 6 of 19 (32%) DDCSs, of which 3 cases harbored *SUZ12* or *EED* alterations in the dedifferentiated component only, suggesting a role for the polycomb repressive complex 2 in dedifferentiation.[45] The demonstration of *H3F3A* mutation in some cases of presumed DDCS with chondroid and giant cell tumor components suggests that these may represent giant cell tumors with cartilage differentiation.[46]

DIFFERENTIAL DIAGNOSIS

As the high-grade component shows histologic and immunohistochemical features of sarcomas of various lineages, imaging correlation is needed for the accurate diagnosis of DDCS in biopsy material. Aberrant cytokeratin expression can be a pitfall and can lead to the misdiagnosis of sarcomatoid carcinoma and affect therapeutic outcome.

PROGNOSIS

The prognosis of DDCS remains dismal with 5-year overall survival of about 18% (range 7%–24%). Metastasis to lung is common. Tumor size (>8 cm), metastasis at the time of diagnosis, and inadequate margin are predictors of poor prognosis.[33]

SECONDARY CHONDROSARCOMA

Secondary CSs arise from a preexisting benign cartilage lesion either central (enchondroma) or peripheral (osteochondroma). Secondary CSs can be syndromic and arise in association with Ollier disease (enchondromatosis), Maffucci syndrome (enchondromas, hemangiomas), and multiple hereditary exostoses (MHE).[4,47] The incidence of malignant transformation is higher in syndromic patients, up to 40% in Ollier disease and 25% in MHE, as is earlier age of onset.[47–49] Imaging features of central secondary CS are similar to those of conventional CS. CSs arising in osteochondromas arise from the cartilage cap with an overall transformation rate of ∼1%.[50] Most common sites are pelvis, scapula, pubic bone, and ribs.[4] Imaging features of malignancy include growth in a skeletally mature patient, erosion and destruction of underlying bone, and large cartilage cap visualized on MRI, of more than 2 cm[14,51] (Fig. 3A and B). Grossly the tumor has a stalk with an irregular cartilage cap, which is covered by a fibrous perichondrium (Fig. 3C).

Histologically, apart from a thickened cartilage cap of more than 2 cm (measured at maximum thickness), soft tissue nodules, invasion of stalk, erosion, and tumor invasion of bone are indicators of malignant transformation. In all cases imaging correlation is necessary and the diagnosis of CS should be based on imaging and histologic features.

Similar to conventional CSs, IDH1/2 mutations are common in tumors arising in patients with Ollier disease (81%) and Maffucci syndrome (77%).[26,49] Secondary CSs arising in osteochondromas show EXT1/2 mutations similar to solitary and hereditary osteochondromas,[52] and malignant transformation is accompanied by genomic instability, severe aneuploidy, and alterations in TP53 and RB1 pathways.[53] Grading is similar to conventional CS. Clinical course depends on the location and the feasibility of adequate resection.[4]

PERIOSTEAL CHONDROSARCOMA

INTRODUCTION

Periosteal CS is a rare variant accounting for less than 2% of all CSs, which arises at the surface of the bone in metaphysis or metadiaphysis closely associated with the periosteum with erosion or invasion of the underlying cortex.[4,54] The tumor presents at the second or third decades of life with a slight male predominance and affects femur as the most common site followed by humerus and rare cases reported in ilium, fibula, and ribs.[4,55] The

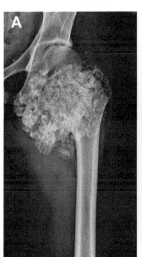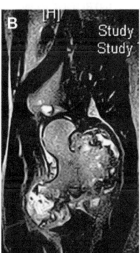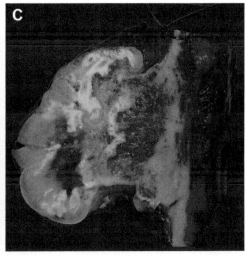

Fig. 3. (A) Chondrosarcoma arising in osteochondroma: AP view of left proximal femur shows a large mass with chondroid-type calcification involving femoral neck. (B) The T2-weighted MRI image shows a corticomedullary continuity (*asterisk*) between the femur and the lesion (T). Irregular thick cartilaginous cap (*arrow*) measuring more than 2 cm in thickness. (C) Gross photograph showing a thick cartilage cap (>2 cm) of a chondrosarcoma arising in an osteochondroma.

clinical course is usually long and indolent, and the prognosis is generally good with a low incidence of metastases (5%–12.2%)[56] with lungs being the most common site and rarely lymph nodes.[56,57]

IMAGING FEATURES

Plain radiographs show a surface soft tissue mass with well-defined borders containing chondroid-type calcifications with underlying cortex, which is irregular, thickened, and eroded (Fig. 4A). On MRI the tumor is lobular with low to intermediate signals on T1-weighted sequences and high signal on T2-weighted sequences typical for cartilage neoplasms. The tumor can invade medullary cavity. The imaging features do not reliably distinguish periosteal chondroma and periosteal CS, and the major difference is the size of the lesion, periosteal CS is larger than 5 cm (mean size 5.3 cm) compared with periosteal chondroma (mean size 2.2 cm).[14,58]

GROSS AND MICROSCOPIC FEATURES

Grossly, the tumor is present at the surface and is covered by a fibrous pseudocapsule and is continuous with the underlying periosteum often eroding or invading the cortex and contains lobules of glistening cartilage (Fig. 4B). Histologically, the tumor is composed of lobules of hyaline cartilage with myxoid changes with variable cellularity and nuclear atypia (Fig. 4C and D). Extension into soft tissue can occur. Although the tumor usually has features of grade 1 or II, grading is not of prognostic significance and hence not applied in periosteal CS.[4,59]

MOLECULAR PATHOLOGY

Mutations of IDH1/2 have been reported in 15% of the cases.[60]

DIFFERENTIAL DIAGNOSIS

The major differential diagnoses are periosteal chondroma and periosteal osteosarcoma. Both periosteal chondroma and periosteal CS have overlapping radiological features. A size greater than 5 cm and invasion of the underlying cortex are criteria for malignancy. Periosteal osteosarcoma, which is often of the chondroblastic type, is an important differential diagnosis with prognostic and therapeutic implications. Osteoid production and deposition by tumor cells is a feature of periosteal osteosarcoma, which also shows more severe atypia of chondrocytes when compared with periosteal CS.[4,61] Secondary peripheral CSs occasionally can be mistaken for periosteal CS. The presence of preexisting osteochondroma and communication into medullary cavity with a stalk are distinguishing features. In parosteal osteosarcoma, a cartilage cap is often seen; however, the tumor has distinctive histologic features of spindle cells admixed with parallel arrangement of well-developed bony trabeculae, which are easily identifiable.

PROGNOSIS

Periosteal CS has a good prognosis with 5-year survival rate of 83%. Patients need long-term follow-up because late metastases have been reported. Wide surgical resection is the treatment of choice.[56]

CLEAR CELL CHONDROSARCOMA

INTRODUCTION

Clear cell CS is a low-grade malignant neoplasm with a characteristic histologic appearance composed of clear cells containing abundant

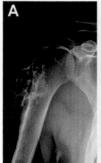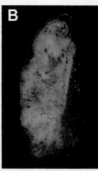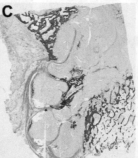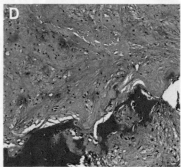

Fig. 4. (A) Periosteal chondrosarcoma: AP view of shoulder radiograph shows a juxtacortical lytic lesion with ring and arc calcifications centered in the humeral cortex. (B) Gross photograph showing a surface cartilage lesion involving cortex and focally extending into medullary cavity. (C) Photomicrograph of periosteal chondrosarcoma showing hyaline cartilage lobules invading cortex and medullary cavity. Lesion is circumscribed at the surface with pseudocapsule Photomicrograph (hematoxylin-eosin, original magnification×10). (D) Photomicrograph of periosteal chondrosarcoma showing cellular cartilage tumor with myxoid changes Photomicrograph (hematoxylin-eosin, original magnification×200).

glycogen.[62,63] A rare tumor accounting for ~2% of all CSs, it affects adults in the third to fifth decades; however, there are reports showing incidence ranging from the second to the ninth decade.[4,63] The disease has a male predominance and typically involves epiphyses of long tubular bone with femur as the common site. Other involved bones include humerus, spine, ribs, and small bones of hands and feet.[4] The 10-year survival is reported to be 89%, and late metastases can occur, necessitating long-term follow-up.[64]

IMAGING FEATURES

Plain radiographs show a lytic lesion located in the epiphyses, which may extend into metaphyses with variable zones of transition; in 20% of cases a thin sclerotic rim can be seen, and in ~30% of cases chondroid type matrix mineralization can be seen[2,14] (**Fig. 5**A). Proximal humerus lesions can have an aggressive radiological appearance. Extension into diaphysis occurs rarely. Extraosseous extension is uncommon.[14,65] MRI is heterogeneous with low to intermediate T1-weighted sequences and high signal intensity in T2-weighted sequences. Heterogeneity is attributed to hemorrhage or mineralization.[14,65]

GROSS AND MICROSCOPIC FEATURES

The tumor does not have the usual appearance of cartilage, is generally well-circumscribed, and can have focal calcifications (**Fig. 5**B). Histologically, the tumor is composed of lobules containing tumor cells with abundant clear cytoplasm and centrally placed nuclei, which are uniform with prominent nucleoli. Admixed among tumor cells are woven bone trabeculae with scattered osteoclast-type giant cells (**Fig. 5**C). Coarse calcifications and areas of hyaline cartilage similar to low-grade conventional CS can be seen. Hemorrhage and secondary aneurysmal bone cystlike changes are present in some cases. Although the gross may appear circumscribed, the tumor can show infiltrative pattern microscopically.[4,63] In very rare instances, a DDCS can arise in a clear cell CS.[66]

MOLECULAR PATHOLOGY

No specific genetic alterations have been reported thus far. No *IDH1/2* mutations have been reported. A single case of Histone *H3F3B K36M* has been reported in a series of 15 cases.[67]

DIFFERENTIAL DIAGNOSIS

The differential diagnoses include chondroblastoma, conventional CS, osteosarcoma, and metastatic clear cell renal cell carcinoma. Chondroblastomas while occurring in the epiphysis do not show the clear cell morphology and reactive bony trabeculae. Although clear cell CS can have areas of low-grade conventional CS,

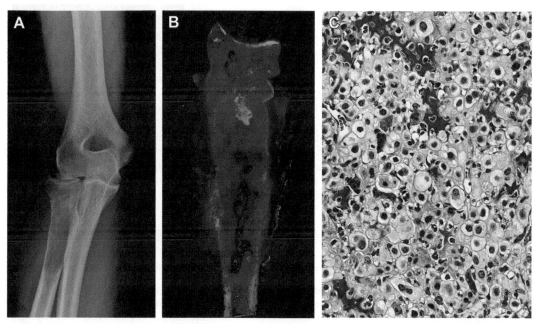

Fig. 5. (*A*) Clear cell chondrosarcoma: AP view of an elbow shows an expansile lytic lesion involving the right proximal radius metaphysis. (*B*) Gross photograph showing an intramedullary cartilage lesion involving epimetaphysis with chalky yellow calcifications. (*C*) Photomicrograph showing clear cells with round nuclei, prominent nuclei interspersed with woven bone trabeculae. Osteoclast-type giant cells are seen Photomicrograph (hematoxylin-eosin, original magnification×200).

rare cases of conventional CS with clear cell change has been reported, which can be a diagnostic challenge necessitating additional molecular workup such as *IDH1/2* mutation analysis.[68] Osteosarcomas are distinguished by neoplastic osteoid and osteoblasts. Clear cell renal carcinoma lack reactive bony trabeculae or chondroid matrix. One must bear in mind that some clear cell CS can show cytokeratin (AE1/AE3 and CK18) positivity.[69]

PROGNOSIS

The disease has an indolent course, but with definite metastatic potential. Overall reported mortality rate is 15%. Lung is the most common site for metastases followed by skeletal sites.[64] En bloc resection with clear margins is the treatment of choice; curettage results in local recurrence up to 86%.[70]

MESENCHYMAL CHONDROSARCOMA

INTRODUCTION

Mesenchymal chondrosarcoma (MC) is a high-grade translocation-associated biphasic malignant neoplasm of bone and soft tissue constituting about 2% of all CSs.[71,72] MC affects adults in the second and third decades; however, it can have wide age distribution with a very slight male preponderance.[4] The tumor commonly affects craniofacial bones (mandible and maxilla), ribs, vertebrae, pelvic bones, and long bones.[73] One-third of the cases occur at extraosseous sites, which include meninges and visceral organs[74] Reported 5- and 10-year survival based on evaluation of 205 patients in the Surveillance, Epidemiology and End Results (SEER) database is 51% and 43%, respectively.[75]

IMAGING FEATURES

The tumor has an aggressive pattern on imaging showing a permeative or moth-eaten bone destruction and periosteal reaction (**Fig. 6**A). In two-thirds of cases chondroid type mineralization is seen.[14] MRI shows more of a heterogeneous signal on T2-weighted sequences unlike the usual hyperintense signal of hyaline cartilage. Extraosseous soft tissue mass is common.[14] A distinct biphasic morphology with a sharp transition zone between calcified and noncalcified component can be seen in some cases.[76]

GROSS AND MICROSCOPIC FEATURES

Grossly the tumors appear circumscribed and show tan-gray and gritty calcifications. Soft tissue involvement is commonly seen. In some cases,

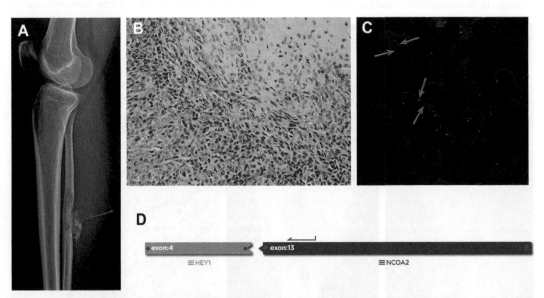

Fig. 6. (*A*) Mesenchymal chondrosarcoma: lateral radiograph shows a destructive lytic lesion with an extraosseous soft tissue mass in the fibula shaft. Calcification is present within the extraosseous soft tissue mass (*arrow*). (*B*) Photomicrograph showing biphasic histology with low-grade cartilage component blending with high-grade round cell component Photomicrograph (hematoxylin-eosin, original magnification×200). (*C*) Fluorescence in situ hybridization study using break-apart probe for NCOA2 showing separation green and red signals (*yellow arrows*) confirming rearrangement of NCOA2 gene. (*D*) Archer FusionPlex targeted RNA sequencing showing an in-frame fusion between *HEY1* exon 4 (NM_012258) and *NCOA2* exon 13 (NM_006540).

cartilaginous component can be prominent and biphasic appearance is grossly visible. Histologically the tumor is composed of 2 components: one composed of small round cells with high nuclear-cytoplasmic ratio (Ewing-like) or primitive-appearing spindle cells in a hemangiopericytic pattern accompanied by a well-differentiated chondroid component composed of hyaline cartilage (**Fig. 6**B). The chondroid component can be seen as islands of cartilage intermingled with round/spindle cell areas or they can be lobulated with clear separation between the two. There are no specific immunohistochemical markers thus far. The tumor can express CD99, S100, and SOX9, which is a marker of cartilage differentiation. Aberrant expression of EMA, desmin, myogenin, and MYOD1 has been reported.[77] Recent reports of positivity for NKX3.1

Table 1
Pertinent clinicopathological and imaging features

Chondrosarcoma Subtype	Age (y)	Common Sites	Radiology	Histology	Molecular
Conventional	30–60	Axial and appendicular skeleton (pelvis, femur, humerus, ribs), rare in small bones of hands and feet	Metaphyseal and diaphyseal Lytic and sclerotic, endosteal scalloping (chondroid-type mineralization ["rings and arcs"]) MRI-high signal T2 weighted	Hyaline cartilage lobules, entrapment. Cortical invasion, myxoid changes	*IDH1/2* mutations in ~50%, *COL2A1* in 37% Other alterations: *TP53, RB1, TERT/ATRX, CDKN2A/B*
Dedifferentiated	60–70	Same as above	Chondroid-type mineralization adjacent to lytic areas, aggressive imaging with cortical destruction, soft tissue extension	Biphasic: well-differentiated cartilage component juxtaposed to high-grade noncartilaginous sarcoma	Same as above
Periosteal	20–30	Femur, humerus, ilium, fibula, ribs	Surface lesion: >5 cm chondroid-type calcifications, cortex thick and eroded	Hyaline cartilage lobules, myxoid changes, atypia	IDH1/2 mutations in 15%
Clear Cell	30–50	Femur, humerus, spine, ribs, small bones of hands and feet	Lytic epiphyseal lesion with variable zones of transition; chondroid-type mineralization	Tumor cells with abundant clear cytoplasm centrally places nuclei with admixed woven bone trabeculae	Not known
Mesenchymal	20–30	Maxilla, mandible, ribs, vertebrae, pelvis, long bones	Aggressive permeative and moth-eaten pattern, periosteal reaction, soft tissue extension	Biphasic small round or primitive spindle cells with admixed well-differentiated cartilage	*Hey1-NCOA2* translocation in ~80% of cases

in these tumors have not been validated in other studies.[78,79]

MOLECULAR PATHOLOGY

The tumor is characterized by a recurrent in-frame fusion between *Hey1* (hairy/enhancer-of-split related with YRPW motif) located at ch8q21.1 and *NCOA2* (nuclear receptor coactivator 2) located at ch8q13.3 in 80% of cases. This chimeric fusion occurs through intrachromosomal deletion between exon 4 of *Hey1* and exon 13 of *NCOA2* where the DNA-binding domain of *Hey1* and the two C-terminal activation domains of *NCOA2* are conserved.[80] This fusion can be detected by fluorescence in situ hybridization, reverse-transcriptase polymerase chain reaction, or RNA sequencing technologies (**Figs. 6**C and D). There is a single case report of an in-frame fusion involving *IRF2BP2* and *CDX1*.[81]

DIFFERENTIAL DIAGNOSIS

In small biopsy material where only the round cell component is present, it can be difficult to distinguish MC from other malignant small blue round cell tumors. As MC is also CD99 positive, molecular studies are needed to confirm the diagnosis. Recently, methylation profiling has successfully shown that MCs cluster separately from other round cell tumors.[82] Differentiation from another biphasic tumor such as DDCS is usually not difficult because DDCS almost always shows abrupt transition of the high nonchondroid sarcomatous component, whereas in MC the chondroid component often blends with the primitive round/spindle cell component. Besides dedifferentiated component of DDCS often shows a pleomorphic sarcoma or osteosarcoma morphology unlike MC.

PROGNOSIS

MC is an aggressive neoplasm with distant metastases reported as late as greater than 20 years. The 5-, 10-, and 20-year event-free survivals are estimated as 45%, 27.2%, and 8.1%, respectively. Wide surgical resection with negative margins is the treatment of choice.[83] The role of chemotherapy in the absence of metastases remains controversial.[84]

SUMMARY

Malignant cartilage tumors are heterogeneous neoplasms with distinctive imaging, pathologic, and molecular characteristics (**Table 1**). Tumor location, extension into soft tissue, and histologic grading are important for prognosis and disease management. Although molecular discoveries have provided better tools for diagnostic accuracy, biological factors influencing prognosis are still unknown with limited treatment options for recurrent and metastatic tumors.

PATHOLOGIC KEY FEATURES

- Low-grade cartilage lesions of long tubular bones are reclassified as ACT and those of axial skeleton remain as CS grade I (CS I)

- Pathologic grading (grades I, II, and III) remains the gold standard for prognosis

- IDH1/2 mutations are seen in ~50% of central and 15% of periosteal CSs and are useful diagnostic markers

- Histologic grading is not applicable for periosteal CSs, and size of tumor (>5 cm) is an important criterion

- Clear cell CS remains an enigma and is the only malignant cartilage tumor with abundant intratumoral woven bone formation

- MS is the only translocation-associated high-grade CS with a biphasic histology and should not be mistaken for DDCS

DISCLOSURE

author has nothing to disclose.

REFERENCES

1. Giuffrida AY, Burgueno JE, Koniaris LG, et al. Chondrosarcoma in the United States (1973 to 2003): an analysis of 2890 cases from the SEER database. J Bone Joint Surg Am 2009;91(5):1063–72.
2. Murphey MD, Walker EA, Wilson AJ, et al. From the archives of the AFIP: imaging of primary chondrosarcoma: radiologic-pathologic correlation. Radiographics 2003;23(5):1245–78.
3. Evans HL, Ayala AG, Romsdahl MM. Prognostic factors in chondrosarcoma of bone: a clinicopathologic analysis with emphasis on histologic grading. Cancer 1977;40(2):818–31.
4. WHO. WHO Classification of tumours of soft tissue and bone. In: Cancer EBaIAfRo, editor. World health organization classification of tumours. 5th edition. Lyon: IARC Press; 2013.
5. Chen JC, Fong YC, Tang CH. Novel strategies for the treatment of chondrosarcomas: targeting integrins. Biomed Res Int 2013;2013:396839.

6. Bjornsson J, McLeod RA, Unni KK, et al. Primary chondrosarcoma of long bones and limb girdles. Cancer 1998;83(10):2105–19.

7. Peterse EFP, van den Akker B, Niessen B, et al. NAD synthesis pathway interference is a viable therapeutic strategy for chondrosarcoma. Mol Cancer Res 2017;15(12):1714–21.

8. Fromm J, Klein A, Baur-Melnyk A, et al. Survival and prognostic factors in conventional central chondrosarcoma. BMC Cancer 2018;18(1):849.

9. Angelini A, Guerra G, Mavrogenis AF, et al. Clinical outcome of central conventional chondrosarcoma. J Surg Oncol 2012;106(8):929–37.

10. Gelderblom H, Hogendoorn PC, Dijkstra SD, et al. The clinical approach towards chondrosarcoma. Oncologist 2008;13(3):320–9.

11. Amary MF, Bacsi K, Maggiani F, et al. IDH1 and IDH2 mutations are frequent events in central chondrosarcoma and central and periosteal chondromas but not in other mesenchymal tumours. J Pathol 2011;224(3):334–43.

12. Guilhamon P, Eskandarpour M, Halai D, et al. Meta-analysis of IDH-mutant cancers identifies EBF1 as an interaction partner for TET2. Nat Commun 2013;4:2166.

13. Tap WD, Villalobos VM, Cote GM, et al. Phase I study of the mutant IDH1 inhibitor ivosidenib: safety and clinical activity in patients with advanced chondrosarcoma. J Clin Oncol 2020;38(15):1693–701.

14. Douis H, Saifuddin A. The imaging of cartilaginous bone tumours. II. Chondrosarcoma. Skeletal Radiol 2013;42(5):611–26.

15. Xu W, Yang H, Liu Y, et al. Oncometabolite 2-hydroxyglutarate is a competitive inhibitor of alpha-ketoglutarate-dependent dioxygenases. Cancer Cell 2011;19(1):17–30.

16. Tarpey PS, Behjati S, Cooke SL, et al. Frequent mutation of the major cartilage collagen gene COL2A1 in chondrosarcoma. Nat Genet 2013;45(8):923–6.

17. Gao L, Hong X, Guo X, et al. Targeted next-generation sequencing of dedifferentiated chondrosarcoma in the skull base reveals combined TP53 and PTEN mutations with increased proliferation index, an implication for pathogenesis. Oncotarget 2016;7(28):43557–69.

18. Lin Y, Seger N, Chen Y, et al. hTERT promoter mutations in chondrosarcomas associate with progression and disease-related mortality. Mod Pathol 2018;31(12):1834–41.

19. Zhu GG, Nafa K, Agaram N, et al. Genomic profiling identifies association of IDH1/IDH2 mutation with longer relapse-free and metastasis-free survival in high-grade chondrosarcoma. Clin Cancer Res 2020;26(2):419–27.

20. Nicolle R, Ayadi M, Gomez-Brouchet A, et al. Integrated molecular characterization of chondrosarcoma reveals critical determinants of disease progression. Nat Commun 2019;10(1):4622.

21. Skeletal Lesions Interobserver Correlation among Expert Diagnosticians Study G. Reliability of histopathologic and radiologic grading of cartilaginous neoplasms in long bones. J Bone Joint Surg Am 2007;89(10):2113–23.

22. Eefting D, Schrage YM, Geirnaerdt MJ, et al. Assessment of interobserver variability and histologic parameters to improve reliability in classification and grading of central cartilaginous tumors. Am J Surg Pathol 2009;33(1):50–7.

23. van Praag Veroniek VM, Rueten-Budde AJ, Ho V, et al. Incidence, outcomes and prognostic factors during 25 years of treatment of chondrosarcomas. Surg Oncol 2018;27(3):402–8.

24. Bindiganavile S, Han I, Yun JY, et al. Long-term outcome of chondrosarcoma: a single institutional experience. Cancer Res Treat 2015;47(4):897–903.

25. Chen L, Long C, Liu J, et al. Prognostic nomograms to predict overall survival and cancer-specific survival in patients with pelvic chondrosarcoma. Cancer Med 2019;8(12):5438–49.

26. Pansuriya TC, van Eijk R, d'Adamo P, et al. Somatic mosaic IDH1 and IDH2 mutations are associated with enchondroma and spindle cell hemangioma in Ollier disease and Maffucci syndrome. Nat Genet 2011;43(12):1256–61.

27. Cleven AHG, Suijker J, Agrogiannis G, et al. IDH1 or -2 mutations do not predict outcome and do not cause loss of 5-hydroxymethylcytosine or altered histone modifications in central chondrosarcomas. Clin Sarcoma Res 2017;7:8.

28. Lugowska I, Teterycz P, Mikula M, et al. IDH1/2 mutations predict shorter survival in chondrosarcoma. J Cancer 2018;9(6):998–1005.

29. Frassica FJ, Unni KK, Beabout JW, et al. Dedifferentiated chondrosarcoma. A report of the clinicopathological features and treatment of seventy-eight cases. J Bone Joint Surg Am 1986;68(8):1197–205.

30. Mitchell AD, Ayoub K, Mangham DC, et al. Experience in the treatment of dedifferentiated chondrosarcoma. J Bone Joint Surg Br 2000;82(1):55–61.

31. Grimer RJ, Gosheger G, Taminiau A, et al. Dedifferentiated chondrosarcoma: prognostic factors and outcome from a European group. Eur J Cancer 2007;43(14):2060–5.

32. Staals EL, Bacchini P, Mercuri M, et al. Dedifferentiated chondrosarcomas arising in preexisting osteochondromas. J Bone Joint Surg Am 2007;89(5):987–93.

33. Strotman PK, Reif TJ, Kliethermes SA, et al. Dedifferentiated chondrosarcoma: a survival analysis of 159 cases from the SEER database (2001-2011). J Surg Oncol 2017;116(2):252–7.

34. Capanna R, Bertoni F, Bettelli G, et al. Dedifferentiated chondrosarcoma. J Bone Joint Surg Am 1988;70(1):60–9.

35. Italiano A, Mir O, Cioffi A, et al. Advanced chondrosarcomas: role of chemotherapy and survival. Ann Oncol 2013;24(11):2916–22.
36. Czerniak B. Dedifferentiated chondrosarcoma. In: Czerniak B, editor. Dorfman and Czerniak's bone tumors. Philadelphia, PA: Elsevier Health Sciences; 2016. p. 510–25.
37. Gambarotti M, Righi A, Frisoni T, et al. Dedifferentiated chondrosarcoma with "adamantinoma-like" features: a case report and review of literature. Pathol Res Pract 2017;213(6):698–701.
38. Jour G, Liu Y, Ricciotti R, et al. Glandular differentiation in dedifferentiated chondrosarcoma: molecular evidence of a rare phenomenon. Hum Pathol 2015; 46(9):1398–404.
39. Zhang Y, Paz Mejia A, Temple HT, et al. Squamous cell carcinoma arising in dedifferentiated chondrosarcoma proved by isocitrate dehydrogenase mutation analysis. Hum Pathol 2014;45(7):1541–5.
40. Staals EL, Bacchini P, Bertoni F. Dedifferentiated central chondrosarcoma. Cancer 2006;106(12): 2682–91.
41. Ropke M, Boltze C, Neumann HW, et al. Genetic and epigenetic alterations in tumor progression in a dedifferentiated chondrosarcoma. Pathol Res Pract 2003;199(6):437–44.
42. Lucas CG, Grenert JP, Horvai A. Targeted Next-Generation Sequencing Identifies Molecular and Genetic Events in Dedifferentiated Chondrosarcoma. Arch Pathol Lab Med 2020;1–9.
43. Dahlin DC, Beabout JW. Dedifferentiation of low-grade chondrosarcomas. Cancer 1971;28(2):461–6.
44. McFarland GB Jr, McKinley LM, Reed RJ. Dedifferentiation of low grade chondrosarcomas. Clin Orthop Relat Res 1977;(122):157–64.
45. Makise N, Sekimizu M, Konishi E, et al. H3K27me3 deficiency defines a subset of dedifferentiated chondrosarcomas with characteristic clinicopathological features. Mod Pathol 2019; 32(3):435–45.
46. Kervarrec T, Collin C, Larousserie F, et al. H3F3 mutation status of giant cell tumors of the bone, chondroblastomas and their mimics: a combined high resolution melting and pyrosequencing approach. Mod Pathol 2017;30(3):393–406.
47. Nielsen GP, Rosenberg AE, Deshpande V, et al. Diagnostic pathology: bone. Philadelphia, PA: Elsevier; 2017.
48. Mazabraud A. Osteogenic exostosis (osteochondroma), multiple exostoses, subungual exostosis, metachondromatosis. In: Pathology of bone tumours. Paris, France: Springer-Verlag Berlin Heidelberg; 1998. p. 63–75.
49. Amary MF, Damato S, Halai D, et al. Ollier disease and Maffucci syndrome are caused by somatic mosaic mutations of IDH1 and IDH2. Nat Genet 2011;43(12):1262–5.
50. Murphey MD, Choi JJ, Kransdorf MJ, et al. Imaging of osteochondroma: variants and complications with radiologic-pathologic correlation. Radiographics 2000;20(5):1407–34.
51. Bernard SA, Murphey MD, Flemming DJ, et al. Improved differentiation of benign osteochondromas from secondary chondrosarcomas with standardized measurement of cartilage cap at CT and MR imaging. Radiology 2010;255(3):857–65.
52. Wuyts W, Schmale GA, Chansky HA, et al. Hereditary multiple osteochondromas. In: Adam MP, Ardinger HH, Pagon RA, et al, editors. GeneReviews® [Internet]. Seattle (WA): University of Washington, Seattle. 1993-2021. p. 1–19.
53. Hameetman L, Bovee JV, Taminiau AH, et al. Multiple osteochondromas: clinicopathological and genetic spectrum and suggestions for clinical management. Hered Cancer Clin Pract 2004;2(4): 161–73.
54. Nojima T, Unni KK, McLeod RA, et al. Periosteal chondroma and periosteal chondrosarcoma. Am J Surg Pathol 1985;9(9):666–77.
55. Bertoni F, Boriani S, Laus M, et al. Periosteal chondrosarcoma and periosteal osteosarcoma. Two distinct entities. J Bone Joint Surg Br 1982;64(3): 370–6.
56. Papagelopoulos PJ, Galanis EC, Mavrogenis AF, et al. Survivorship analysis in patients with periosteal chondrosarcoma. Clin Orthop Relat Res 2006;448: 199–207.
57. Matsumoto K, Hukuda S, Ishizawa M, et al. Parosteal (juxtacortical) chondrosarcoma of the humerus associated with regional lymph node metastasis. A case report. Clin Orthop Relat Res 1993;(290):168–73.
58. Chaabane S, Bouaziz MC, Drissi C, et al. Periosteal chondrosarcoma. AJR Am J Roentgenol 2009; 192(1):W1–6.
59. Kenan S, Abdelwahab IF, Klein MJ, et al. Lesions of juxtacortical origin (surface lesions of bone). Skeletal Radiol 1993;22(5):337–57.
60. Cleven AH, Zwartkruis E, Hogendoorn PC, et al. Periosteal chondrosarcoma: a histopathological and molecular analysis of a rare chondrosarcoma subtype. Histopathology 2015;67(4):483–90.
61. Hall RB, Robinson LH, Malawar MM, et al. Periosteal osteosarcoma. Cancer 1985;55(1):165–71.
62. Unni KK, Dahlin DC, Beabout JW, et al. Chondrosarcoma: clear-cell variant. A report of sixteen cases. J Bone Joint Surg Am 1976;58(5):676–83.
63. Czerniak B, Dorfman H. Bone tumors. 2nd edition. Philadelphia, PA: Elsevier Health Sciences; 2016.
64. Itala A, Leerapun T, Inwards C, et al. An institutional review of clear cell chondrosarcoma. Clin Orthop Relat Res 2005;440:209–12.
65. Collins MS, Koyama T, Swee RG, et al. Clear cell chondrosarcoma: radiographic, computed tomographic, and magnetic resonance findings in 34

patients with pathologic correlation. Skeletal Radiol 2003;32(12):687–94.

66. Kalil RK, Inwards CY, Unni KK, et al. Dedifferentiated clear cell chondrosarcoma. Am J Surg Pathol 2000; 24(8):1079–86.

67. Behjati S, Tarpey PS, Presneau N, et al. Distinct H3F3A and H3F3B driver mutations define chondroblastoma and giant cell tumor of bone. Nat Genet 2013;45(12):1479–82.

68. Lam SW, van Langevelde K, Suurmeijer AJH, et al. Conventional chondrosarcoma with focal clear cell change: a clinicopathological and molecular analysis. Histopathology 2019;75(6):843–52.

69. Matsuura S, Ishii T, Endo M, et al. Epithelial and cartilaginous differentiation in clear cell chondrosarcoma. Hum Pathol 2013;44(2):237–43.

70. Bjornsson J, Unni KK, Dahlin DC, et al. Clear cell chondrosarcoma of bone. Observations in 47 cases. Am J Surg Pathol 1984;8(3):223–30.

71. Bertoni F, Picci P, Bacchini P, et al. Mesenchymal chondrosarcoma of bone and soft tissues. Cancer 1983;52(3):533–41.

72. Nakashima Y, Unni KK, Shives TC, et al. Mesenchymal chondrosarcoma of bone and soft tissue. A review of 111 cases. Cancer 1986;57(12):2444–53.

73. Cesari M, Bertoni F, Bacchini P, et al. Mesenchymal chondrosarcoma. An analysis of patients treated at a single institution. Tumori 2007;93(5):423–7.

74. Frezza AM, Cesari M, Baumhoer D, et al. Mesenchymal chondrosarcoma: prognostic factors and outcome in 113 patients. A European Musculoskeletal Oncology Society study. Eur J Cancer 2015; 51(3):374–81.

75. Schneiderman BA, Kliethermes SA, Nystrom LM. Survival in mesenchymal chondrosarcoma varies based on age and tumor location: a survival analysis of the SEER database. Clin Orthop Relat Res 2017; 475(3):799–805.

76. Ghafoor S, Hameed MR, Tap WD, et al. Mesenchymal chondrosarcoma: imaging features and clinical findings. Skeletal Radiol 2021;50(2):333–41.

77. Folpe AL, Graham RP, Martinez A, et al. Mesenchymal chondrosarcomas showing immunohistochemical evidence of rhabdomyoblastic differentiation: a potential diagnostic pitfall. Hum Pathol 2018;77:28–34.

78. Yoshida KI, Machado I, Motoi T, et al. NKX3-1 Is a useful immunohistochemical marker of EWSR1-NFATC2 sarcoma and mesenchymal chondrosarcoma. Am J Surg Pathol 2020;44(6):719–28.

79. Chen W, Hornick JL, Fletcher CDM. NKX3.1 immunoreactivity is not identified in mesenchymal chondrosarcoma: a 25-case cohort study. Histopathology 2021;78(2):334–7.

80. Wang L, Motoi T, Khanin R, et al. Identification of a novel, recurrent HEY1-NCOA2 fusion in mesenchymal chondrosarcoma based on a genome-wide screen of exon-level expression data. Genes Chromosomes Cancer 2012;51(2):127–39.

81. Nyquist KB, Panagopoulos I, Thorsen J, et al. Whole-transcriptome sequencing identifies novel IRF2BP2-CDX1 fusion gene brought about by translocation t(1;5)(q42;q32) in mesenchymal chondrosarcoma. PLoS One 2012;7(11):e49705.

82. Koelsche C, Hartmann W, Schrimpf D, et al. Array-based DNA-methylation profiling in sarcomas with small blue round cell histology provides valuable diagnostic information. Mod Pathol 2018;31(8): 1246–56.

83. Xu J, Li D, Xie L, et al. Mesenchymal chondrosarcoma of bone and soft tissue: a systemic review of 107 patients in the past 20 years. PLoS One 2015; 7:10–7.

84. Mendenhall WM, Reith JD, Scarborough MT, et al. Mesenchymal chondrosarcoma. Int J Part Ther 2016;3(2):300–4.

Notochordal Tumors

Roberto Tirabosco, MD[a],*, Paul O'Donnell, MD[b],
Adrienne M. Flanagan, MD, PhD[a],[c]

KEYWORDS
- Bone • Spine • Base of skull • Notochordal tumors • Chordoma • Brachyury

- Notochordal tumors comprise a spectrum of neoplasms with variable biological behavior, ranging from benign to highly aggressive tumors, usually arising in the axial skeleton.
- Notochordal tumors have a phenotype that recapitulates the embryonic notochord, characterized by the dual expression of cytokeratins and brachyury. In addition, poorly differentiated chordoma is defined by the loss of SMARCB1 expression.
- Benign notochordal tumors are usually found incidentally on imaging, whereas malignant notochordal tumors commonly present as a large painful mass with site-related neurologic symptoms.
- Surgery is the main treatment option for malignant notochordal tumors, with or without neoadjuvant or adjuvant treatment.

ABSTRACT

This review provides an overview of the spectrum of tumors showing notochordal differentiation. This spectrum encompasses benign entities that are mostly discovered incidentally on imaging, reported as benign notochordal cell tumor, usually not requiring surgical intervention; slowly growing and histologically low-grade tumors referred to as conventional chordoma but associated with a significant metastatic potential and mortality; and more aggressive disease represented by histologically higher-grade tumors including dedifferentiated chordoma, a high-grade biphasic tumor characterized by a conventional chordoma juxtaposed to a high-grade sarcoma, usually with a spindle or pleomorphic cell morphology, and associated with a poor prognosis and poorly differentiated chordoma.

OVERVIEW

Notochordal tumors comprise a group of rare bone neoplasms commonly arising within the axial skeleton, from the clivus to the sacrococcygeal vertebrae. As a group, they are defined by a phenotype that recapitulates the embryonic notochord (**Fig. 1**). The current World Health Organization (WHO) classification of soft tissue and bone tumors subdivides notochordal tumors into 4 main categories, based on morphologic features and biological behavior: benign notochordal cell tumor (BNCT), conventional chordoma, poorly differentiated chordoma, and dedifferentiated chordoma.[1] Regardless of their histologic subtype, all notochordal tumors are characterized by the coexpression of cytokeratins and brachyury, encoded by *TBXT*, a transcription factor required for notochordal development.[2] Brachyury is the diagnostic hallmark of the notochordal tumor group and is the single most helpful marker in the differential diagnostic process, which includes chondrosarcoma, metastatic carcinoma, myoepithelial tumors, and meningioma.[3] In addition, a recently added variant, namely, poorly differentiated chordoma, is defined by the loss of SMARCB1 expression.[4–7] A clinicopathological overview of the different types of notochordal tumors is depicted in **Table 1**.

[a] Department of Histopathology, Royal National Orthopaedic Hospital, Brockley Hill, Stanmore, Middlesex HA7 4LP, UK; [b] Department of Radiology, Royal National Orthopaedic Hospital, Brockley Hill, Stanmore, Middlesex HA7 4LP, UK; [c] UCL Cancer Institute, University College London, 72 Huntley Street, London WC1 E 6DD, UK
* Corresponding author.
E-mail address: roberto.tirabosco@nhs.net

Surgical Pathology 14 (2021) 619–643
https://doi.org/10.1016/j.path.2021.06.006
1875-9181/21/

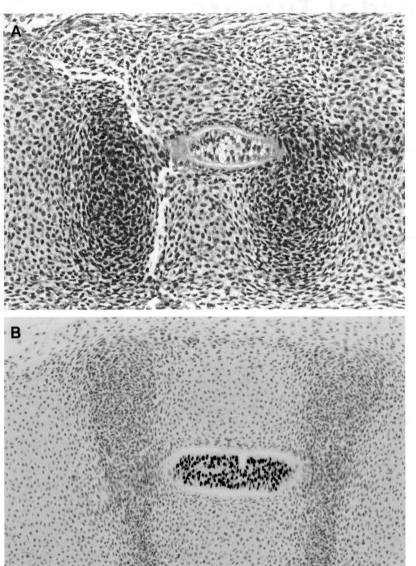

Fig. 1. Human embryo. (*A*) Microphotograph showing the embryonic notochord, highlighted in (*B*) by Brachyury immunostain.

BENIGN NOTOCHORDAL CELL TUMOR

INTRODUCTION

BNCT is an intraosseous neoplasm showing notochordal differentiation, occurring at the base of skull and along the spine, with no preferential location.[8] BNCT is usually asymptomatic and found incidentally on imaging in adults, although it has been rarely described in children. The actual frequency is not known, but it has been reported as high as 20% in a Japanese autopsy study.[9] BNCT may also be found in association with

conventional chordoma and may be multicentric along the spine.[10]

IMAGING

BNCTs (**Fig. 2**) are usually occult on radiographs but may show vertebral body sclerosis, more likely to be seen in large lesions or the cervical spine: rarely, there is the appearance of an ivory vertebra. There is frequently sclerosis in the central vertebral body on computed tomography (CT), but no destruction of the medullary bone or cortex.[11] T1-weighted MRI shows a well-demarcated

Table 1
Clinicopathological overview of notochordal tumors

Type	Age	Histology	Immunoprofile	Treatment	Prognosis
BNCT	Any age but more frequent in adults	Adipocyticlike cells. No myxoid stroma. No multilobular architecture. No osteolysis	Cytokeratins and brachyury positive	None (most cases). Clinical surveillance	Excellent
Conventional chordoma	Any age but more frequent in adults	Cords/nests of epithelioid cells with vacuolated and eosinophilic cytoplasm. Multilobular architecture. Bone destruction and soft tissue invasion	Cytokeratins and brachyury positive	Resection and neo/adjuvant therapy	Frequent local recurrence and significant metastatic potential. Median survival time of 7 y
Poorly differentiated chordoma	Any age but more frequent in children	Epithelioid/rhabdoid cells, solid pattern. No physaliphorous cells. Little or no myxoid stroma. Tumor necrosis	Cytokeratins and brachyury positive. Loss of SMARCB1	Resection and neo/adjuvant therapy	Poor
Dedifferentiated chordoma	Adult	Biphenotypic tumor with features of conventional chordoma and high-grade sarcoma	Cytokeratins and brachyury positive in the conventional component	Resection and neo/adjuvant therapy	Extremely poor

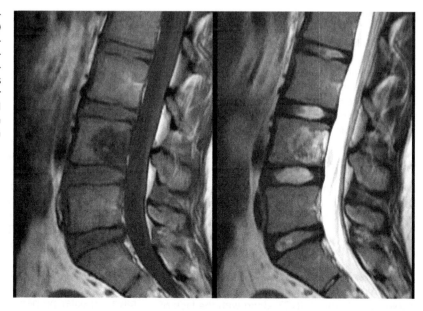

Fig. 2. BNCT. Sagittal T1- (*left*) and T2- (*right*) weighted magnetic resonance images of the lumbar spine. A well-defined, lobular lesion is seen at the posterior aspect of the vertebral body, hypointense on T1- and hyperintense on T2-weighted images.

lesion, which is predominantly low in signal but may contain foci of fat[12]; fluid-sensitive magnetic resonance sequences show heterogeneous hyperintensity. The lesion is classically completely intramedullary, with no extraosseous tumor. No enhancement is seen after contrast administration; there is no activity within the lesion on technetium isotope (methylene diphosphonate [MDP]) bone scans.[13] Difficult-to-classify lesions with atypical features,[14] and BNCTs showing extraosseous tumor[15] and enhancement,[16] have been reported.

GROSS FEATURES

BNCT is an ill-defined, intramedullary tumor usually of small size, not associated with bone destruction or expansion. However, gross specimens of BNCT are uncommon, because most do not require surgical intervention.

MICROSCOPIC FEATURES

BNCT may be difficult to recognize microscopically, because it resembles fatty marrow that could be also entrapped within the tumor itself. BNCT is composed of a mixture of large adipocytelike cells and nonvacuolated cells with eosinophilic cytoplasm, pinpoint nuclei, and no mitotic activity. Tumor cells are usually back-to-back, with no intervening myxoid matrix or fibrous septa. A lobular architecture, which is so characteristic of conventional chordoma, is not a feature seen in BNCT (**Fig.3**). In addition, there is no host bone entrapment, although focal bone resorption can be seen or short trabeculae of woven bone may be intermingled within the tumor (**Fig. 4**).[17] Distinguishing BNCT from early transition to chordoma can be challenging and has given rise to the term "atypical notochordal cell tumor." Most consider that if the tumor invades surrounding soft tissue it is not compatible with a diagnosis of BNCT. However, this point is debated because there are some examples of large BNCTs that have remained stable for a long period.[14]

IMMUNOHISTOCHEMISTRY

BNCT has the same immunoprofile as conventional chordoma, namely, coexpression of cytokeratins and brachyury.

DIFFERENTIAL DIAGNOSIS

The main differential diagnosis is conventional chordoma. The distinction is based on the bland cytologic features of BNCT along with the lack of extracellular myxoid matrix, multilobular configuration, and host bone entrapment.

BNCT should not be mistaken for notochordal rests (vestiges), microscopic foci of vestigial notochordal cells found incidentally within intervertebral disk.[18] These structures are not considered to be related to ecchordosis physaliphora spheno-occipitalis, which is an extra-osseous residual notochordal embryonic tissue located in the clivus region, found incidentally in about 2% on autopsy and imaging studies, but occasionally associated with site-related neurologic symptoms.[19]

PROGNOSIS

BNCT is a benign tumor with an excellent prognosis that does not need surgical intervention in most cases. Some BNCTs may progress to conventional chordoma, but the true incidence is not known.

PATHOLOGIC KEY FEATURES OF BENIGN NOTOCHORDAL CELL TUMOR

- Intraosseous tumor with no soft tissue invasion
- Adipocyteslike cells with back-to-back pattern
- Lack of myxoid stroma
- Lack of multilobular architecture
- No osteolysis
- Coexpression of cytokeratins and brachyury

CONVENTIONAL CHORDOMA

INTRODUCTION

Conventional chordoma is a malignant tumor representing the most common entity of the notochordal family.[20] Conventional chordoma is rare, with an incidence of 0.08 of 100,000 per year and a male to female ratio of 1.8:1. Conventional chordoma is a tumor presenting most commonly between the fifth to seventh decades, although it may occur at any age. The site of origin adheres to the notochordal anatomy with minor differences in frequency along the axis: 32% base of skull, 32.8% mobile spine, and 29.2% sacrococcygeal region.[21,22] Tumors in children and young adults have a greater propensity to occur at the base of

Fig. 3. BNCT. (*A*) The tumor is composed of large adipocyticlike cells intermingled with islands of hematopoietic and fatty marrow. (*B*) The tumor cells are back-to-back with no intervening myxoid matrix and (*C*) may be difficult to distinguish from fatty marrow cells.

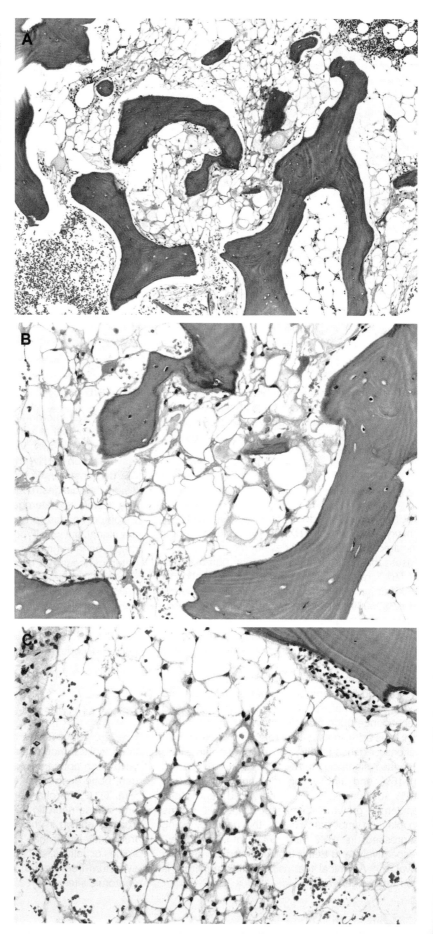

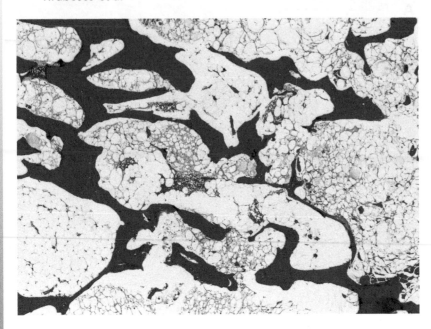

Fig. 4. BNCT. The tumor is seen within the medullary canal with appositional bone and focal resorption.

skull and upper cervical vertebrae. Extra-axial and extraskeletal chordomas have been reported rarely.[3,23–25] Patients with conventional chordoma commonly present with pain and site-related neurologic symptoms.

PATHOGENESIS

The hallmark of chordoma is the expression of brachyury, encoded by *TBXT*, a transcription factor required for notochordal development: in 27% of cases, this is associated with copy number gain of *TBXT*, recapitulating the tandem duplication of *TBXT* of familial chordoma.[2,26–28] The association of rs2305089 in *TBXT* in patients with chordoma makes a strong case that this single-nucleotide polymorphism critically contributes to the development of chordoma.[29] Brachyury also acts as a master regulator of an oncogenic transcriptional network encompassing diverse signaling pathways, including components of the cell cycle and extracellular matrix.[30] Finally, growth arrest and senescence upon silencing of *TBXT* in chordoma cell lines adds to its critical role.[26] In addition, mutations of genes involved in the phosphoinositide 3-kinase signaling pathway have been reported in 16% and inactivating mutations of *LYST* in 10% of cases.[27] Phosphorylated and total epidermal growth factor receptor (EGFR) seems to play an important role in the disease, being expressed in 47% and 67% of chordomas, respectively, and EGFR inhibitors reduce cell survival.[31,32] A clinical trial using EGFR inhibitors is currently underway.

IMAGING

Conventional chordomas (**Fig. 5**) are destructive midline tumors that are often large at presentation, having grown slowly. Visualization on radiographs may be hampered by the sacral or spinal location. CT demonstrates a low-density expansile lytic lesion, cortical destruction, and bone fragments.[33] The lesion is heterogeneous in signal on T1-weighted images, predominantly intermediate to low signal, but with hyperintensity owing to hemorrhage, bone fragments, and mucin.[34] The lesion is heterogeneous but largely hyperintense on fluid-sensitive sequences, with low signal septation. Following contrast administration, there is enhancement, usually low level and heterogeneous, often with septal/honeycomb morphology.[33] Low activity/avidity is seen on technetium isotope (MDP) bone[13]/PET scans.[35]

GROSS FEATURES

Grossly, conventional chordoma is a multilobulated, solid tumor with a gelatinous, white-gray to yellow-tan appearance, associated with a significant bone destruction and extraosseous invasion (**Fig. 6**). Cystic change containing mucous pools and diffuse necrotic areas are common findings. Tumors arising in the sacrococcygeal region are frequently larger than those located in the mobile spine or clivus, most likely due to a longer symptom-free period in view of the particular anatomic site.

Fig. 5. Conventional chordoma. Sagittal T2-weighted magnetic resonance image shows a lobular, heterogeneous hyperintense mass extending from S2 to the distal coccyx, with a large extraosseous component. The intraspinal tumor shows more marked cranial extension to the level of the S1 vertebra (*arrow*).

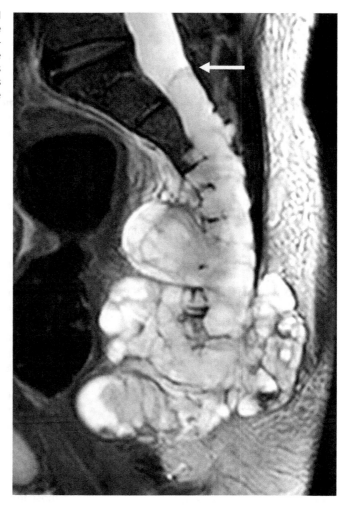

Fig. 6. Conventional chordoma. (*A, B*) Sacrectomy specimens showing large multilobulated, gelatinous tumors, destroying the sacrum and the invading soft tissue.

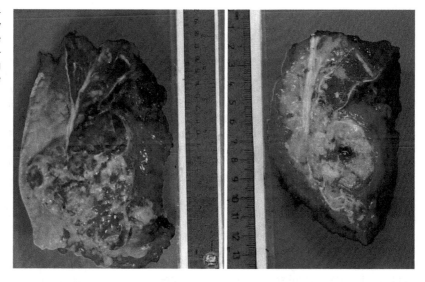

MICROSCOPIC FEATURES

On scanning view, conventional chordoma is a multilobulated tumor crossed by fibrous septa with a variable amount of myxoid stroma, ranging from minimal to large pools of mucinous material, forming pseudocysts, with a characteristic light basophilic appearance (**Fig. 7**). The tumor is composed of large epithelioid cells with vacuolated, sometimes bubbly, cytoplasm, called physaliphorous cells, and admixed with smaller cells with eosinophilic cytoplasm, arranged in cords, nests, and solid areas (**Fig. 8**). Although most tumors have a monotonous appearance, there may be a considerable cytologic variation, including significant nuclear atypia with pleomorphism, bizarre nuclei, and even cellular spindling, with cells arranged in short fascicles mimicking a low-grade myxoid spindle cell sarcoma (**Fig. 9**). Some tumors lack the classical chordoid or nested architecture, and the cells are closely packed forming a pseudoalveolar pattern reminiscent of a renal cell carcinoma. Mitotic activity is generally low, and tumor necrosis may be present.

In some tumors, the characteristic myxoid matrix may have the features of hyaline cartilage resembling a chondrosarcoma. This variant is known as chondroid chordoma (**Fig. 10**).[36,37]

IMMUNOHISTOCHEMISTRY

The essential diagnostic immunoprofile of conventional chordoma is the coexpression of cytokeratins and brachyury, whereas the immunostain for EMA and S100 is variable (**Fig. 11**).

An important point to remember is that specimens decalcified with an acid-based protocol (nitric or formic acid) may be falsely negative for brachyury. Therefore, for diagnostic confirmation, an ethylenediaminetetraacetic acid-based decalcification should be used in biopsy specimen.

DIFFERENTIAL DIAGNOSIS

Conventional chordoma must be distinguished from metastatic carcinoma, chondrosarcoma, and myoepithelial tumors occurring in bone. The discovery of brachyury has greatly helped in such distinction, being an extremely specific and sensitive marker.

The vertebrae are common metastatic sites for carcinomas. Correlation with the clinical history and imaging is essential. However, cancers of unknown primary do happen, and imaging may show a single tumor site. In most cases, the histologic features are typically those of a carcinoma, and the diagnosis is straightforward. Tumors that most likely are confused for chordoma are metastases from mucinous adenocarcinoma and renal cell carcinoma. To date, only a subset of carcinoma types have been reported in the literature as being immunoreactive for brachyury.[38]

Chondrosarcoma, the second most frequent primary bone sarcoma, is also to be considered in the differential diagnostic process, especially against chondroid chordoma.[39] Chondrosarcoma is a malignant cartilage-forming tumor most frequently arising in the long tubular bones and hip bones but rarely also involving the axial skeleton and base of skull. Chondrosarcoma may have similar radiological and gross appearance to chordoma; histologically, it is composed of round, stellate, and spindle-shaped chondrocytes set within a hyaline or myxoid matrix. The cytologic features, cellularity, and quality of matrix (hyaline vs myxoid) differ depending on the histologic grade (low vs high grade). In difficult cases, immunohistochemistry proves to be very helpful, because chondrosarcoma does not express cytokeratins and brachyury. S100 immunostain is of no use because both tumors are positive. Furthermore, approximately 70% of central chondrosarcomas harbor an *IDH1/2* mutation, a genetic alteration never found in chordoma.[40–42]

A myoepithelial tumor occurring in bone (primary and metastatic) is another neoplasm to be considered in the differential diagnosis. Myoepithelial tumors comprise a spectrum of neoplasms that share morphologic features and immunoprofile with salivary glands and their cutaneous counterpart, the vast majority of which are benign and most frequently arise in the soft tissue, and are usually referred to as myoepithelioma and mixed tumor. Primary malignant myoepithelial tumors arising in bone have been described and are usually referred to as malignant myoepithelial tumor or a myoepithelial carcinoma.[43] The diagnosis of myoepithelial tumor is not easy because a vast range of cytologic and architectural features characterize them. Furthermore, they coexpress cytokeratins and S100 in most cases. Therefore, once again the positivity for brachyury represents the ultimate distinguishing marker, especially for those sharing a striking morphologic similarity to chordoma, which in the past were reported as "parachordoma."[3,44]

Finally, chordoid meningioma may resemble conventional chordoma. This tumor is composed of cords and trabeculae of epithelioid cells with variable cytoplasmic vacuolation, resembling physaliphorous cells, set within a mucinous stroma. Areas of more typical meningioma are often present and provide a helpful diagnostic clue. Chordoid meningioma is usually classified as WHO central nervous system grade 2. Diffuse

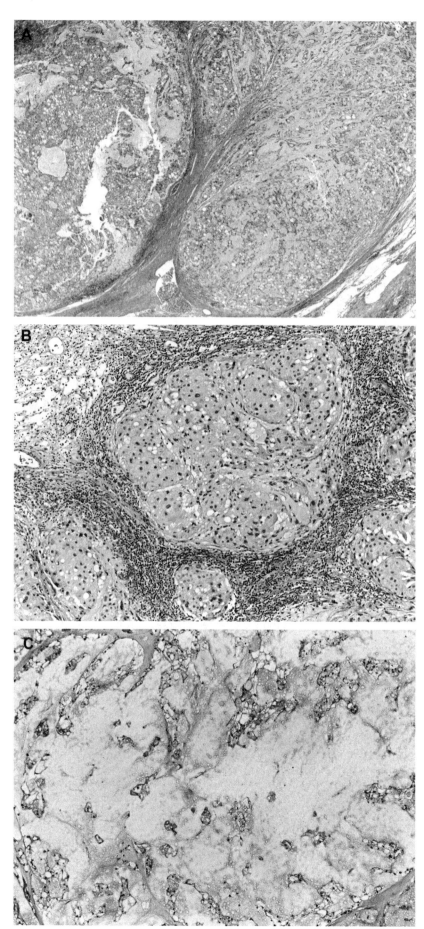

Fig. 7. Conventional chordoma. (*A*) The tumor is characterized by a multilobulated pattern with fibrous septa. (*B*) Note the perilobular, intratumoral lymphocytic infiltrate, a common finding in chordoma. (*C*) Large pools of extracellular mucin with the characteristic light basophilic appearance.

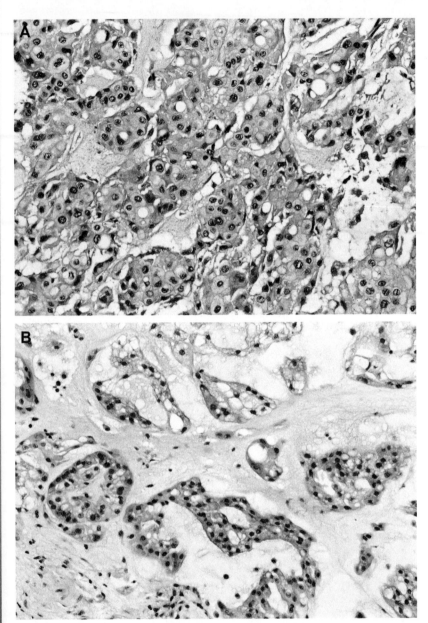

Fig. 8. Conventional chordoma. (*A*) Tumor cells are typically arranged in cords, (*B*) nests, and

and strong EMA immunostaining is the rule, but there is no expression of cytokeratins and brachyury.[45]

PROGNOSIS

Conventional chordoma, although morphologically not a high-grade tumor, has an overall median survival of 7 years and significant metastatic potential. The reason for the poor outcome is accounted for by the high incidence of incomplete surgical resection, especially for the cases arising at the base of skull and mobile spine, where complete surgery with wide margins is in most cases not achievable. Sacrococcygeal chordomas are often large at presentation, and marginal excision can often only be achieved unless the most radical of operations is undertaken. Local recurrence is frequent. Most common metastatic sites include the lung, bone, and subcutaneous tissue.[46–49]

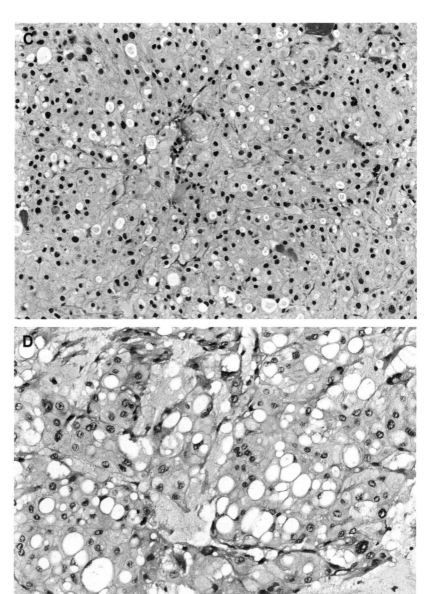

Fig. 8. (*continued*). (*C*) solid areas. (*D*) The hallmark cells of conventional chordoma have intracytoplasmic vacuolation with a bubbly appearance (physaliphorous cells).

PATHOLOGIC KEY FEATURES OF CONVENTIONAL CHORDOMA

- Large tumor with soft tissue invasion
- Multilobular architecture with intervening fibrous septa
- Epithelioid cells with vacuolated or eosinophilic cytoplasm arranged in cords, nests, and solid areas
- Variable amount of myxoid stroma
- Coexpression of cytokeratins and brachyury

DIFFERENTIAL DIAGNOSIS OF CONVENTIONAL CHORDOMA

- Metastatic carcinoma, especially mucinous adenocarcinoma and renal cell carcinoma
- Chondrosarcoma
- Myoepithelial tumor
- Chordoid meningioma

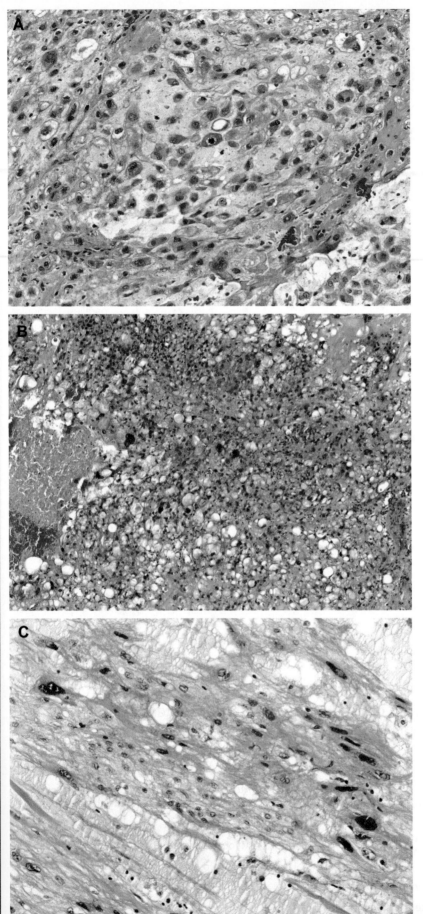

Fig. 9. Conventional chordoma. (*A*) Significant cytologic atypia may be seen in some cases, along with atypical mitoses. (*B*) Severe nuclear pleomorphism, solid arrangement, and tumor necrosis, mimicking a metastatic carcinoma. (*C*) Cellular spindling and fascicular arrangement may also be present.

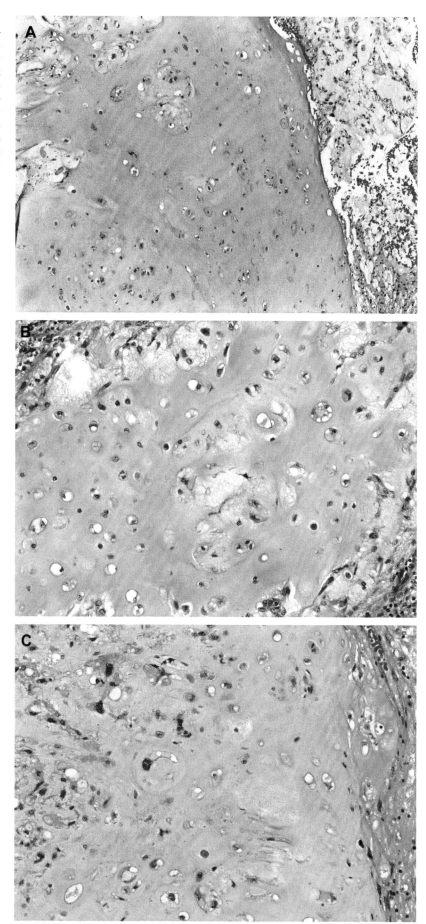

Fig. 10. Chondroid chordoma. (*A*) This chordoma variant is characterized by diffuse hyaline matrix resembling chondrosarcoma. Areas of conventional chordoma may be admixed. (*B*) Tumor cells have cytologic features similar to chondrocytes and (*C*) may have significant nuclear atypia.

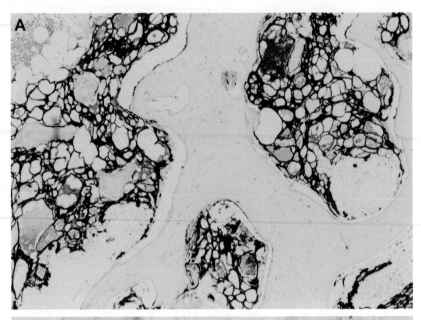

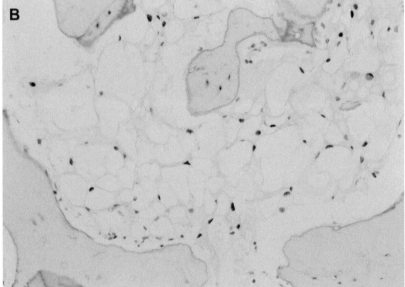

Fig. 11. Conventional chordoma. (*A*) Tumor cells highlighted by cytokeratins (MNF116) and (*B*) brachyury.

PITFALLS OF CONVENTIONAL CHORDOMA

- False-negative brachyury immunostain on acid-based decalcified samples (nitric/formic acid)
- Expression of SMARCB1 (INI-1) can be lost in rare cases of conventional chordoma

POORLY DIFFERENTIATED CHORDOMA

INTRODUCTION

Poorly differentiated chordoma is the most recent type of notochordal tumor added to the WHO classification,[4] and only a small number of cases have been reported in the literature. This tumor most frequently affects the base of skull and cervical vertebrae and most commonly arises in children and young adults with a female to male ratio of

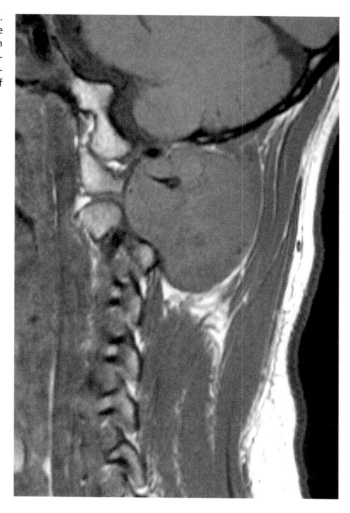

Fig. 12. Poorly differentiated chordoma. Sagittal T1-weighted magnetic resonance image of the cervical spine. Large mass in the left posterior paraspinal region, abutting the skull base and the articular processes of C1 and C2. The neural arch of C1 is engulfed by tumor.

2:1.[5–7,37,50–54] The usual clinical presentation of these tumors is headache and site-related neurologic symptoms.

PATHOGENESIS

Poorly differentiated chordoma is characterized by loss of SMARCB1 (INI-1) expression that is related to heterozygous or homozygous deletion of *SMARCB1* gene, which can be detected by fluorescence in situ hybridization (FISH).[5–7] Codeletion of the nearby *EWSR1* gene has been described in a subset of cases, and this is shown with a complex FISH pattern, which is not similar to the typical *EWSR1* break-apart seen in Ewing sarcoma.[55]

IMAGING

There are few reports of the imaging features of poorly differentiated chordomas (**Fig. 12**): they overlap with those of conventional tumors, especially on radiographs and CT. Diffuse relative hypointensity on fluid-sensitive sequences, rather than a focal low-signal mass, which suggests a dedifferentiated chordoma (see later discussion), may be seen.[7,56] Contrast enhancement and diffusion-weighted imaging (DWI) were unable to distinguish poorly differentiated from conventional chordomas in one study,[56] although the former may show restricted diffusion on DWI suggesting a cellular tumor.[7]

GROSS FEATURES

Most tumors measure about 5 cm at the time of presentation with a range of 2 to greater than 10 cm.[5,6,51] Literature on the gross appearance is lacking because en bloc excision is rarely performed due to the anatomic site. The tumor is destructive and may be well demarcated and multilobulated, as described in conventional

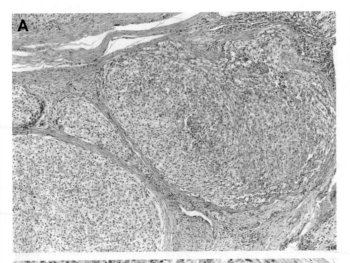

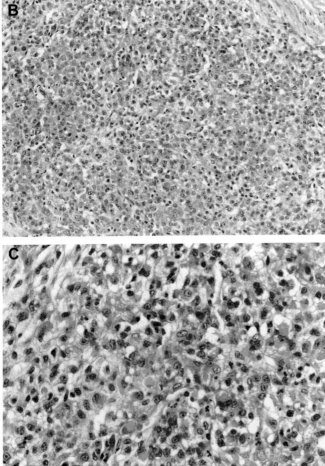

Fig. 13. Poorly differentiated chordoma. (A) Tumor is crossed by fibrous septa into multiple lobules. (B) Note the solid growth pattern with no intervening myxoid stroma. (C) Tumor cells are typically epithelioid with frequent rhabdoid and signet-ring cytoplasmic features.

chordoma.[50] In our experience, poorly differentiated chordoma presents as a lobulated, solid, and firm mass with no discernible myxoid component, almost always invading the soft tissue.

MICROSCOPIC FEATURES

Poorly differentiated chordoma is a solid tumor composed of epithelioid cells with frequent

Fig. 14. Poorly differentiated chordoma. (*A*) Brachyury-positive immunostain and (*B*) complete loss of SMARCB1 expression, which is retained in the background lymphocytes.

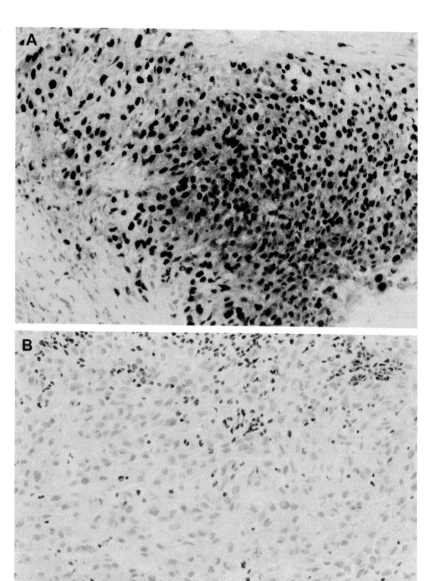

rhabdoid and signet-ring appearance, round to ovoid nuclei, and mild to moderate pleomorphism. The typical physaliphorous cells that characterize conventional chordoma are not seen. Tumor cells are arranged in sheets and nests with little or no intervening myxoid stroma. Mitoses are easily identified, and tumor necrosis may be substantial (**Fig. 13**).

IMMUNOHISTOCHEMISTRY

In addition to the characteristic notochordal immunoprofile, the hallmark of poorly differentiated chordoma is the complete loss of SMARCB1 expression (**Fig. 14**).[5–7] Of note, loss of SMARCB1 expression has been recently reported in a sacral conventional chordoma.[57]

DIFFERENTIAL DIAGNOSIS

The tumors that may have similar appearance to poorly differentiated chordoma are metastatic poorly differentiated carcinoma, malignant rhabdoid tumor (MRT), and rhabdoid meningioma. Metastatic carcinoma has been discussed in the previous section.

MRT is a very rare, highly malignant tumor mainly affecting infants and children, morphologically and genetically identical to MRT arising in the kidney and brain. Extrarenal and extracerebral MRTs usually arise in the deep, axial soft tissue of the neck and paraspinal, retroperitoneal, pelvic, and perineal regions.

MRT is composed of sheets or trabeculae of rhabdoid cells, many of them showing the characteristic juxtanuclear periodic acid-Schiff-positive, diastase-resistant inclusions. Most tumors express cytokeratins and EMA and typically show complete loss of SMARCB1 expression. Brachyury is not expressed.

Rhabdoid meningioma is a subtype of meningioma defined by the presence of rhabdoid cells. In line with the meningothelial differentiation, rhabdoid meningiomas express EMA but are negative for cytokeratins and brachyury. There are a few reports describing *SMARCB1* mutations in meningioma.[58]

PROGNOSIS

In view of the particular anatomic location, complete excision is rarely achieved and the treatment is generally a combination of surgery, neoadjuvant and/or adjuvant radiotherapy, and chemotherapy. There is no literature on the impact of adjuvant therapies on this tumor subtype, but poorly differentiated chordoma has a worse prognosis than conventional chordoma.[5,37,51,59]

PATHOLOGIC KEY FEATURES OF POORLY DIFFERENTIATED CHORDOMA

- Base of skull and cervical vertebrae. Rarely arising in other sections of spine, including sacrococcygeal region
- Epithelioid cells with rhabdoid and signet-ring features, arranged in cohesive solid areas or compact trabeculae
- Absence of physaliphorous cells
- Lack or only focal myxoid stroma
- Coexpression of cytokeratins and brachyury
- Complete loss of SMARCB1 (INI-1) expression

DIFFERENTIAL DIAGNOSIS OF POORLY DIFFERENTIATED CHORDOMA

- Metastatic poorly differentiated carcinoma
- MRT
- Rhabdoid meningioma

PITFALLS OF POORLY DIFFERENTIATED CHORDOMA

- Codeletion of *EWSR1* gene may result in an abnormal, complex FISH pattern
- Expression of SMARCB1 (INI-1) can be lost in rare cases of conventional chordoma

DEDIFFERENTIATED CHORDOMA

INTRODUCTION

Dedifferentiated chordoma is a rare and aggressive subtype of notochordal tumor with only case reports and small series published to date[57,60–62]; it is a high-grade, biphasic tumor defined by the presence of a conventional chordoma associated with a high-grade sarcoma, and it may be present *de novo* or at a site of a previously excised chordoma. This tumor arises in axial locations similar to those of other notochordal tumors but most frequently in the sacrococcygeal region. The clinical presentation is comparable to that of other types of chordoma, but symptom progression is more rapid.

IMAGING

Dedifferentiated chordomas (**Fig. 15**) are indistinguishable from conventional tumors on radiographs and CT. There may be a biphasic appearance on fluid-sensitive MRI sequences, the conventional component showing the typical lobular morphology and hyperintensity (see earlier discussion), and the high-grade tumor, a demarcated, relatively hypointense mass.[60] Homogeneous enhancement of viable tumor, central necrosis, and increased avidity for fludeoxyglucose on PET studies[61] may also indicate a dedifferentiated component.

GROSS FEATURES

The typical gross specimen of dedifferentiated chordoma is a large tumor mass with a well-demarcated biphasic appearance: the gross features of a conventional chordoma are associated with a fleshy, solid tumor, frequently with large areas of necrosis. Diffuse bone destruction and extension into soft tissue is the rule (**Fig. 16**). The mass can be calcified in cases of osteosarcomatous differentiation.

Fig. 15. Dedifferentiated chordoma. Axial T2-weighted magnetic resonance (MR) image (*top*) shows a large hyperintense mass arising from the sacrum (conventional chordoma) with a distinct, well-defined, low-signal region antero-laterally on the left (dedifferentiated component, *arrows*). Axial T1 fat-saturated MR image after contrast injection (*lower* image) shows intense enhancement of the high-grade tumor. A central area that does not enhance and is hyperintense on the T2-weighted image is consistent with necrosis (*asterisk*). The conventional chordoma shows poor enhancement.

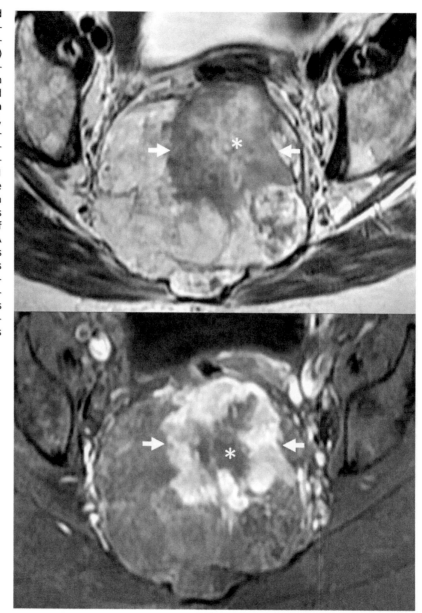

MICROSCOPIC FEATURES

Dedifferentiated chordoma shows the histologic features of conventional chordoma, including the chondroid variant, juxtaposed with a high-grade sarcoma. The 2 components are usually abruptly separated, but they can be intermingled. The high-grade component is classified most frequently as a spindle or pleomorphic cell sarcoma, not otherwise specified, but it can display more specific lines of differentiation, such as an osteosarcomatous or rhabdomyosarcomatous phenotype (**Fig. 17**).

IMMUNOHISTOCHEMISTRY

The classical notochordal immunoprofile is not expressed by the dedifferentiated component, although focal cytokeratin immunostain may be present. The specific line of differentiation, for example, rhabdomyoblastic, may be confirmed by positive immunostain for desmin and myogenin (**Fig. 18**).

DIFFERENTIAL DIAGNOSIS

The differential diagnosis includes dedifferentiated chondrosarcoma, osteosarcoma, and undifferentiated

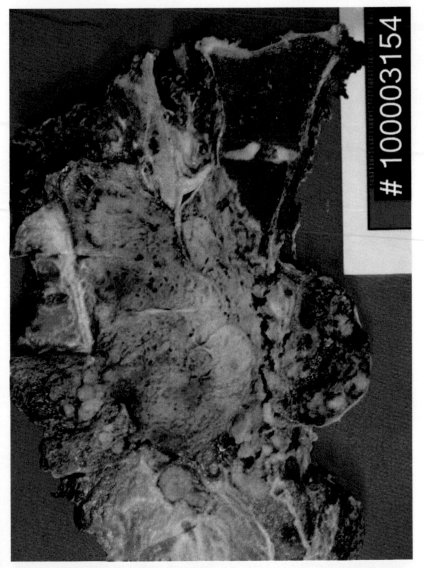

Fig. 16. Dedifferentiated chordoma. Sacrectomy specimen showing a large tumor destroying the sacrum and extending into soft tissue, composed of a conventional chordoma (anterior aspect) and a fleshy, solid, and largely necrotic high-grade sarcoma (posterior aspect).

pleomorphic sarcoma of bone. Imaging is essential in this diagnostic process, because the pathologic specimen, usually a biopsy, may lack the well-differentiated notochordal component. In addition, a high-grade sarcoma diagnosed at the site of a previously excised conventional chordoma should raise the suspicion of dedifferentiated chordoma. However, to this regard, one should be aware of the clinical history, especially the knowledge of previous radiotherapy at this site and the time interval, to exclude a de novo radiotherapy-induced sarcoma.

PROGNOSIS

Dedifferentiated chordoma is an aggressive tumor with a poor outcome and a survival of less than 2 years. Surgical excision is the main treatment option as the effect of radiotherapy and/or chemotherapy is negligible.

PATHOLOGIC KEY FEATURES OF DEDIFFERENTIATED CHORDOMA

- Biphasic tumor composed of a conventional chordoma and a high-grade sarcoma, usually of spindle or pleomorphic type
- Most frequently arising in sacrococcygeal region as a large destructive mass
- The typical notochordal immunoprofile is absent in the dedifferentiated component
- Poor prognosis

Fig. 17. Dedifferentiated chordoma. (*A*) The high-grade sarcoma component and the conventional chordoma are juxtaposed and sharply separated. (*B*) Most frequently, the high-grade component is represented by a spindle or pleomorphic sarcoma, NOS, but (*C*) specific lineage, that is, rhabdomyoblastic differentiation, may be seen.

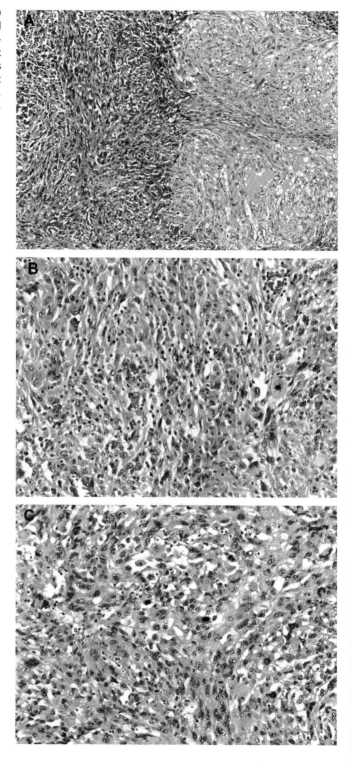

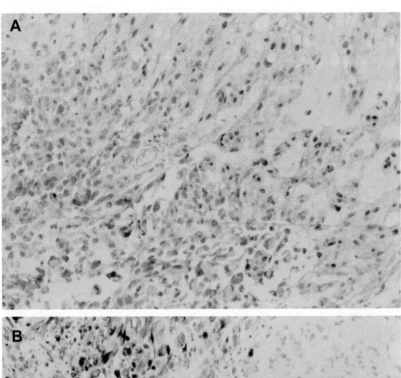

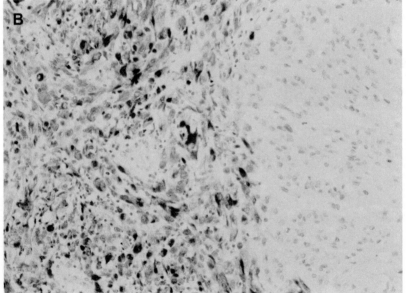

Fig. 18. Dedifferentiated chordoma. (*A*) Brachyury is expressed only in the conventional chordoma component. (*B*) Rhabdomyoblastic differentiation highlighted by desmin positivity.

DIFFERENTIAL DIAGNOSIS OF DEDIFFERENTIATED CHORDOMA

- Dedifferentiated chondrosarcoma
- Osteosarcoma
- Undifferentiated pleomorphic sarcoma of bone

DISCLOSURE

The authors have nothing to disclose.

REFERENCES

1. Notochordal tumours. In: WHO Classification of tumours editorial board. Soft tissue and bone tumours. 5th edition. IARC; 2020. p. 449–57.
2. Vujovic S, Henderson S, Presneau N, et al. Brachyury, a crucial regulator of notochordal

development, is a novel biomarker for chordomas. J Pathol 2006;209(2):157–65.

3. Tirabosco R, Mangham DC, Rosenberg AE, et al. Brachyury expression in extra-axial skeletal and soft tissue chordomas: a marker that distinguishes chordoma from mixed tumor/myoepithelioma/parachordoma in soft tissue. Am J Surg Pathol 2008; 32(4):572–80.

4. Nielsen GP, Dickson BC, Tirabosco R. WHO Classification of tumours editorial board. Poorly differentiated chordoma. In: Soft tissue and bone tumours. 5th edition. IARC; 2020. p. 456–7.

5. Owosho AA, Zhang L, Rosenblum MK, et al. High sensitivity of FISH analysis in detecting homozygous SMARCB1 deletions in poorly differentiated chordoma: a clinicopathologic and molecular study of nine cases. Genes Chromosomes Cancer 2018; 57(2):89–95.

6. Antonelli M, Raso A, Mascelli S, et al. SMARCB1/INI1 involvement in pediatric chordoma: a mutational and immunohistochemical analysis. Am J Surg Pathol 2017;41(1):56–61.

7. Mobley BC, McKenney JK, Bangs CD, et al. Loss of SMARCB1/INI1 expression in poorly differentiated chordomas. Acta Neuropathol 2010;120(6):745–53.

8. Yamaguchi T, Inwards CY, Tirabosco R. WHO Classification of tumours editorial board. Benign notochordal cell tumour. In: Soft tissue and bone tumours. 5th edition. IARC; 2020. p. 449–50.

9. Yamaguchi T, Suzuki S, Ishiiwa H, et al. Intraosseous benign notochordal cell tumours: overlooked precursors of classic chordomas? Histopathology 2004; 44(6):597–602.

10. Deshpande V, Nielsen GP, Rosenthal DI, et al. Intraosseous benign notochord cell tumors (BNCT): further evidence supporting a relationship to chordoma. Am J Surg Pathol 2007;31(10):1573–7.

11. Yamaguchi T, Iwata J, Sugihara S, et al. Distinguishing benign notochordal cell tumors from vertebral chordoma. Skeletal Radiol 2008;37(4):291–9.

12. Lalam R, Cassar-Pullicino V, McClure J, et al. Entrapped intralesional marrow: a hitherto undescribed imaging feature of benign notochordal cell tumor. Skeletal Radiol 2012;41(6):725–31.

13. Abdulrehman A, Hornicek F, Schwab J, et al. Chordoma arising from benign multifocal notochordal tumors. Skeletal Radiol 2017;46(12):1745–52.

14. Carter J, Wenger D, Rose P, et al. Atypical notochordal cell tumors: a series of notochordal-derived tumors that defy current classification schemes. Am J Surg Pathol 2017;41(1):39–48.

15. Nishigushi T, Mochizuki K, Ohsawa M, et al. Differentiating benign notochordal cell tumors from chordomas: radiographic features on MRI, CT, and tomography. AJR Am J Roentgenol 2011;196(3): 644–50.

16. Kreshak J, Larousserie F, Picci P, et al. Difficulty distinguishing benign notochordal cell tumor from chordoma further suggests a link between them. Cancer Imaging 2014;14(1):4.

17. Amer HZM, Hameed M. Intraosseous benign notochordal cell tumor. Arch Pathol Lab Med 2010; 134(2):283–8.

18. Yamaguchi T, Suzuki S, Ishiiwa H, et al. Benign notochordal cell tumors. A comparative histological study of benign notochordal cell tumors, classic chordomas and notochordal vestiges of fetal intervertebral discs. Am J Surg Pathol 2004;28(6): 756–61.

19. Mehnert F, Beschorner R, Küker W, et al. Retroclival ecchordosis physaliphora: MR imaging and review of the literature. AJNR Am J Neuroradiol 2004; 25(10):1851–5.

20. Tirabosco R, O'Donnell PG, Yamaguchi T. WHO Classification of tumours editorial board. Conventional chordoma. In: Soft tissue and bone tumours. 5th edition. IARC; 2020. p. 451–3.

21. McMaster ML, Goldstein AM, Bromley CM, et al. Chordoma: incidence and survival patterns in the United States, 1973-1995. Cancer Causes Control 2001;12(1):1–11.

22. Mukherjee D, Chaichana KL, Gokaslan ZL, et al. Survival of patients with malignant primary osseous spinal neoplasms: results from the Surveillance, Epidemiology, and End Results (SEER) database from 1973 to 2003. J Neurosurg Spine 2011;14(2): 143–50.

23. Righi A, Sbaraglia M, Gambarotti M, et al. Extra-axial chordoma: a clinicopathologic analysis of six cases. Virchows Arch 2018;472(6):1015–20.

24. Balogh P, O'Donnell P, Lindsay D, et al. Extra-axial skeletal poorly differentiated chordoma: a case report. Histopathology 2020;76(6):924–7.

25. Lauer SR, Edgar MA, Gardner JM, et al. Soft tissue chordomas. A clinicopathologic analysis of 11 cases. Am J Surg Pathol 2013;37(5):719–26.

26. Presneau N, Shalaby A, Ye H, et al. Role of the transcription factor T (brachyury) in the pathogenesis of sporadic chordoma: a genetic and functional-based study. J Pathol 2011;223(3):327–35.

27. Tarpey PS, Behjati S, Young MD, et al. The driver landscape of sporadic chordoma. Nat Commun 2017;8(1):890.

28. Yang XR, Ng D, Alcorta DA, et al. T (brachyury) gene duplication confers major susceptibility to familial chordoma. Nat Genet 2009;41(11):1176–8.

29. Pillay N, Plagnol V, Tarpey PS, et al. A common single-nucleotide variant in T is strongly associated with chordoma. Nat Genet 2012;44(11):1185–7.

30. Nelson AC, Pillay N, Henderson S, et al. An integrated functional genomics approach identifies the regulatory network directed by brachyury (T) in chordoma. J Pathol 2012;228(3):274–85.

31. Shalaby A, Presneau N, Ye H, et al. The role of epidermal growth factor receptor in chordoma pathogenesis: a potential therapeutic target. J Pathol 2011;223(3):336–46.

32. Scheipl S, Barnard M, Cottone L, et al. EGFR inhibitors identified as a potential treatment for chordoma in a focused compound screen. J Pathol 2016;239(3):320–34.

33. Sung M, Lee G, Kang H, et al. Sacrococcygeal chordoma: MR imaging in 30 patients. Skeletal Radiol 2005;34(2):87–94.

34. Murphey M, Andrews C, Flemming D, et al. From the archives of the AFIP. Primary tumors of the spine: radiologic pathologic correlation. Radiographics 1996;16(5):1131–58.

35. Park S, Kim H. F-18 FDG PET/CT evaluation of sacrococcygeal chordoma. Clin Nucl Med 2008;33(12):906–8.

36. Rosenberg AE, Brown GA, Bhan AK, et al. Chondroid chordoma–a variant of chordoma. A morphologic and immunohistochemical study. Am J Clin Pathol 1994;101(1):36–41.

37. Hoch BL, Nielsen GP, Liebsch NJ, et al. Base of skull chordomas in children and adolescents: a clinicopathologic study of 73 cases. Am J Surg Pathol 2006;30(7):811–8.

38. Miettinen M, Wang Z, Lasota J, et al. Nuclear Brachyury expression is consistent in chordoma, common in germ cell tumors and small cell carcinomas, and rare in other carcinomas and sarcomas: an immunohistochemical study of 5229 cases. Am J Surg Pathol 2015;39(10):1305–12.

39. Bovee JVMG, Bloem JL, Flanagan AM, et al. WHO Classification of tumours editorial board. Central chondrosarcoma, grades 2and 3. In: Soft tissue and bone tumours. 5th edition. IARC; 2020. p. 375–8.

40. Amary MF, Bacsi K, Maggiani F, et al. IDH1 and IDH2 mutations are frequent events in central chondrosarcoma and central and periosteal chondromas but not in other mesenchymal tumours. J Pathol 2011;224(3):334–43.

41. Amary MF, Damato S, Halai D, et al. Ollier disease and Maffucci syndrome are caused by somatic mosaic mutations of IDH1 and IDH2. Nat Genet 2011;43(12):1262–5.

42. Pansuriya TC, van Eijk R, d'Adamo P, et al. Somatic mosaic IDH1 and IDH2 mutations are associated with enchondroma and spindle cell hemangioma in Ollier disease and Maffucci syndrome. Nat Genet 2011;43(12):1256–61.

43. Kurzawa P, Kattapuram S, Hornicek FJ, et al. Primary myoepithelioma of bone. A report of 8 cases. Am J Surg Pathol 2013;37(7):960–8.

44. Folpe AL, Agoff SN, Willis J, et al. Parachordoma is immunohistochemically and cytogenetically distinct from axial chordoma and extraskeletal myxoid chondrosarcoma. Am J Surg Pathol 1999;23(9):1059–67.

45. Sangoi AR, Dulai MS, Beck AH, et al. Distinguishing chordoid meningiomas from their histologic mimics: an immunohistochemical evaluation. Am J Surg Pathol 2009;33(5):669–81.

46. Bergh P, Kindblom LG, Gunterberg B, et al. Prognostic factors in chordoma of the sacrum and mobile spine: a study of 39 patients. Cancer 2000;88(9):2122–34.

47. Boari N, Gagliardi F, Cavalli A, et al. Sacral chordoma: long-term outcome of a large series of patients surgically treated at two reference centers. Spine (Phila Pa 1976) 2016;41(12):1049–57.

48. Frezza AM, Botta L, Trama A, et al. Chordoma: update on disease, epidemiology, biology and medical therapies. Curr Opin Oncol 2019;31(2):114–20.

49. Radaelli S, Fossati P, Stacchiotti S, et al. The sacral chordoma margin. Eur J Surg Oncol 2020;46(8):1415–22.

50. Rekhi B, Kosemehmetoglu K, Rane S, et al. Poorly differentiated chordomas showing loss of INI1/SMARCB1: a report of 2 rare cases with diagnostic implications. Int J Surg Pathol 2018;26(7):637–43.

51. Shih AR, Cote GM, Chebib I, et al. Clinicopathologic characteristics of poorly differentiated chordoma. Mod Pathol 2018;31(8):1237–45.

52. Buccoliero AM, Caporalini C, Scagnet M, et al. A diagnostic pitfall: atypical teratoid rhabdoid tumor versus dedifferentiated/poorly differentiated chordoma: analysis of a mono-institutional series. Appl Immunohistochem Mol Morphol 2019;27(2):147–54.

53. Cha YJ, Hong CK, Kim DS, et al. Poorly differentiated chordoma with loss of SMARCB1/INI1 expression in pediatric patients: a report of two cases and review of the literature. Neuropathology 2018;38(1):47–53.

54. Renard C, Pissaloux D, Decouvelaere AV, et al. Non-rhabdoid pediatric SMARCB1-deficient tumors: overlap between chordomas and malignant rhabdoid tumors? Cancer Genet 2014;207(9):384–9.

55. Huang SC, Zhang L, Sung YS, et al. Secondary EWSR1 gene abnormalities in SMARCB1-deficient tumors with 22q11-12 regional deletions: Potential pitfalls in interpreting EWSR1 FISH results. Genes Chromosomes Cancer 2016;55(10):767–76.

56. Yeom K, Lober R, Mobley B, et al. Diffusion-weighted MRI: distinction of skull base chordoma from chondrosarcoma. AJNR Am J Neuroradiol 2013;34(5):1056–61.

57. Hung YP, Diaz-Perez JA, Cote GM, et al. Dedifferentiated chordoma: clinicopathologic and molecular characteristics with integrative analysis. Am J Surg Pathol 2020;44(9):1213–23.

58. van den Munckhof P, Christiaans I, Kenter SB, et al. Germline SMARCB1 mutation predisposes to multiple meningiomas and schwannomas with

preferential location of cranial meningiomas at the falx cerebri. Neurogenetics 2012;13(1):1–7.

59. Hasselblatt M, Thomas C, Hovestadt V, et al. Poorly differentiated chordoma with SMARCB1/INI1 loss: a distinct molecular entity with dismal prognosis. Acta Neuropathol 2016;132(1):149–51.

60. Hanna S, Tirabosco R, Amin A, et al. Dedifferentiated chordoma: a report of four cases arising 'de novo'. J Bone Joint Surg Br 2008;90(5):652–6.

61. Kato S, Gasbarrini A, Ghermandi R, et al. Spinal chordomas dedifferentiated to osteosarcoma: a report of two cases and a literature review. Eur Spine J 2016;25(Suppl 1):251–6.

62. Asioli S, Zoli M, Guaraldi F, et al. Peculiar pathological, radiological and clinical features of skull-base dedifferentiated chordomas. Results from a referral centre case-series and literature review. Histopathology 2020;76(5):731–9.

Vascular Tumors of Bone
Updates and Diagnostic Pitfall

Yin P. Hung, MD, PhD[a,b]

KEYWORDS

- Hemangioma • Epithelioid hemangioma • Pseudomyogenic hemangioendothelioma
- Epithelioid hemangioendothelioma • Angiosarcoma

Key Points

- Primary vascular tumors of bone include hemangioma, epithelioid hemangioma, pseudomyogenic hemangioendothelioma, epithelioid hemangioendothelioma, and angiosarcoma.
- Primary vascular tumors of bone are classified based on cytologic and architectural assessment, including whether well-formed vascular channels are present.
- Epithelioid hemangioma of bone can extend into soft tissue and be mistaken for angiosarcoma. Protuberant epithelioid cells and round circumscribed borders are diagnostic clues.
- Pseudomyogenic hemangioendothelioma and most epithelioid hemangioendotheliomas (except those with *YAP1-TFE3* fusion) lack well-formed vascular channels.
- Cytokeratin expression is common in vascular tumors and may lead to confusion with metastatic carcinoma.

ABSTRACT

Vascular tumors of bone can be diagnostically challenging because of their rarity and histologic overlap with diverse mimics. Vascular tumors of bone can be categorized as benign (hemangioma), intermediate-locally aggressive (epithelioid hemangioma), intermediate-rarely metastasizing (pseudomyogenic hemangioendothelioma), and malignant (epithelioid hemangioendothelioma and angiosarcoma). Recurrent genetic alterations have been described, such as *FOSB* rearrangements in pseudomyogenic hemangioendothelioma and a subset of epithelioid hemangiomas; *CAMTA1* or *TFE3* rearrangements in epithelioid hemangioendothelioma. This review discusses the clinical, histologic, and molecular features of vascular tumors of bone, along with diagnostic pitfalls and strategies for avoidance.

OVERVIEW

Vascular tumors comprise less than 2% of all bone tumors and overlap with diverse entities radiologically and histologically. On imaging, the presence of multiple osseous lesions in an anatomic region may indicate a vascular tumor, in addition to other diagnoses, such as metastatic carcinoma and multiple myeloma. Microscopically, as vascular tumors can show epithelioid histology and express cytokeratins, they can be mistaken for metastatic carcinoma.[1] Correct diagnosis requires recognition of their vascular nature.

The literature on vascular tumors of bone can be confusing to peruse because of evolving nomenclature over the years. Compared with their soft tissue counterparts, vascular tumors of bone have fewer diagnostic categories. Vascular tumors of bone can be categorized into the following: benign (hemangioma), intermediate-locally aggressive (epithelioid hemangioma), intermediate-rarely metastasizing (pseudomyogenic hemangioendothelioma), and malignant (epithelioid hemangioendothelioma and angiosarcoma) **(Table 1)**. Historically, the terms "hemangioma," "hemangioendothelioma," and "angiosarcoma" designated tumors that were benign, of intermediate biological potential, and malignant, respectively. However, currently, the term

---

[a] Department of Pathology, Massachusetts General Hospital, 55 Fruit Street, Boston, MA, USA; [b] Harvard Medical School, Boston, MA, USA
E-mail address: yphung@mgh.harvard.edu

Surgical Pathology 14 (2021) 645–663
https://doi.org/10.1016/j.path.2021.06.007

Table 1
Overview of Vascular Tumors of Bone

	Hemangioma	Epithelioid Hemangioma	Pseudomyogenic Hemangioendothelioma	Epithelioid Hemangioendothelioma	Angiosarcoma
Biological Potential	Benign	Intermediate-locally aggressive	Intermediate- rarely metastasizing	Malignant	
Clinical features — Prevalence	Common (~10%)	Rare (≤ 1 in 1,000,000)			
% of patients with multifocal presentation	<20	~20	>90	>50	>50
% 5-y overall survival	100		>95	~75	<40
Radiographic features	Lytic ("corduroy"-like)		Lytic to mixed lytic-sclerotic		Lytic and aggressive
Histologic features — Border	Smooth	Smooth	Infiltrative and ragged	Infiltrative and ragged	Infiltrative and ragged
Lobulation	Yes	Yes	No	No	No
Vasoformation	Yes	Yes	No	Usually no[a]	Variable
Cytologic features	Spindled	Epithelioid	Spindled-to-epithelioid	Epithelioid-to-spindled	
Necrosis	Uncommon	Occasional	Occasional	Occasional	Frequent
Immunohisto-chemistry — Cytokeratins	None	Positive in a subset of all vascular tumors			None
Diagnostic markers for distinction	None	FOSB (in a subset of tumors)	FOSB	CAMTA1 (rarely TFE3)	None
Recurrent genetic mutations	None	*FOS* (rarely *FOSB*) rearrangement	*FOSB* rearrangement	*WWTR1-CAMTA1* (rarely *YAP1-TFE3* or other) fusion	Diverse

[a] Although most epithelioid hemangioendotheliomas lack vasoformative features, well-formed vascular channels are present in a small subset of tumors (that harbor the *YAP1-TFE3* fusion).

"hemangioendothelioma of bone" should not be used, as it denotes not a single entity but rather an admixture of epithelioid hemangioma, epithelioid hemangioendothelioma, and others.[2,3]

Recurrent genetic alterations have been identified in vascular tumors, such as *FOS* and *FOSB* rearrangements in a subset of epithelioid hemangiomas, *FOSB* rearrangement in pseudomyogenic hemangioendothelioma, and *WWTR1-CAMTA1* and *YAP1-TFE3* fusions in epithelioid hemangioendothelioma. Translated from these findings, immunohistochemical and molecular tools have been devised to aid the diagnosis of vascular tumors. Nevertheless, as bone tumors are often decalcified during processing, technical failures in ancillary studies are common and compound the diagnostic challenge. To preserve tumor DNA and antigenicity, the use of EDTA-based in lieu of acid-based decalcification should be considered when available.

HEMANGIOMA

OVERVIEW

Hemangioma of bone is benign and often asymptomatic, although it may rarely lead to symptoms such as neurologic deficits.[4,5] Although typically not sampled, given its high prevalence (approximately 10%), hemangioma is the most common vascular tumor encountered in orthopedic pathology.[6] Patients present with single or multiple hemangiomas, which are located in the spine (**Fig. 1**A), skull, or long bones.[5,7,8]

GROSS FEATURES

Hemangioma is situated in the medullary cavity and displays a spongelike appearance with hemorrhage (see **Fig. 1**B). Its border is delineated by variably sclerotic bone.

MICROSCOPIC FEATURES

Hemangioma of bone comprises 2 subtypes: cavernous and capillary, although both patterns can be present in individual tumors. Gaping vascular spaces are present in cavernous hemangiomas (see **Fig. 1**C), whereas capillary hemangiomas display lobules of capillaries and small vessels (see **Fig. 1**D). The endothelial cells are bland (see **Fig. 1**E). Reactive woven bone may be present at the edge.

DIAGNOSIS

On radiographs and computed tomographic imaging, hemangioma appears lucent, imparting a polka-dot or "corduroy"-like appearance (see **Fig. 1**A). On MRI, it appears hyperintense on fluid-sensitive sequences.[9,10] Hemangioma can be recognized by its radiologic appearance and seldom requires tissue sampling to establish a diagnosis. In patients with unusual presentation/imaging or a history of malignancy, tissue sampling may be considered to exclude mimics. Although seldom required, immunohistochemistry for vascular markers, such as ERG, FLI1, CD34, and CD31 (see **Fig. 1**F), can be used to highlight the endothelial cells.

DIFFERENTIAL DIAGNOSIS

In biopsies, hemangioma may be erroneously deemed nondiagnostic, as tissue may be scant and ignored. Other considerations include angiomatosis, arteriovenous malformation, epithelioid hemangioma, and angiosarcoma.

Skeletal angiomatosis, as characterized by multiple cystic bone lesions, can be subdivided into regional, disseminated (cystic angiomatosis), and aggressive subtypes.[11] Aggressive angiomatosis is associated with massive osteolysis/Gorham-Stout syndrome.[12] Microscopically, angiomatosis appears indistinguishable from hemangioma. Their distinction requires clinical and radiologic correlation. Similarly, as hemangioma histologically overlaps with arteriovenous malformation, their distinction requires radiologic and angiographic correlation.

Epithelioid hemangioma may be confused with hemangioma. In epithelioid hemangioma, at least 50% of tumor cells appear epithelioid, whereas in hemangiomas, endothelial cells are banal, with epithelioid cytomorphology confined to a small fraction of cells.

Angiosarcoma can be spindled, reminiscent of capillary hemangioma. The distinction can be challenging in select cases, including small biopsies. While hemangioma is circumscribed and lobulated with bland cytology, angiosarcoma is infiltrative and overtly malignant. Clinical and radiologic correlation can be helpful.

MOLECULAR FEATURES

EWSR1-NFATC1 fusion has been reported in a hemangioma of bone.[13] No recurrent alterations have been reported to date.

PROGNOSIS

Hemangioma is benign and does not require treatment in most cases. Symptomatic patients may be managed by intralesional curettage, arterial embolization, or other conservative measures.

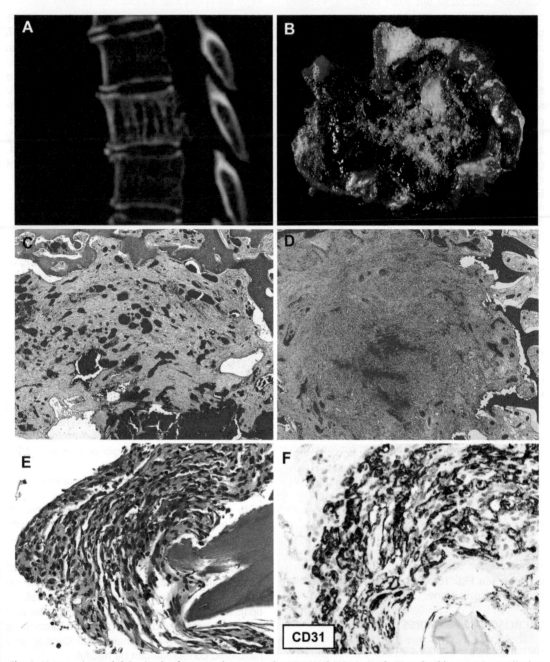

Fig. 1. Hemangioma. (*A*) Sagittal reformatted computed tomographic image of a vertebral hemangioma displays a polka-dot or "corduroy"-like appearance. (*B*) Gross photograph of a vertebral hemangioma shows a smooth delineated border. (*C*) A cavernous hemangioma demonstrates gaping vascular spaces (hematoxylin-eosin, original magnification ×40). (*D*) A capillary hemangioma shows circumscription and lobules of capillaries (hematoxylin-eosin, original magnification ×40). (*E*) A biopsy of a hemangioma reveals compressed fragments of bland vascular proliferation and bone (hematoxylin-eosin, original magnification ×400). (*F*) Diffuse immunoreactivity for CD31 is present (original magnification ×400).

Key Features of Hemangioma

- Benign, common, and often asymptomatic
- Capillary or cavernous histologic types
- Bland endothelial cells

Pitfall of Diagnosing Hemangioma

- It can be tricky to recognize a hemangioma in biopsies, in which "empty"-appearing spaces are seen along with fragments of disrupted spicules, fibrous tissue, and marrow elements. Radiologic correlation and noticing the endothelial cells at the edge of the vascular spaces aid the correct diagnosis.

Differential Diagnosis of Hemangioma

- Angiomatosis
  - Distinctive radiologic appearance
- Arteriovenous malformation
  - Distinct radiologic and angiographic appearance
- Epithelioid hemangioma
  - At least 50% of endothelial cells protuberant-epithelioid
- Angiosarcoma
  - Infiltrative and overtly malignant

EPITHELIOID HEMANGIOMA

OVERVIEW

As a vascular tumor of intermediate biological potential (locally aggressive), epithelioid hemangioma of bone shares similar pathologic features with its soft tissue counterparts, although soft tissue epithelioid hemangiomas are considered benign.[14] Epithelioid hemangioma of bone involves typically the long bones of the appendicular skeleton. Patients can present incidentally, with localized pain, or with pathologic fracture.[15,16]

GROSS FEATURES

Epithelioid hemangioma appears cystic with hemorrhage, with a delineated border. Epithelioid hemangioma of bone can break through the cortex and extend to the adjacent soft tissue.[17]

MICROSCOPIC FEATURES

Epithelioid hemangioma displays a smooth circumscribed border, a lobular configuration, and well-formed vasculature (**Fig. 2**A, B). The vascular channels are lined by protuberant to hobnailed epithelioid cells, with eosinophilic cytoplasm and occasional intracytoplasmic vacuoles (see **Fig. 2**C). A subset of tumors displays atypical features, such as hypercellularity, mild to moderate cytologic pleomorphism, and necrosis; yet, these are not pathognomonic of malignancy.[18] A subset of tumors (so-called hemorrhagic epithelioid and spindle cell hemangioma of bone) demonstrates predominantly spindle cells with focal (rather than diffuse) vasoformation.[19] Reactive woven bone and osteoclast-type giant cells can be present.[16]

DIAGNOSIS

Radiographically, epithelioid hemangioma shows a sharp sclerotic border and a lytic to mixed lytic-sclerotic center. Epithelioid hemangioma appears generally hyperintense on fluid-sensitive sequences on MRI.[20]

Definitive diagnosis requires tissue sampling. Although its histologic diagnosis is typically straightforward, immunohistochemistry and molecular testing can aid in challenging cases, such as those with subtle vasoformation. Immunohistochemistry for smooth muscle actin and ERG/CD31 can be used to highlight the pericytes and the endothelial cells, respectively (see **Fig. 2**D, E, F). A subset of epithelioid hemangiomas harbors rearrangements involving *FOS* or *FOSB*, which can be interrogated via fluorescence in situ hybridization or other methods.

DIFFERENTIAL DIAGNOSIS

Epithelioid hemangioma of bone can be difficult to diagnose, with less than 20% of tumors correctly recognized initially in 1 series.[21] Mimics include metastatic carcinoma, hemangioma, pseudomyogenic hemangioendothelioma, epithelioid hemangioendothelioma, and angiosarcoma.[22]

Although cytokeratins can be expressed in both epithelioid hemangioma and metastatic carcinoma, the latter is overtly malignant. Vascular markers can be used to confirm the diagnosis of epithelioid hemangioma.

Distinction between epithelioid hemangioma and hemangioma is important, given the lower risk of local recurrence in the latter. In hemangioma, endothelial cells are small and inconspicuous, although a small fraction may be epithelioid. In epithelioid hemangioma, at least 50% of endothelial cells are epithelioid with abundant cytoplasm.

There is histologic and molecular overlap between pseudomyogenic hemangioendothelioma and epithelioid hemangioma. Diffuse FOSB expression, which is diagnostic of pseudomyogenic hemangioendotheliomas, can be seen in a subset of epithelioid hemangiomas. Nearly all pseudomyogenic hemangioendotheliomas harbor *FOSB* fusion, typically to *SERPINE1* or *ACTB* and rarely to *WWTR1* or *CLTC*. In contrast, a minor subset of epithelioid hemangiomas harbors *FOSB* fusion to partners such as *ZFP36* or *WWTR1*, the latter suggesting genetic overlap. Nonetheless, distinction should be straightforward based on architectural and cytologic features: Epithelioid hemangioma contains bona fide vascular channels, whereas pseudomyogenic hemangioendothelioma is not vasoformative. Epithelioid

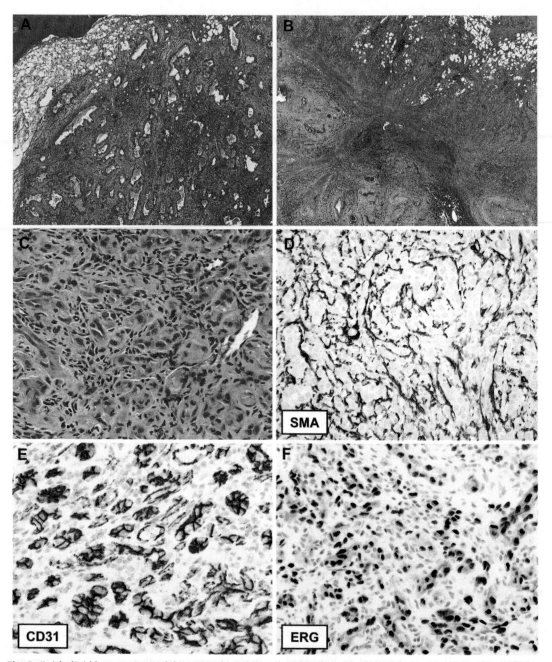

Fig. 2. Epithelioid hemangioma. (*A*) A smooth circumscribed border with variably conspicuous arterioles is characteristic (hematoxylin-eosin, original magnification ×20). (*B*) Epithelioid hemangioma of bone occasionally extends to soft tissues (hematoxylin-eosin, original magnification ×20). (*C*) The endothelial cells are hobnailed and arranged in nests, with well-formed vascular channels (hematoxylin-eosin, original magnification ×400). (*D*) Immunohistochemistry for smooth muscle actin highlights the pericytes (original magnification ×400). (*E*) CD31 is expressed by the tumor cells (original magnification ×400). (*F*) ERG immunohistochemistry highlights the plump nuclei (original magnification ×400).

hemangioma is epithelioid, whereas pseudomyogenic hemangioendothelioma is generally spindled.

Unlike epithelioid hemangioma, most epithelioid hemangioendotheliomas do not show well-formed vascular channels and instead display anastomosing cords of cells with variable vacuolation and myxohyaline stroma. CAMTA1 immunohistochemistry can aid the distinction, with nuclear staining in greater than 80% of epithelioid hemangioendothelioma but absent in epithelioid hemangioma.

Epithelioid hemangioma occasionally appears cellular, solid, and "infiltrative" with extension to soft tissue, raising a concern for epithelioid angiosarcoma. Nevertheless, epithelioid hemangioma retains a round circumscribed border, lobulation, and overt vasoformation. Its hobnailed endothelial cells do not display severe cytologic atypia.

Epithelioid hemangioma may be obscured by florid inflammation and resembles reactive conditions, such as osteomyelitis. However, the latter lacks epithelioid endothelial cells.

MOLECULAR FEATURES

Gene rearrangements in *FOS* and, less commonly, *FOSB* are present in a subset of epithelioid hemangiomas, including those of bone primary.[21,23,24] *ZFP36-FOSB* fusion has been reported in those with prominent spindle-cell component or atypical histologic features.[18,25]

PROGNOSIS

Epithelioid hemangioma can be locally aggressive but very rarely metastasizes. Treatment options include intralesional curettage, surgical resection, arterial embolization, and radiotherapy.

Key Features of Epithelioid Hemangioma

- Vascular tumor of intermediate biological potential (locally aggressive/rarely metastasizing)
- Circumscribed border and lobulation
- Well-formed vascular channels with protuberant epithelioid cells
- FOS or FOSB rearrangements in a subset of cases

Pitfall of Diagnosing Epithelioid Hemangioma

- Epithelioid hemangioma can break through cortical bone and extend into soft tissues. Such "infiltrative" behavior may be mistaken for angiosarcoma. Helpful clues include a round circumscribed border and hobnailed epithelioid tumor cells.

Differential Diagnosis of Epithelioid Hemangioma

- Metastatic carcinoma
  - Overtly malignant
  - Negative for vascular markers (except ERG in a subset of prostatic carcinomas)
- Hemangioma
  - Banal endothelial cells

- Epithelioid histology in a minority (<50%) of endothelial cells
- Pseudomyogenic hemangioendothelioma
  - No vasoformation
  - Rhabdomyoblast-like cells
  - Positive for FOSB in most cases
- Epithelioid hemangioendothelioma
  - No vasoformation (except cases with *YAP1-TFE3* fusion)
  - Myxohyaline stroma, anastomosing cords, vacuolation
  - Positive for CAMTA1 in most cases
- Angiosarcoma
  - Ill-defined border
  - Vasoformative features variable, ranging from conspicuous to absent
  - Overtly malignant

PSEUDOMYOGENIC HEMANGIOENDOTHELIOMA

OVERVIEW

Pseudomyogenic hemangioendothelioma (or epithelioid sarcoma-like hemangioendothelioma) is a distinctive vascular tumor of intermediate biological potential (intermediate-rarely metastasizing) that presents predominantly in the extremities of young adults, with multiple nodules in a regional distribution (**Fig. 3**A).[26–28] Although most tumors involve soft tissue, pseudomyogenic hemangioendothelioma with exclusive bone involvement (such as appendicular skeleton) has been reported.[29] Symptoms include progressive localized pain and/or pathologic fracture.

GROSS FEATURES

Pseudomyogenic hemangioendothelioma displays multiple discrete circumscribed nodules, often involving multiple bones in an anatomic region.[29]

MICROSCOPIC FEATURES

Pseudomyogenic hemangioendothelioma is not vasoformative (see **Fig. 3**B, C, D). It displays sheets to fascicles of plump spindled to epithelioid cells, some harboring abundant cytoplasm and mimicking rhabdomyoblasts (see **Fig. 3**D).[28] Cytoplasmic eosinophilia can be accentuated in decalcified specimens. Conspicuous mitoses, necrosis, and severe cytologic atypia are typically absent. Tumors may be obscured by intermixed reactive woven bone (see **Fig. 3**B), osteoclast-like giant cells (see **Fig. 3**C), and hemorrhage. A neutrophilic inflammatory background is uncommon among cases arising in bone.[29]

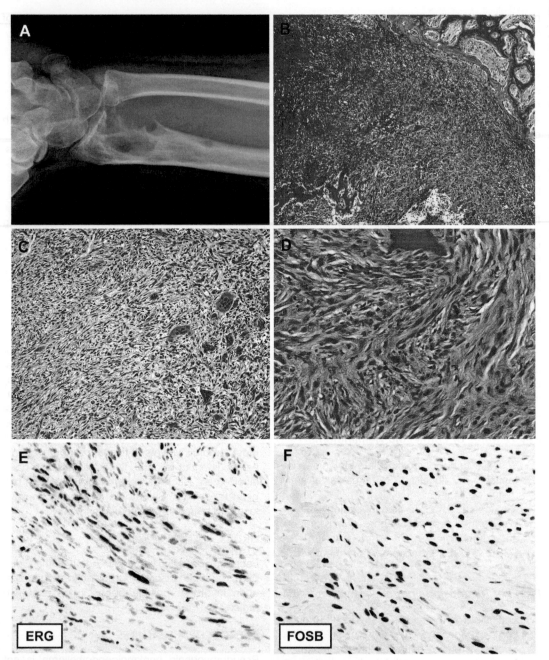

Fig. 3. Pseudomyogenic hemangioendothelioma. (*A*) Radiograph shows a multicystic-lytic meta-epiphyseal lesion and a small lucency in the diaphyseal cortex of the radius. (*B*) Pseudomyogenic hemangioendothelioma displays sheets and fascicles of spindled cells with no vasoformation. Reactive woven bone is present (hematoxylin-eosin, original magnification ×100). (*C*) Tumor cells intermingle with osteoclast-like giant cells (hematoxylin-eosin, original magnification ×200). (*D*) Tumor cells show characteristic rhabdomyoblast-like morphology with abundant eosinophilic cytoplasm (hematoxylin-eosin, original magnification ×400). (*E*) ERG immunohistochemistry highlights the elongated nuclei (original magnification ×400). (*F*) Diffuse nuclear FOSB staining is present in most cases, including this example (original magnification ×400).

DIAGNOSIS

Radiographically, pseudomyogenic hemangioendothelioma appears as multiple delineated lytic to mixed lytic-sclerotic lesions, involving one or several bones in an anatomic distribution (see **Fig. 3**A). On MRI, pseudomyogenic hemangioendothelioma is typically hyperintense on fluid-sensitive sequences.[29]

Definitive diagnosis requires tissue sampling. By immunohistochemistry, pseudomyogenic hemangioendothelioma expresses cytokeratins, most commonly AE1/AE3 cocktail.[28] Expression of ERG (see **Fig. 3**E) and FLI1 is present in greater than 90% of cases. CD31 immunoreactivity is noted in a subset, whereas CD34 is generally negative. FOSB is a sensitive marker for pseudomyogenic hemangioendothelioma,[30,31] with nuclear staining in greater than 95% of cases (see **Fig. 3**F),[31] although its performance can be suboptimal after decalcification. Fluorescence in situ hybridization testing and/or next-generation sequencing can also be used to assess for *FOSB* rearrangement.[32]

DIFFERENTIAL DIAGNOSIS

Differential diagnosis includes epithelioid sarcoma, epithelioid hemangioendothelioma, angiosarcoma, and other sarcomas.

Epithelioid sarcoma and pseudomyogenic hemangioendothelioma resemble each other, both presenting in the extremities of young adults and expressing cytokeratins.[26–28] In epithelioid sarcoma, tumor cells are infiltrative, occasionally in single files and associated with geographic necrosis, imparting a "granuloma-like" appearance; tumor cells lack the rhabdomyoblast-like cytomorphology as in pseudomyogenic hemangioendothelioma. Select immunohistochemical tools aid distinction. CD34 and EMA are expressed in a subset of epithelioid sarcomas but are absent in most pseudomyogenic hemangioendotheliomas. Nearly all epithelioid sarcomas show complete loss of INI1 expression,[33] whereas INI1 expression is intact in pseudomyogenic hemangioendothelioma.[28] Unlike pseudomyogenic hemangioendothelioma, epithelioid sarcoma lacks diffuse FOSB immunoreactivity.[31]

Distinction between epithelioid hemangioendothelioma and pseudomyogenic hemangioendothelioma can be difficult. Epithelioid hemangioendothelioma displays intracytoplasmic vacuoles and myxohyaline background, which are not seen in pseudomyogenic hemangioendothelioma. Most epithelioid hemangioendotheliomas are positive for CAMTA1 and negative for FOSB; conversely, pseudomyogenic hemangioendothelioma is positive for FOSB and negative for CAMTA1.

Angiosarcoma can mimic pseudomyogenic hemangioendothelioma. Angiosarcomas show variable but sometimes overt vasoformation, whereas vasoformative features are uniformly absent in pseudomyogenic hemangioendothelioma. Angiosarcoma typically lacks significant FOSB expression.

The rhabdomyoblast-like morphology of pseudomyogenic hemangioendothelioma may be confused with spindle-cell rhabdomyosarcoma or leiomyosarcoma. Pseudomyogenic hemangioendothelioma lacks bona fide myogenic differentiation and is negative for desmin, myogenin, and myoD1.

Pseudomyogenic hemangioendothelioma can be obscured by reactive woven bone and osteoclast-like giant cells, thereby mimicking osteoblastoma, giant cell tumor of bone, or fibrous dysplasia. These mimics are radiographically distinctive and lack rhabdomyoblast-like cells or evidence of endothelial differentiation.

MOLECULAR FEATURES

Pseudomyogenic hemangioendothelioma harbors recurrent chromosomal translocations,[34] resulting in rearrangements involving *FOSB*, which is fused to *SERPINE1* or *ACTB*, rarely *WWTR1* or *CLTC*.[32,35–38] The oncogenic fusion places the transactivation domain of FOSB under the control of a constitutively active promoter.

PROGNOSIS

Pseudomyogenic hemangioendothelioma of bone behaves similarly as its soft tissue counterpart. It is generally locally aggressive but indolent. The rate of local recurrence is ~30% to 60%, but the risk of distant metastases is less than 6%.[28,39]

It is primarily managed by wide surgical resection, including amputation in select patients. Data on the efficacy of radiotherapy and chemotherapy remain limited. Targeted therapy is under clinical investigation.[40]

Key Features of Pseudomyogenic Hemangioendothelioma

- Vascular tumor of intermediate biological potential (locally aggressive/rarely metastasizing)
- Generally, multiple nodules in an anatomic region
- No vasoformative features
- Sheets of plump rhabdomyoblast-like cells

- Positive for AE1/AE3, ERG, CD31, and FOSB in most cases

Pitfall of Diagnosing Pseudomyogenic Hemangioendothelioma

- It may be obscured by intermixed reactive woven bone and osteoclast-like giant cells, mimicking osteoblastoma and other bone tumors. Helpful clues include rhabdomyoblast-like cells.

Differential Diagnosis of Pseudomyogenic Hemangioendothelioma

- Epithelioid sarcoma
  - Prominent necrosis with "granuloma-like" appearance
  - Loss of INI1 expression
- Epithelioid hemangioendothelioma
  - Myxohyaline stroma, anastomosing cords, vacuolation
  - Positive for CAMTA1 in greater than 80% of cases
- Angiosarcoma
  - Presence of vasoformative features in a subset of tumors
  - Overtly malignant, with severe cytologic atypia and multilayering
  - Lacks diffuse FOSB expression
- Rhabdomyosarcoma
  - Positive for desmin, myoD1, and myogenin
  - Negative for vascular markers
- Metastatic carcinoma
  - Lacks rhabdomyoblast-like cells
  - Negative for vascular markers (except ERG in a subset of prostatic carcinomas)
- Other primary bone tumors
  - Distinctive radiographic appearance
  - Lacks rhabdomyoblast-like cells

EPITHELIOID HEMANGIOENDOTHELIOMA

OVERVIEW

Epithelioid hemangioendothelioma presents with a wide age range and involves soft tissue/viscera and rarely bone exclusively.[41] Primary skeletal epithelioid hemangioendothelioma presents in a multifocal fashion in greater than 50% of cases, affecting typically long bones and less frequently axial skeleton. Symptoms include progressive localized pain with variable swelling.[42,43]

GROSS FEATURES

It displays single to multiple nodules in the cortex and/or medulla.

MICROSCOPIC FEATURES

Epithelioid cells are arranged in anastomosing cords to strands, in a myxoid to hyaline background (Fig. 4A, B). Intracytoplasmic vacuoles are often present (so-called blister cells), although the extent may be focal. In bone, epithelioid hemangioendothelioma can be obscured by osteoclast-like giant cells and reactive woven bone.

Most epithelioid hemangioendotheliomas do not harbor bona fide vascular channels, except those with YAP1-TFE3 fusion. YAP1-TFE3 fusion-positive epithelioid hemangioendothelioma displays a nested pattern, voluminous eosinophilic cytoplasm, and a fibrocollagenous background that lacks the myxohyaline matrix (see Fig. 4C).[44] Vasoformation is generally present, albeit with variable extent (including absent in 1 case).[45]

About 30% of epithelioid hemangioendotheliomas demonstrates pleomorphism, conspicuous mitoses, and geographic necrosis; such overtly malignant appearance (see Fig. 4D) overlaps with that of angiosarcoma. So-called malignant epithelioid hemangioendothelioma, these tumors may be more aggressive.

DIAGNOSIS

Radiographically, epithelioid hemangioendothelioma is characterized by solitary or multiple lytic to mixed lytic-sclerotic lesions. Definitive diagnosis requires tissue sampling.

Nearly all epithelioid hemangioendotheliomas express CD31 (see Fig. 4E), ERG, and FLI1. CD34 immunoreactivity is common. Nuclear CAMTA1 staining is present in greater than 80% of epithelioid hemangioendothelioma (see Fig. 4F), corresponding to those with WWTR1-CAMTA1 fusion,[46,47] and is specific. In addition, fluorescence in situ hybridization or other methods can be used to assess for CAMTA1 rearrangement.[48]

TFE3-rearranged epithelioid hemangioendothelioma lacks nuclear CAMTA1 staining but instead shows diffuse strong nuclear TFE3 expression. Of note, patchy weak TFE3 staining is nonspecific. Fluorescence in situ hybridization testing or other methods can be used to interrogate for TFE3 and/or YAP1 rearrangements.[44,49]

DIFFERENTIAL DIAGNOSIS

Epithelioid hemangioendothelioma is one of the master mimickers with resemblance to diverse tumors: metastatic carcinomas, other vascular tumors (epithelioid hemangioma, pseudomyogenic hemangioendothelioma, and angiosarcoma), and

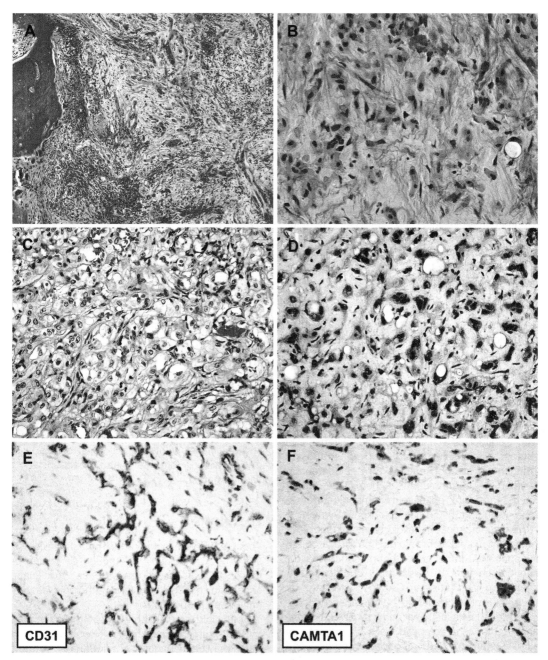

Fig. 4. Epithelioid hemangioendothelioma. (*A*) At low magnification, tumor cells may be obscured by hemorrhage (hematoxylin-eosin, original magnification ×100). (*B*) For most epithelioid hemangioendotheliomas (those with *WWTR1-CAMTA1* fusion), histologic features include myxohyaline stroma, a reticular arrangement, and intracytoplasmic vacuoles (hematoxylin-eosin, original magnification ×400). (*C*) *YAP1-TFE3* fusion-positive epithelioid hemangioendothelioma displays a nested architecture, well-formed vasculature, and voluminous cytoplasm (hematoxylin-eosin, original magnification ×400). (*D*) A subset of epithelioid hemangioendotheliomas appears overtly malignant with marked pleomorphism (hematoxylin-eosin, original magnification ×400). (*E*) CD31 immunoreactivity is present in most cases (original magnification ×400). (*F*) Nuclear CAMTA1 staining, indicative of *CAMTA1* rearrangement, is present in most cases (original magnification ×400).

other mesenchymal tumors (extraskeletal myxoid chondrosarcoma, myoepithelial tumors, chondromyxoid fibroma, chordoma, and others).

Given its epithelioid morphology and cytokeratin immunoreactivity, epithelioid hemangioendothelioma is not infrequently mistaken for metastatic carcinoma.[50,51] Diagnostic clues include myxo-hyaline matrix, which is uncommon among metastatic carcinomas. Immunoreactivity for ERG is present in epithelioid hemangioendothelioma but absent in most carcinomas (except a subset of prostatic carcinomas).[52]

Unlike most epithelioid hemangioendotheliomas, epithelioid hemangioma is consistently vasoformative, with well-formed vascular channels lined by hobnailed endothelial cells. Epithelioid hemangioma does not show nuclear CAMTA1 expression, which is characteristic of most epithelioid hemangioendotheliomas.

The distinction between pseudomyogenic hemangioendothelioma and epithelioid hemangioendothelioma can be difficult, as both vascular tumors lack vasoformation. Epithelioid hemangioendothelioma does not display the rhabdomyoblast-like cytomorphology of pseudomyogenic hemangioendothelioma. CAMTA1 nuclear staining is absent in pseudomyogenic hemangioendothelioma, whereas diffuse FOSB expression is present in greater than 90% of pseudomyogenic hemangioendothelioma but less than 10% of epithelioid hemangioendotheliomas.

The distinction between angiosarcoma and so-called malignant epithelioid hemangioendothelioma can be problematic. The presence of vasoformative features strongly favors angiosarcoma over epithelioid hemangioendothelioma. In contrast, myxohyaline matrix and anastomosing arrangement are not features for angiosarcoma. Positive CAMTA1 immunohistochemistry supports the diagnosis of epithelioid hemangioendothelioma, including the so-called malignant variant.

The distinction of epithelioid hemangioendothelioma from extraskeletal myxoid chondrosarcoma, myoepithelial tumors, and other mesenchymal tumors can be aided by select tools. Endothelial differentiation and nuclear CAMTA1 staining, as present in most epithelioid hemangioendotheliomas, are absent in these mimics. EWSR1 rearrangements characteristic of a subset of extraskeletal myxoid chondrosarcomas and myoepithelial tumors have not been described in epithelioid hemangioendothelioma.

Epithelioid hemangioendothelioma may mimic chondromyxoid fibroma, as both show reticular architecture with myxoid background. Distinction should be straightforward, given their distinct radiologic and cytologic features. Chondromyxoid fibroma is a solitary circumscribed eccentric lesion typically involving a long bone. Unlike epithelioid hemangioendothelioma, chondromyxoid fibroma displays delicate spindle cells.

Epithelioid hemangioendothelioma may be confused with conventional-type chordoma, as both harbor epithelioid cells embedded within myxoid matrix. The cytoplasm in chordoma appears multivacuolated and bubbly (so-called physaliferous cells), unlike the univacuolated cells in epithelioid hemangioendothelioma. Although both tumors can express cytokeratins, chordoma is positive for T-brachyury, a specific marker for notochordal differentiation, whereas epithelioid hemangioendothelioma is negative for T-brachyury and expresses vascular markers.

Epithelioid hemangioendothelioma can be obscured by hemorrhage, reactive woven bone, and osteoclast-like giant cells, mimicking fibrous dysplasia, giant cell tumor of bone, and other bone tumors. Helpful clues include anastomosing cords of epithelioid cells and myxohyaline matrix, along with judicious use of endothelial markers.

MOLECULAR FEATURES

WWTR1-CAMTA1 fusion is present in greater than 80% of epithelioid hemangioendotheliomas.[53,54] Alternate fusions include YAP1-TFE3, rarely WWTR1-MAML2 and WWTR1-ACTL6A.[44,55] Except those with YAP1-TFE3 fusion[44] (including those occurring in bone),[56] epithelioid hemangioendotheliomas (with WWTR1 fusions) demonstrate classic histology characterized by myxohyaline stroma and absence of vasoformation.

PROGNOSIS

Local recurrence is common. The risk of metastases is ~20% to 30%.[41] Although pertaining primarily to soft tissue cases, risk stratification schemata based on clinicopathologic features have been proposed.[57,58]

Epithelioid hemangioendothelioma is managed by wide surgical resection.[59] Nonsurgical candidates may be managed by radiotherapy, cytotoxic chemotherapy, or a combination thereof.[41]

Key Features of Epithelioid Hemangioendothelioma

- Malignant vascular tumor, with better outcome than angiosarcoma
- No vasoformative features (except those with YAP1-TFE3 fusion)
- Myxohyaline matrix, anastomosing cords of cells, intracytoplasmic vacuoles
- Positive for CAMTA1 in greater than 80% of cases

Pitfall of Diagnosing Epithelioid Hemangioendothelioma

- Given its epithelioid morphology and cytokeratin expression, epithelioid hemangioendothelioma can be mistaken for metastatic carcinoma. Helpful clues include myxohyaline stroma and intracytoplasmic vacuoles, which can be focal.

Differential Diagnosis of Epithelioid Hemangioendothelioma

- Metastatic carcinoma
  - No myxohyaline matrix
  - Negative for CD34 and CD31 in most cases
  - Negative for ERG (except a subset of prostatic carcinomas)
- Epithelioid hemangioma
  - Well-formed vascular channels lined by plump endothelial cells
  - Positive for FOSB in a subset of cases
- Pseudomyogenic hemangioendothelioma
  - Rhabdomyoblast-like spindled cells
  - Positive for FOSB in most cases
- Angiosarcoma
  - Vasoformative features variable, ranging from conspicuous to absent
  - Overtly malignant, with prominent nucleoli
- Extraskeletal myxoid chondrosarcoma
  - Reticular arrangement of uniform cells
  - Positive for *NR4A3* rearrangement
- Myoepithelial tumors
  - Myoepithelial immunophenotype
  - Positive for *EWSR1* rearrangement in a subset of cases
- Chondromyxoid fibroma
  - Solitary eccentric lytic lesion
  - Delicate bland spindle cells
- Chordoma
  - Physaliferous cells with multivacuolated cytoplasm
  - Positive for T-brachyury

ANGIOSARCOMA

OVERVIEW

Primary angiosarcoma of bone accounts for less than 5% of all angiosarcomas, presents typically in the elderly, and involves most commonly long tubular bones of extremities, followed by pelvis and axial skeleton (**Fig. 5**A).[60] Approximately half of the patients present with multifocal disease.

GROSS FEATURES

Angiosarcoma is friable, destructive, and hemorrhagic, with ill-defined borders. Extraosseous extension is common.

MICROSCOPIC FEATURES

More than 90% of primary angiosarcoma of bone demonstrates epithelioid histology (see **Fig. 5**B, C).[61,62] Angiosarcoma of exclusively spindle-cell histology rarely arises in bone and may suggest metastasis from elsewhere. Angiosarcoma shows an ill-defined border and permeative sheetlike growth (see **Fig. 5**B), along with necrosis and hemorrhage. Cytologically, tumor cells are overtly malignant, with eosinophilic to amphophilic cytoplasm, vesicular nuclei, and prominent macronuclei (see **Fig. 5**C). Vasoformative features are variable and range from diffuse to focal. Tumor cells at the edge of the vascular spaces can exhibit multilayering.

DIAGNOSIS

Radiographically, angiosarcoma appears aggressive and lytic, with ill-defined borders and frequent cortical destruction. Definitive diagnosis requires tissue sampling.

Cytokeratin expression is present in ~70% of angiosarcomas and may lead to confusion with metastatic carcinoma (see **Fig. 5**D). Most angiosarcomas express CD31 (see **Fig. 5**E), ERG (see **Fig. 5**F), and FLI1, although the extent of staining can be limited in some tumors. CD34 expression is present in ~40% of tumors. D2-40 immunoreactivity indicative of lymphatic differentiation is seen in ~30% of tumors.

DIFFERENTIAL DIAGNOSIS

Primary angiosarcoma of bone can be mistaken for metastatic carcinoma (**Fig. 6**A, B), metastatic angiosarcoma from elsewhere (see **Fig. 6**C, D), melanoma, epithelioid sarcoma (proximal-type), histiocytic sarcoma, Kaposi sarcoma (see **Fig. 6**E, F), epithelioid hemangioma, pseudomyogenic hemangioendothelioma, and epithelioid hemangioendothelioma.

Both metastatic carcinoma and angiosarcoma show overlapping radiologic features, epithelioid histology, and express cytokeratins.[63] Distinction can be aided by endothelial markers, which are expressed in angiosarcomas but not carcinomas (aside from ERG expression in a subset of prostatic carcinomas).

The prominent macronucleoli in angiosarcoma may be reminiscent of those in metastatic

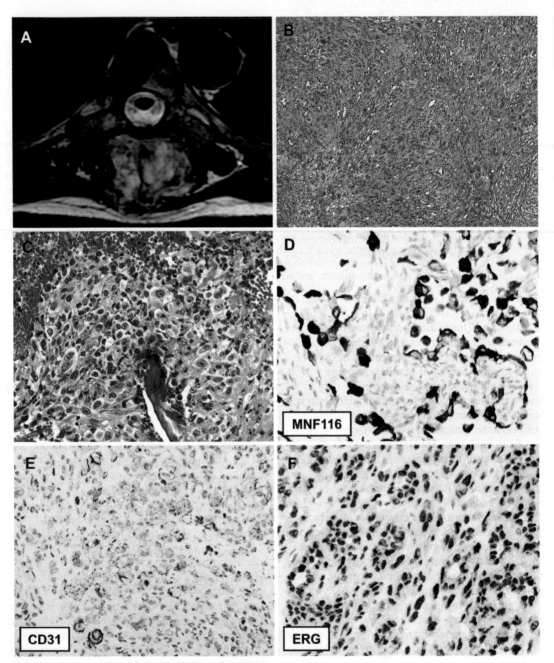

Fig. 5. Angiosarcoma. (*A*) Axial T2-weighted MRI of a vertebral angiosarcoma shows hyperintense signals in bone and posterior soft tissues. (*B*) Angiosarcoma displays an infiltrative sheetlike growth with variable vasoformation, including channels lined by malignant cells in this example (hematoxylin-eosin, original magnification ×100). (*C*) Primary angiosarcoma of bone frequently appears epithelioid, with moderate cytoplasm and macronucleoli (hematoxylin-eosin, original magnification ×400). (*D*) Immunoreactivity for cytokeratins (such as MNF116) in angiosarcomas may lead to confusion with metastatic carcinoma (original magnification ×400). (*E*) CD31 immunoreactivity can be variable, including focal extent in this example (original magnification ×400). (*F*) ERG immunohistochemistry highlights the nuclei of malignant cells (original magnification ×400).

melanoma. Unlike angiosarcoma, metastatic melanoma lacks expression of endothelial markers and expresses melanocytic markers, such as S-100 protein, SOX10, and HMB45.

Epithelioid sarcoma and epithelioid angiosarcoma show morphologic and immunophenotypic overlap, including CD34 expression. Depending on the antibody clone used, ERG expression has

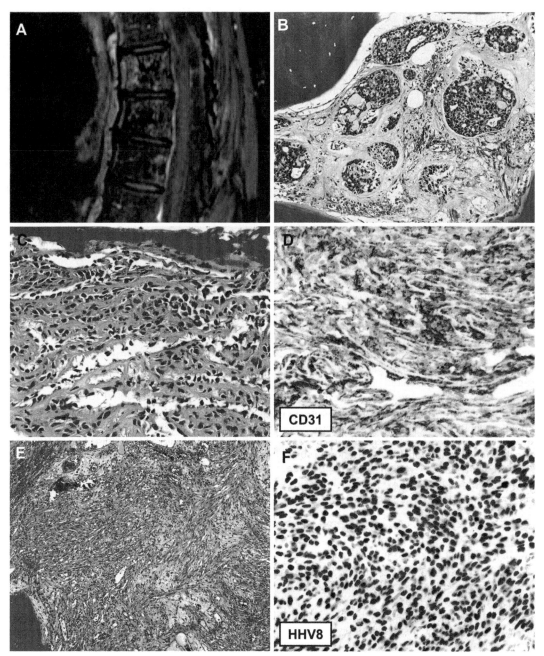

Fig. 6. Select mimics of primary vascular tumors of bone. (*A*) Sagittal postcontrast T1-weighted MRI shows mixed lytic-sclerotic lesions across 3 vertebrae; differentials include metastasis and primary vascular tumor. (*B*) A biopsy on the bone lesions in (*A*) reveals metastatic adenoid cystic carcinoma of tracheal primary (hematoxylin-eosin, original magnification ×200). (*C*) This spindle-cell angiosarcoma represents a metastasis from bladder primary (hematoxylin-eosin, original magnification ×400). (*D*) Immunohistochemistry for CD31 is positive (original magnification ×400). (*E*) Kaposi sarcoma replaces the native marrow elements and mimics spindle-cell angiosarcoma. Diagnostic clues include overlapping fascicles in a "sieve"-like pattern and the lack of cytologic atypia (hematoxylin-eosin, original magnification ×100). (*F*) HHV8 immunoreactivity confirms the diagnosis of Kaposi sarcoma (original magnification ×400).

been reported in epithelioid sarcoma, leading to diagnostic confusion.[64,65] Epithelioid sarcoma involves primarily soft tissue and rarely bone exclusively.[66] Epithelioid sarcoma lacks CD31 immunoreactivity and shows complete loss of INI1 in nearly all cases.[33]

Epithelioid hemangioma of bone occasionally extends to soft tissues and may exhibit cytologic atypia, necrosis, and/or conspicuous mitoses. Unlike angiosarcoma, epithelioid hemangioma shows a circumscribed border with lobular configuration; its hobnailed endothelial cells lack malignant cytologic features. Immunohistochemical stain for smooth muscle actin and vascular markers can be used to highlight the orderly architecture in epithelioid hemangioma. Rearrangements involving *FOS* or *FOSB* are present in a subset of epithelioid hemangiomas and absent in angiosarcomas.

Pseudomyogenic hemangioendothelioma appears spiculated and may be confused with angiosarcoma. Pseudomyogenic hemangioendothelioma lacks vasoformation, whereas most angiosarcomas display bona fide vascular channels and are overtly malignant. Also, the rhabdomyoblast-like cells and diffuse strong FOSB expression are characteristic of most pseudomyogenic hemangioendotheliomas.

A subset of epithelioid hemangioendothelioma appears overtly malignant, with considerable histologic overlap with angiosarcoma. In these so-called malignant epithelioid hemangioendotheliomas, myxohyaline stroma, anastomosing configuration, and nuclear CAMTA1 expression can generally be identified.

CD31 are expressed in histiocytes and a subset of histiocytic sarcoma, leading to diagnostic confusion with angiosarcoma.[67] Nevertheless, histiocytic sarcoma lacks ERG expression and is positive for other histiocytic markers: CD163, PU.1, or CD68.[68,69]

Rarely, Kaposi sarcoma involves the musculoskeletal system[70] and resembles spindle-cell angiosarcoma. Microscopically, overlapping fascicles of uniform bland cells with a "sieve"-like appearance are characteristic. Hyaline globules, although not entirely specific, can be a helpful clue. Overtly malignant cytology and hyperchromasia are absent. Immunohistochemistry for human herpesvirus 8 (HHV8) aid the definitive diagnosis.

MOLECULAR FEATURES

Similar to its soft tissue counterparts,[71,72] angiosarcoma of bone shows karyotypic and genetic diversity.[73,74] Both simple and complex aberrations with multiple chromosomal gains and losses have been reported.[74] Amplification of *MYC* is present in a subset of skeletal angiosarcomas and does not necessarily indicate a history of radiation treatment.[74]

PROGNOSIS

The prognosis is dismal for skeletal angiosarcomas, with a 5-year overall survival of less than 40%.[62] Patients may be managed by wide surgical resection (including amputation), chemotherapy, radiotherapy, or a combination thereof.[75]

Key Features of Angiosarcoma

- Malignant vascular tumor with a dismal prognosis
- Predominantly epithelioid histology for skeletal primary
- Variable vasoformative features
- Amphophilic cytoplasm, macronucleoli, overtly malignant

Pitfall of Diagnosing Angiosarcoma

- Cytokeratin expression is frequent in angiosarcomas and can lead to confusion with metastatic carcinoma. Helpful clues for angiosarcoma include lack of marked pleomorphism, amphophilic cytoplasm, macronucleoli, and vasoformation.
- Metastatic angiosarcoma to bone can show spindle cells with variable cytologic atypia and minimal/subtle multilayering.
- Hemangioma and epithelioid hemangioma may be mistaken for angiosarcoma when extending to soft tissues. However, they show smooth circumscribed borders and lack malignant cytologic features.

Differential Diagnosis of Angiosarcoma

- Metastatic carcinoma
  - Negative for CD34 and CD31 in most cases
  - Negative for ERG (except a subset of prostatic carcinomas)
- Metastatic melanoma
  - Packets of cells with conspicuous nucleoli
  - Positive for melanocytic markers
- Epithelioid sarcoma
  - Involves soft tissue and rarely bone exclusively
  - Loss of INI1 expression in most cases
- Histiocytic sarcoma
  - Positive for histiocytic markers CD163, PU.1, and/or others
  - Negative for ERG
- Kaposi sarcoma
  - Overlapping fascicles of uniform cells with a "sieve"-like appearance
  - Positive for HHV8
- Epithelioid hemangioma

- o Smooth circumscribed border and lobulation
- o Hobnailed endothelial cells
- o May exhibit cytologic atypia, necrosis, and/or conspicuous mitoses
- o *FOS* or *FOSB* rearrangements in a subset of cases
- Pseudomyogenic hemangioendothelioma
  - o No vasoformative features
  - o Spindled cells with rhabdomyoblast-like morphology
  - o Positive for AE1/AE3, ERG, and FOSB in most cases
- Epithelioid hemangioendothelioma
  - o Myxohyaline stroma, anastomosing cords, vacuolation
  - o Positive for CAMTA1 in most cases

DISCLOSURE

No disclosure.

ACKNOWLEDGMENTS

I thank Dr G. Petur Nielsen, who generously allowed me to photograph his consult cases for some of the illustrations; and Mayerling R. Dada and Linda M. Arini at the Massachusetts General Hospital for administrative support.

REFERENCES

1. Gray MH, Rosenberg AE, Dickersin GR, et al. Cytokeratin expression in epithelioid vascular neoplasms. Hum Pathol 1990;21(2):212–7.

2. Evans HL, Raymond AK, Ayala AG. Vascular tumors of bone: a study of 17 cases other than ordinary hemangioma, with an evaluation of the relationship of hemangioendothelioma of bone to epithelioid hemangioma, epithelioid hemangioendothelioma, and high-grade angiosarcoma. Hum Pathol 2003; 34(7):680–9.

3. Boriani S, Cecchinato R, Righi A, et al. Primary vascular bone tumors in the spine: a challenge for pathologists and spine oncology surgeons. Eur Spine J 2019;28(6):1502–11.

4. Robbins LR, Fountain EM. Hemangioma of cervical vertebras with spinal-cord compression. N Engl J Med 1958;258(14):685–7.

5. Fox MW, Onofrio BM. The natural history and management of symptomatic and asymptomatic vertebral hemangiomas. J Neurosurg 1993;78(1): 36–45.

6. Righi A, Sbaraglia M, Gambarotti M, et al. Primary vascular tumors of bone: a monoinstitutional morphologic and molecular analysis of 427 cases with emphasis on epithelioid variants. Am J Surg Pathol 2020;44(9):1192–203.

7. Dorfman HD, Steiner GC, Jaffe HL. Vascular tumors of bone. Hum Pathol 1971;2(3):349–76.

8. McAllister VL, Kendall BE, Bull JW. Symptomatic vertebral haemangiomas. Brain 1975;98(1):71–80.

9. Kaleem Z, Kyriakos M, Totty WG. Solitary skeletal hemangioma of the extremities. Skeletal Radiol 2000;29(9):502–13.

10. Wenger DE, Wold LE. Benign vascular lesions of bone: radiologic and pathologic features. Skeletal Radiol 2000;29(2):63–74.

11. Verbeke SL, Bovee JV. Primary vascular tumors of bone: a spectrum of entities? Int J Clin Exp Pathol 2011;4(6):541–51.

12. Gorham LW, Stout AP. Massive osteolysis (acute spontaneous absorption of bone, phantom bone, disappearing bone); its relation to hemangiomatosis. J Bone Joint Surg Am 1955;37-A(5):985–1004.

13. Arbajian E, Magnusson L, Brosjo O, et al. A benign vascular tumor with a new fusion gene: EWSR1-NFATC1 in hemangioma of the bone. Am J Surg Pathol 2013;37(4):613–6.

14. Rosai J, Gold J, Landy R. The histiocytoid hemangiomas. A unifying concept embracing several previously described entities of skin, soft tissue, large vessels, bone, and heart. Hum Pathol 1979;10(6): 707–30.

15. O'Connell JX, Kattapuram SV, Mankin HJ, et al. Epithelioid hemangioma of bone. A tumor often mistaken for low-grade angiosarcoma or malignant hemangioendothelioma. Am J Surg Pathol 1993; 17(6):610–7.

16. Nielsen GP, Srivastava A, Kattapuram S, et al. Epithelioid hemangioma of bone revisited: a study of 50 cases. Am J Surg Pathol 2009;33(2):270–7.

17. Errani C, Zhang L, Panicek DM, et al. Epithelioid hemangioma of bone and soft tissue: a reappraisal of a controversial entity. Clin Orthop Relat Res 2012;470(5):1498–506.

18. Antonescu CR, Chen HW, Zhang L, et al. ZFP36-FOSB fusion defines a subset of epithelioid hemangioma with atypical features. Genes Chromosomes Cancer 2014;53(11):951–9.

19. Keel SB, Rosenberg AE. Hemorrhagic epithelioid and spindle cell hemangioma: a newly recognized, unique vascular tumor of bone. Cancer 1999;85(9): 1966–72.

20. Schenker K, Blumer S, Jaramillo D, et al. Epithelioid hemangioma of bone: radiologic and magnetic resonance imaging characteristics with histopathological correlation. Pediatr Radiol 2017;47(12):1631–7.

21. Tsuda Y, Suurmeijer AJH, Sung YS, et al. Epithelioid hemangioma of bone harboring FOS and FOSB gene rearrangements: a clinicopathologic and molecular study. Genes Chromosomes Cancer 2021; 60(1):17–25.

22. Cone RO, Hudkins P, Nguyen V, et al. Histiocytoid hemangioma of bone: a benign lesion which may mimic angiosarcoma. Report of a case and review of literature. Skeletal Radiol 1983;10(3):165–9.

23. van IDG, de Jong D, Romagosa C, et al. Fusion events lead to truncation of FOS in epithelioid hemangioma of bone. Genes Chromosomes Cancer 2015;54(9):565–74.

24. Huang SC, Zhang L, Sung YS, et al. Frequent FOS gene rearrangements in epithelioid hemangioma: a molecular study of 58 cases with morphologic reappraisal. Am J Surg Pathol 2015;39(10):1313–21.

25. Keil F, Dietmaier W, Hoffstetter P, et al. ZFP36-FOSB fusion in a haemorrhagic epithelioid and spindle cell haemangioma of bone: is there a family of FOSB-rearranged vascular neoplasms of the bone? Histopathology 2020;76(3):490–3.

26. Mirra JM, Kessler S, Bhuta S, et al. The fibroma-like variant of epithelioid sarcoma. A fibrohistiocytic/myoid cell lesion often confused with benign and malignant spindle cell tumors. Cancer 1992;69(6):1382–95.

27. Billings SD, Folpe AL, Weiss SW. Epithelioid sarcoma-like hemangioendothelioma. Am J Surg Pathol 2003;27(1):48–57.

28. Hornick JL, Fletcher CD. Pseudomyogenic hemangioendothelioma: a distinctive, often multicentric tumor with indolent behavior. Am J Surg Pathol 2011;35(2):190–201.

29. Inyang A, Mertens F, Puls F, et al. Primary pseudomyogenic hemangioendothelioma of bone. Am J Surg Pathol 2016;40(5):587–98.

30. Sugita S, Hirano H, Kikuchi N, et al. Diagnostic utility of FOSB immunohistochemistry in pseudomyogenic hemangioendothelioma and its histological mimics. Diagn Pathol 2016;11(1):75.

31. Hung YP, Fletcher CD, Hornick JL. FOSB is a useful diagnostic marker for pseudomyogenic hemangioendothelioma. Am J Surg Pathol 2017;41(5):596–606.

32. Zhu G, Benayed R, Ho C, et al. Diagnosis of known sarcoma fusions and novel fusion partners by targeted RNA sequencing with identification of a recurrent ACTB-FOSB fusion in pseudomyogenic hemangioendothelioma. Mod Pathol 2019;32(5):609–20.

33. Hornick JL, Dal Cin P, Fletcher CD. Loss of INI1 expression is characteristic of both conventional and proximal-type epithelioid sarcoma. Am J Surg Pathol 2009;33(4):542–50.

34. Trombetta D, Magnusson L, von Steyern FV, et al. Translocation t(7;19)(q22;q13)-a recurrent chromosome aberration in pseudomyogenic hemangioendothelioma? Cancer Genet 2011;204(4):211–5.

35. Walther C, Tayebwa J, Lilljebjorn H, et al. A novel SERPINE1-FOSB fusion gene results in transcriptional up-regulation of FOSB in pseudomyogenic

haemangioendothelioma. J Pathol 2014;232(5):534–40.

36. Agaram NP, Zhang L, Cotzia P, et al. Expanding the spectrum of genetic alterations in pseudomyogenic hemangioendothelioma with recurrent novel ACTB-FOSB gene fusions. Am J Surg Pathol 2018;42(12):1653–61.

37. Panagopoulos I, Lobmaier I, Gorunova L, et al. Fusion of the genes WWTR1 and FOSB in pseudomyogenic hemangioendothelioma. Cancer Genomics Proteomics 2019;16(4):293–8.

38. Bridge JA, Sumegi J, Royce T, et al. A novel CLTC-FOSB gene fusion in pseudomyogenic hemangioendothelioma of bone. Genes Chromosomes Cancer 2021;60(1):38–42.

39. Sun Y, Zhao M, Lao IW, et al. The clinicopathological spectrum of pseudomyogenic hemangioendothelioma: report of an additional series with review of the literature. Virchows Arch 2020;477(2):231–40.

40. van IDGP, Sleijfer S, Gelderblom H, et al. Telatinib is an effective targeted therapy for pseudomyogenic hemangioendothelioma. Clin Cancer Res 2018;24(11):2678–87.

41. Lau K, Massad M, Pollak C, et al. Clinical patterns and outcome in epithelioid hemangioendothelioma with or without pulmonary involvement: insights from an internet registry in the study of a rare cancer. Chest 2011;140(5):1312–8.

42. Tsuneyoshi M, Dorfman HD, Bauer TW. Epithelioid hemangioendothelioma of bone. A clinicopathologic, ultrastructural, and immunohistochemical study. Am J Surg Pathol 1986;10(11):754–64.

43. Kleer CG, Unni KK, McLeod RA. Epithelioid hemangioendothelioma of bone. Am J Surg Pathol 1996;20(11):1301–11.

44. Antonescu CR, Le Loarer F, Mosquera JM, et al. Novel YAP1-TFE3 fusion defines a distinct subset of epithelioid hemangioendothelioma. Genes Chromosomes Cancer 2013;52(8):775–84.

45. Puls F, Niblett A, Clarke J, et al. YAP1-TFE3 epithelioid hemangioendothelioma: a case without vasoformation and a new transcript variant. Virchows Arch 2015;466(4):473–8.

46. Shibuya R, Matsuyama A, Shiba E, et al. CAMTA1 is a useful immunohistochemical marker for diagnosing epithelioid haemangioendothelioma. Histopathology 2015;67(6):827–35.

47. Doyle LA, Fletcher CD, Hornick JL. Nuclear expression of CAMTA1 distinguishes epithelioid hemangioendothelioma from histologic mimics. Am J Surg Pathol 2016;40(1):94–102.

48. Anderson T, Zhang L, Hameed M, et al. Thoracic epithelioid malignant vascular tumors: a clinicopathologic study of 52 cases with emphasis on pathologic grading and molecular studies of WWTR1-CAMTA1 fusions. Am J Surg Pathol 2015;39(1):132–9.

49. Flucke U, Vogels RJ, de Saint Aubain Somerhausen N, et al. Epithelioid hemangioendothelioma: clinicopathologic, immunohistochemical, and molecular genetic analysis of 39 cases. Diagn Pathol 2014;9:131.

50. Weiss SW, Enzinger FM. Epithelioid hemangioendothelioma: a vascular tumor often mistaken for a carcinoma. Cancer 1982;50(5):970–81.

51. Dail DH, Liebow AA, Gmelich JT, et al. Intravascular, bronchiolar, and alveolar tumor of the lung (IVBAT). An analysis of twenty cases of a peculiar sclerosing endothelial tumor. Cancer 1983;51(3):452–64.

52. Miettinen M, Wang ZF, Paetau A, et al. ERG transcription factor as an immunohistochemical marker for vascular endothelial tumors and prostatic carcinoma. Am J Surg Pathol 2011;35(3):432–41.

53. Tanas MR, Sboner A, Oliveira AM, et al. Identification of a disease-defining gene fusion in epithelioid hemangioendothelioma. Sci Transl Med 2011;3(98):98ra82.

54. Errani C, Zhang L, Sung YS, et al. A novel WWTR1-CAMTA1 gene fusion is a consistent abnormality in epithelioid hemangioendothelioma of different anatomic sites. Genes Chromosomes Cancer 2011;50(8):644–53.

55. Suurmeijer AJH, Dickson BC, Swanson D, et al. Variant WWTR1 gene fusions in epithelioid hemangioendothelioma-a genetic subset associated with cardiac involvement. Genes Chromosomes Cancer 2020;59(7):389–95.

56. Zhang HZ, Dong L, Wang SY, et al. TFE3 rearranged epithelioid hemangioendothelioma of bone: a clinicopathological, immunohistochemical and molecular study of two cases. Ann Diagn Pathol 2020;46:151487.

57. Deyrup AT, Tighiouart M, Montag AG, et al. Epithelioid hemangioendothelioma of soft tissue: a proposal for risk stratification based on 49 cases. Am J Surg Pathol 2008;32(6):924–7.

58. Rosenbaum E, Jadeja B, Xu B, et al. Prognostic stratification of clinical and molecular epithelioid hemangioendothelioma subsets. Mod Pathol 2020; 33(4):591–602.

59. Angelini A, Mavrogenis AF, Gambarotti M, et al. Surgical treatment and results of 62 patients with epithelioid hemangioendothelioma of bone. J Surg Oncol 2014;109(8):791–7.

60. Carter JH, Dickerson R, Needy C. Angiosarcoma of bone: a review of the literature and presentation of a case. Ann Surg 1956;144(1):107–17.

61. Deshpande V, Rosenberg AE, O'Connell JX, et al. Epithelioid angiosarcoma of the bone: a series of 10 cases. Am J Surg Pathol 2003;27(6):709–16.

62. Verbeke SL, Bertoni F, Bacchini P, et al. Distinct histological features characterize primary angiosarcoma of bone. Histopathology 2011;58(2):254–64.

63. Fletcher CD, Beham A, Bekir S, et al. Epithelioid angiosarcoma of deep soft tissue: a distinctive tumor readily mistaken for an epithelial neoplasm. Am J Surg Pathol 1991;15(10):915–24.

64. Miettinen M, Wang Z, Sarlomo-Rikala M, et al. ERG expression in epithelioid sarcoma: a diagnostic pitfall. Am J Surg Pathol 2013;37(10):1580–5.

65. Stockman DL, Hornick JL, Deavers MT, et al. ERG and FLI1 protein expression in epithelioid sarcoma. Mod Pathol 2014;27(4):496–501.

66. Raoux D, Peoc'h M, Pedeutour F, et al. Primary epithelioid sarcoma of bone: report of a unique case, with immunohistochemical and fluorescent in situ hybridization confirmation of INI1 deletion. Am J Surg Pathol 2009;33(6):954–8.

67. McKenney JK, Weiss SW, Folpe AL. CD31 expression in intratumoral macrophages: a potential diagnostic pitfall. Am J Surg Pathol 2001;25(9):1167–73.

68. Hornick JL, Jaffe ES, Fletcher CD. Extranodal histiocytic sarcoma: clinicopathologic analysis of 14 cases of a rare epithelioid malignancy. Am J Surg Pathol 2004;28(9):1133–44.

69. Hung YP, Lovitch SB, Qian X. Histiocytic sarcoma: new insights into FNA cytomorphology and molecular characteristics. Cancer Cytopathol 2017;125(8): 604–14.

70. Caponetti G, Dezube BJ, Restrepo CS, et al. Kaposi sarcoma of the musculoskeletal system: a review of 66 patients. Cancer 2007;109(6):1040–52.

71. Huang SC, Zhang L, Sung YS, et al. Recurrent CIC gene abnormalities in angiosarcomas: a molecular study of 120 cases with concurrent investigation of PLCG1, KDR, MYC, and FLT4 gene alterations. Am J Surg Pathol 2016;40(5):645–55.

72. Painter CA, Jain E, Tomson BN, et al. The Angiosarcoma Project: enabling genomic and clinical discoveries in a rare cancer through patient-partnered research. Nat Med 2020;26(2):181–7.

73. Verbeke SL, Bertoni F, Bacchini P, et al. Active TGF-beta signaling and decreased expression of PTEN separates angiosarcoma of bone from its soft tissue counterpart. Mod Pathol 2013;26(9):1211–21.

74. Verbeke SL, de Jong D, Bertoni F, et al. Array CGH analysis identifies two distinct subgroups of primary angiosarcoma of bone. Genes Chromosomes Cancer 2015;54(2):72–81.

75. Young RJ, Brown NJ, Reed MW, et al. Angiosarcoma. Lancet Oncol 2010;11(10):983–91.

Intra-Articular Tumors

Marta Sbaraglia, MD[a,b], Marco Gambarotti, MD[c], Gianluca Businello, MD[a,b], Alberto Righi, MD[c], Matteo Fassan, MD[a,b], Angelo P. Dei Tos, MD[a,b],*

KEYWORDS
- Bone • Articular space • Joint diseases • Mesenchymal tumors • Synovial chondromatosis
- Tenosynovial giant cell tumors

ABSTRACT

The intra-articular space is a relatively rare site of occurrence of neoplastic diseases. The 2 distinct groups of clinicopathologic entities that exhibit an almost exclusive tropism for the joints are represented by synovial chondromatosis and tenosynovial giant cell tumors (TGCT). Synovial chondromatosis is a locally aggressive chondrogenic neoplasm that very rarely can show malignant behavior. TGCT occur in 2 main variants, the localized variant and the more locally aggressive diffuse type. Malignant TCGT is exceedingly rare and is characterized by significant rates of both local recurrence and metastatic spread.

OVERVIEW

The intra-articular space represents a relatively rare site of occurrence of neoplastic diseases. Paradoxically, synovial sarcoma, of which its label might indicate a distinct relationship with synovium-lined anatomic sites, only exceptionally occurs primarily within the joint. Consequently, this review focuses on 2 distinct groups of clinicopathologic entities exhibiting almost exclusive intra-articular tropism, represented by synovial chondromatosis and tenosynovial giant cell tumor (TGCT), including the exceedingly rare malignant forms of both entities.

SYNOVIAL CHONDROMATOSIS

Synovial chondromatosis represents a locally aggressive neoplasm composed of nodules of hyaline cartilage. It involves the joint space and the subsynovial tissue.[1] The extra-articular forms involve the tenosynovial tissue (tenosynovial chondromatosis). It is a rare neoplasm that affects approximately 1.8 cases per 1 million person-years. It mainly occurs in adults between the third and the fifth decades of life, with a male-to-female ratio of 2:1.[2] Any joint can be affected, including the temporomandibular and intervertebral joints, although it most frequently arises in the knee (60%–70% of cases) followed by other large joints. Local pain, swelling, and mechanical joint impairment are the most frequent presenting signs and symptoms.[2]

On plain radiographs, it generally appears as a lobulated calcified mass with chondroid-type mineralization and calcification or as multiple ossified nodules generally homogeneous in size and shape[3] (Fig. 1). Computed tomographic scan is helpful in identifying the calcifications. MRI generally shows lobulated areas of low-signal intensity because of calcifications and ossifications, with T2 hyperintensity owing to cartilage, or fatty signal owing to bone marrow, with peripheral contrast enhancement.[3]

Grossly, synovial chondromatosis generally consists of multiple whitish nodules with a smooth to irregular surface (Fig. 2). Histologically, it is composed of nodules of mature hyaline cartilage, surrounded by connective fibrous tissue or synovial tissue. The nodules contain mildly atypical chondrocytes, typically arranged in clusters (Fig. 3A, B).[4] Binucleation can occur. Older lesions may show calcifications or peripheral endochondral ossification. From the molecular standpoint in approximately 50% of cases, fibronectin 1 (*FN1*)–activin receptor 2A (*ACVR2A*) and *ACVR2A-FN1* fusion genes are present, whereas

a Department of Pathology, Azienda Ospedale-Università Padova, Padua, Italy; b Department of Medicine, University of Padua School of Medicine, Padua, Italy; c Unit of Surgical Pathology, Istituto Ortopedico Rizzoli, Bologna, Italy
* Corresponding author. Department of Medicine, University of Padua School of Medicine, Padua, Italy.
E-mail address: angelo.deitos@unipd.it

Surgical Pathology 14 (2021) 665–677
https://doi.org/10.1016/j.path.2021.06.008

surgpath.theclinics.com

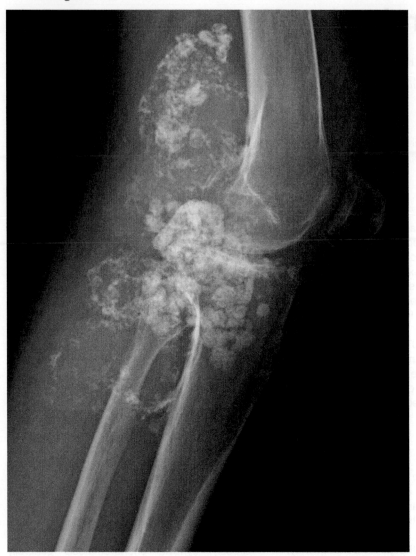

Fig. 1. A radiograph of the knee shows multiple well-defined distinctive intra-articular and extra-articular radiopaque masses composed of small calcified/ossified bodies.

IDH1/2 mutations are consistently absent.[5–7] It is still unclear whether the oncogenic driver is represented by *FN1* or *ACRV2A*, as both fusions are predicted to be "in frame." Interestingly, both genes are involved in the development of other benign tumors, such as leiomyomas of the gastrointestinal tract[8] and calcifying aponeurotic fibroma.[9]

Synovial chondromatosis is a locally aggressive tumor that recurs in 15% to 20% of cases.[2] Surgical excision is the treatment of choice. Importantly, synovial chondromatosis should be distinguished from multiple osteochondral loose bodies in the setting of degenerative joint disease.[6] The latter is characterized by concentric layers of cartilage with uniformly distributed chondrocytes, lacking the typical clustering of synovial chondromatosis, and by contrast, tends not to exhibit local aggressiveness.

KEY POINTS

- Locally aggressive intra-articular chondrogenic neoplasm.

- Distinctive arrangement of chondrocytes in clusters.

- Characterized molecularly by *FN1-ACBVRA2* and *ACVR2A-FN1* fusion genes.

- Local recurrences in approximately 20% of cases.

SYNOVIAL CHONDROSARCOMA

Synovial chondrosarcoma is an exceedingly rare malignant tumor, with only 61 cases reported in the literature to date. It may arise as a primary neoplasm or secondary to a benign, typically long-standing, or

Fig. 2. Grossly, synovial chondromatosis is composed of multiple nodules, whitish in color, generally similar in size and shape.

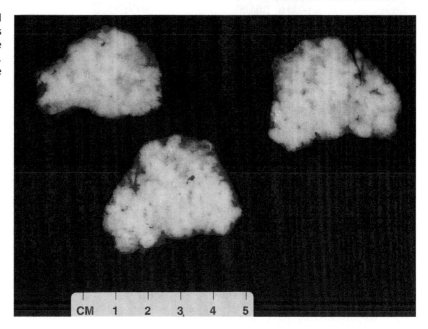

locally recurrent synovial chondromatosis.[4,10] The median age at diagnosis is 51 years old (range: 19–79 years).[4,11–15] The hip is the joint most commonly affected, followed by the knee, the temporomandibular joint, elbow, wrist, ankle, shoulder, metacarpophalangeal joints, and lumbar spine.

Three clinical presentations are recognized for synovial chondrosarcoma: (1) synovial chondrosarcoma in patients with a history of preexisting synovial chondromatosis, but without areas of chondromatosis at the time of diagnosis of synovial chondrosarcoma; (2) synovial chondrosarcoma with preexisting history and histologic evidence of chondromatosis associated with the chondrosarcomatous areas; and (3) synovial chondrosarcoma diagnosed without prior history or histologic evidence of synovial chondromatosis.[10,11] The last represents an ultrarare condition accounting for approximately 10% of the synovial chondrosarcomas reported in the literature.[4,10–15]

Malignant progression from synovial chondromatosis to synovial chondrosarcoma is usually suspected in the presence of a sudden worsening of pain or a rapid recurrence after complete resection of a synovial chondromatosis. The incidence of malignant transformation of synovial chondromatosis has been reported to be around 2.5%, based on the 2 largest studies published in the literature.[4,13]

Radiologically, the differential diagnosis between synovial chondromatosis and synovial chondrosarcoma can be challenging because aggressive features, such as periarticular cortical erosion, extra-articular soft tissue extension, and intramedullary infiltration, can only be found in a minority of cases (**Fig. 4**).[3,10–12,16]

Macroscopically, synovial chondrosarcoma appears as a cartilaginous and myxoid mass with invasion into adjacent periarticular soft tissues or underlying bone (**Fig. 5**).

Morphologically, features that favor malignancy over synovial chondromatosis are hypercellularity, loss of chondrocyte clustering, myxoid change of the extracellular matrix, peripheral spindling of tumor cells, presence of chondrocyte necrosis, and permeation of bony trabeculae in a "filling up" pattern, as opposed to the "pushing" pattern of synovial chondromatosis (see **Fig. 3**C–F). The above criteria, proposed by Bertoni and colleagues[10] (**Table 1**), have been adopted by many investigators[4,13,16–18] and seem most useful when associated with both clinical and radiologic aggressive findings. It must be emphasized that the presence of cytologic atypia does not contribute to the distinction between synovial chondromatosis and synovial chondrosarcoma, as it can be seen in both conditions.

Synovial chondrosarcoma shares with synovial chondromatosis the same *FN1-ACVR2A* fusion, in keeping with an early initiating molecular pathogenetic event. This fusion has been detected by whole-genome sequencing,[6,19] and *FN1* and/or *ACVR2A* gene rearrangements have been confirmed to be present in both synovial chondromatosis and synovial chondrosarcoma.[1,6,19,20] As a consequence, molecular genetics does not help in the establishing malignancy in synovial cartilaginous neoplasms. More recently, a novel *KMT2A-BCOR* in-frame gene fusion has been detected by targeted RNA sequencing in a case of a dedifferentiated

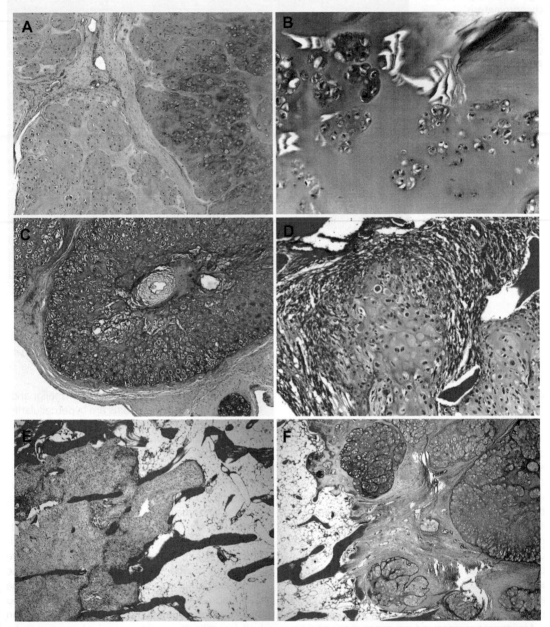

Fig. 3. Microscopically, synovial chondromatosis is characterized by multiple hypocellular nodules of cartilaginous tissue covered by subsynovial connective tissue (A) [hematoxylin-eosin stain, original magnification x 20]. Clusters of chondrocytes with low-grade nuclei on abundant chondroid matrix is a typical feature. Slightly enlarged and binucleation of chondrocytes is frequently seen (B) [hematoxylin-eosin stain, original magnification x 20]. Synovial chondrosarcoma is relatively more hypercellular with a variable degree of chondrocyte atypia. Myxoid change is a common feature (C) [hematoxylin-eosin stain, original magnification x 20]. At the periphery, tumor cells exhibit more spindle cell morphology (D) [hematoxylin-eosin stain, original magnification x 20]. Invasion pattern is different as synovial chondrosarcoma shows "filling" pattern (E) [hematoxylin-eosin stain, original magnification x 20] compared with "pushing" pattern of synovial chondromatosis (F) [hematoxylin-eosin stain, original magnification x 20].

chondrosarcoma with areas of osteosarcoma, arising in the background of a synovial chondromatosis, therefore leading to a diagnosis of dedifferentiated synovial chondrosarcoma.[5] As also mentioned for synovial chondromatosis,[7] *IDH1*

and *IDH2* gene mutations are absent in synovial chondrosarcoma,[1,4] underlining the existence of a distinct molecular pathogenesis. Although many synovial chondrosarcomas reported in literature have behaved as low-grade conventional

Fig. 4. Coronal gadolinium chelate–enhanced fat-suppressed MRI of synovial chondrosarcoma of hip joint.

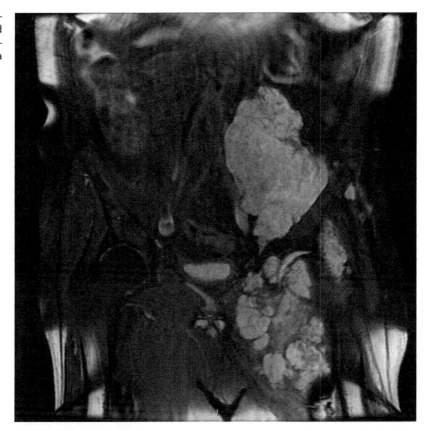

Fig. 5. Macroscopically, synovial chondrosarcoma shows a gray-white gelatinous mass originated on articular surface shows invasion into periarticular soft tissue and minimal permeation of underlying cortex.

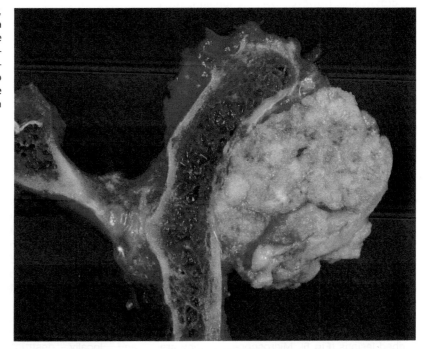

Table 1
Comparison between histologic features of synovial chondromatosis and synovial chondrosarcoma

Histologic Features	Synovial Chondromatosis	Synovial Chondrosarcoma
Chondrocyte arrangement pattern	Cluster	Sheets
Quality of stroma	Chondroid	Chondroid to myxoid
Cellularity	Usually hypocellular	Hypercellular with spindling of tumor cells at periphery
Presence of necrosis	No	Yes
Bony permeation pattern	Pushing pattern	"Filling up" pattern

chondrosarcomas, metastasis, mainly to the lungs, can develop in approximately 25% to 30% of patients. A wide surgical treatment is recommended for disease control. Recurrence rate, however, is high, especially in patients with inadequate surgery.[4,10,11,14]

KEY POINTS

- Synovial chondrosarcoma can be either primary neoplasm or secondary to synovial chondromatosis.

- Permeation of bone is the most useful morphologic diagnostic criteria (see **Table 1**).

- Complete molecular overlap with synovial chondromatosis.

- Clinical behavior is similar to low-grade chondrosarcoma. However, systemic spread is reported in approximately one-third of cases.

TENOSYNOVIAL GIANT CELL TUMORS

The label TGCT includes distinct lesions usually occurring in the synovia of joints, bursae, and tendon sheaths. On the basis of anatomic site (intra-articular vs extra-articular) and growth pattern (circumscribed or infiltrative), 2 different subtypes of TGCT (localized vs diffuse) have been identified, and despite sharing a common pathogenesis, are characterized by different clinical presentation and biological behavior.[21]

Localized TGCT most often occurs in fingers or wrists (85% of cases). Those rare cases arising within large joints have shown the tendency to exhibit an equally indolent clinical behavior.[21] The incidence of localized-type TGCT is approximately 5 times higher than diffuse-type TGCT with almost 29 cases per 1 million person-years. Clinically, the localized TGCT results in a small painless mass. Localized-type TGCTs are circumscribed lesions (**Fig 6**). Microscopically, they are composed of a heterogeneous cell population set in a variably collagenized stroma: (1) mononuclear cells, (2) multinucleated osteoclast-like giant cells, (3) foamy macrophages, (4) inflammatory cells. Hemosiderin is variably present (**Fig. 7**). The proportion of those components is heterogeneous and is different in each TGCT subtype. Mononuclear cells can be further subdivided in 2 populations: (1) small histiocyte-like cells with pale cytoplasm and round/reniform nuclei and (2) epithelioid cells with amphophilic cytoplasm and round, vesicular nuclei[1] (**Fig. 8**). Mitotic activity can be brisk, but atypical figures are usually absent. In the localized variant, multinucleated giant cells and hemosiderin are usually promptly recognized, although some tumors may be less represented, therefore representing a diagnostic challenge. Foamy macrophages typically aggregate at the periphery of the nodules.[22–24]

Diffuse TGCTs, in the past also named "pigmented villonodular tenosynovitis," typically involve large joints, such as the knee (75% of cases) and the hip (16%), with an intra-articular localization.[25] The tumor affects middle-aged adults with a peak of incidence between the fourth and fifth decades, with a slight prevalence in women.[26] Clinically, diffuse TGCT is frequently associated with pain, swelling, and functional limitation of the affected joint. Diffuse-type TGCT is characterized by an infiltrative growth pattern and frequently presents cleftlike spaces and pseudopapillary projections (**Fig. 9**). In contrast to the localized type, in diffuse TGCT, multinucleated giant cells are less numerous, and in approximately 20% of cases, they are totally absent or extremely rare[24,27,28] (**Fig. 10**). Foamy histiocytes are most often abundant (**Fig. 11**). Foci of necrosis may be appreciated mostly in larger lesions. Rarely, foci of chondroid metaplasia are observed in tumors occurring within the temporomandibular joint.

Compared with the localized subtype, the diffuse TGCT subtype exhibits a more aggressive and locally destructive behavior. Multiple

Fig. 6. Localized TGCT. A synovium-lined well-circumscribed contour is observed (hematoxylin-eosin stain, original magnification x 20).

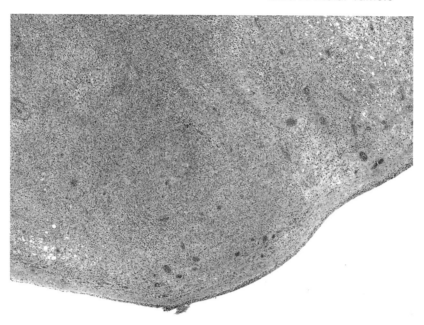

recurrences may be observed leading to major functional loss.[27] Immunohistochemically, in both localized and diffuse variants, histiocyte-like cells express CD68, CD163, and CD45, whereas larger mononuclear cells express clusterin and in up to 80% of cases desmin.

From the genetic standpoint, trisomies of chromosomes 5 and 7 and translocations involving the region of chromosome 1p11-13 with the region of the chromosome 2q37 have been identified.[29] In detail, this translocation leads to the fusion of

COL6A3 with CSF1 (located at 1p13), leading to overexpression and secretion of CSF1.[30] CFS1 recruits nonneoplastic monocyte and macrophages expressing CSF1 receptor, thus promoting their survival, proliferation, and differentiation.[29] Interestingly, in the context of a TGCT, only a small population of cells (ranging between 2% and 16%) actually carries the t(1,2) translocation and is actually neoplastic. The identification of CSF1 rearrangement may be diagnostically helpful in selected cases, for example, when dealing with

Fig. 7. Localized TGCT is composed of a variable mixture of osteoclast-like giant cells, mononuclear cells, foamy histiocytes, and hemosiderin deposits (hematoxylin-eosin stain, original magnification x 20).

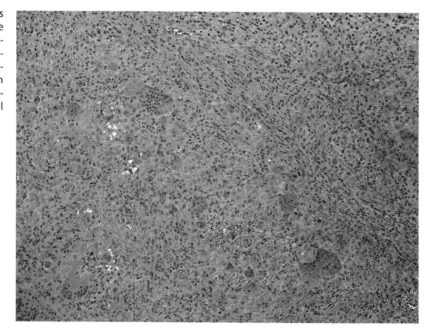

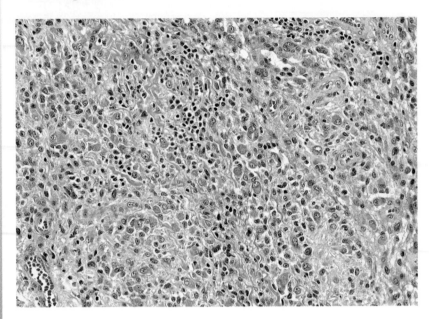

Fig. 8. Mononuclear cells are represented by small histiocyte-like cells with pale cytoplasm and round/reniform nuclei and epithelioid cells with amphophilic cytoplasm and round, vesicular nuclei (hematoxylin-eosin stain, original magnification x 20).

tumors lacking the distinctive cytomorphological features of the TGCT (ie, in the case of the absence of multinucleated giant cells). It should also be considered to confirm the diagnosis when TGCT exceptionally occurs in an extra-articular location. Most often these lesions are localized in the periarticular soft tissues; however, they can also present as intramuscular or subcutaneous lesions.

MALIGNANCY IN TENOSYNOVIAL GIANT CELL TUMOR

Malignant TGCT is exceedingly rare with only 50 cases reported in the literature. These cases affect adults (50–60 years) and occur typically in the lower limbs, especially around the knees, followed by the hip, ankle, and pelvic area (**Fig. 12**A, B). Interestingly, malignant TGCT may arise de novo or develop after multiple recurrences of conventional TGCT.[31–35]

Malignant TGCTs are characterized by the coexistence of a benign TGCT with morphologically malignant areas. The latter component is generally characterized by the presence of sheets or nodules of enlarged mononuclear cells with large nuclei and prominent nucleoli, associated with areas showing an overtly spindled morphology (**Fig. 13**). High proliferative activity is usually observed often associated with the

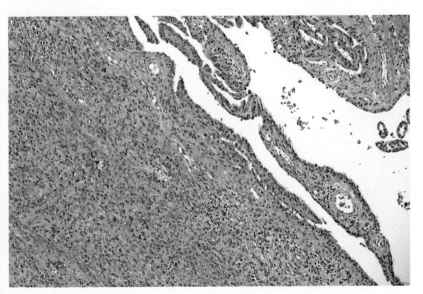

Fig. 9. Diffuse TGCT. The presence of papillary and pseudopapillary projections justifies the old terminology "pigmented villonodular synovitis." (hematoxylin-eosin stain, original magnification x 20)

Fig. 10. Diffuse TGCT. Osteoclast-like multinucleated giant cells can be poorly represented (hematoxylin-eosin stain, original magnification x 20).

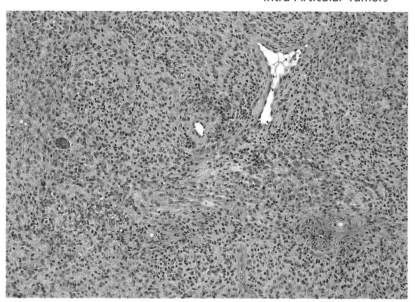

presence of atypical mitotic figures and large foci of necrosis. Furthermore, areas resembling undifferentiated pleomorphic sarcoma and myxofibrosarcoma may also be seen.[31–35]

In summary, from the clinical standpoint, localized TGCT is usually benign, even if in approximately 4% to 30% of cases, local nondestructive recurrences are described.[22–24,36] Diffuse TGCT is characterized by a higher recurrence rate (40%–60% of cases) that may cause a severe joint function impairment.[37] Metastasis to lungs and lymph nodes from morphologically benign tumors has been rarely described.[38] In stark contrast, malignant TGCT shows an aggressive clinical behavior, with both high metastatic (50% of cases) and mortality rates (approximately 30% of patients).[31,32,33,34,35] Surgical treatment is the gold standard in primary and recurrent TGCTs. Dysregulation of the CSF1/CSF1R pathway represents an opportunity for molecularly targeted therapies, and CSF1 inhibitors, such as nilotinib, imatinib, pexidartinib, emactuzumab, and cabrilazimab, are currently used in unresectable or metastasizing TGCTs.[39–42]

Fig. 11. Diffuse TGCT. Foamy histiocytes can be numerous (hematoxylin-eosin stain, original magnification x 20).

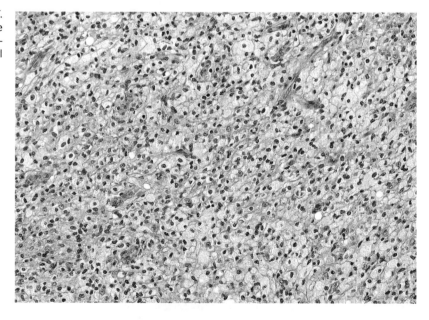

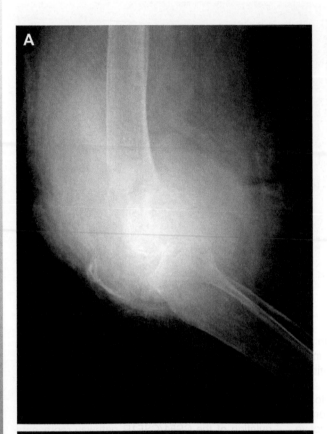

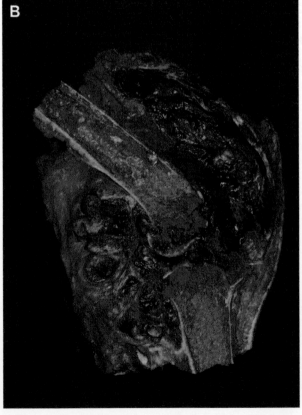

Fig. 12. Malignant TGCT. A knee radiograph projection shows a voluminous, destructive mass (*A*). Grossly, the lesion involves the entire knee joint. Areas of hemorrhage and necrosis are visible (*B*).

Fig. 13. Malignant TGCT. Neoplastic cells exhibits striking spindled morphology, overt nuclear atypia, and brisk mitotic activity (hematoxylin-eosin stain, original magnification x 20).

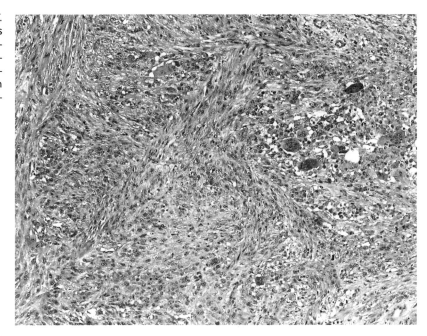

KEY POINTS

- TGCT can be either localized or diffuse.

- The diffuse variant tends to affect large joints and is locally far more aggressive than the localized one.

- Microscopically, TGCT is composed of a variable combination of mononuclear and multinucleated giant cell population.

- Molecularly, a *COL6A3-CSF1* gene fusion is present.

- CSF1 upregulation allows successful target therapy with anti CFS1 compounds.

- Malignant TGCT is very rare and clinically aggressive.

SUMMARY

Intra-articular tumors are mostly represented by synovial chondromatosis and TGCT. They both represent morphologically and molecularly distinct clinicopathologic entities that can lead to significant locoregional morbidity. Malignant transformation can occur in both conditions; however, it represents an exceedingly rare condition. Unfortunately, molecular pathology does not allow distinction between benign/locally aggressive forms and malignant ones. Diagnosis in fact only relies on morphologic criteria that

nonetheless need to be evaluated in context with radiologic imaging as well as clinical presentation. Importantly, the elucidation of the molecular mechanisms underlying the development of TCGT has been translated into a successful therapeutic opportunity represented by CSF1 inhibitors. Extreme rarity certainly hampers diagnostic accuracy. It is therefore recommended that challenging cases are referred to expert centers or expert networks.

DISCLOSURE

The authors have nothing to disclose.

REFERENCES

1. Flanagan AM, Bloem JL, Cates JMM, et al. Synovial chondromatosis. In: WHO classification of tumours editorial board. Soft tissue and bone tumoursvol. 3, 5th edition. Lyon, France: International Agency for Research on Cancer; 2020. WHO classification of tumours series.
2. Neumann JA, Garrigues GE, Brigman BE, et al. Synovial chondromatosis. JBJS Rev 2016;4(5), 01874474-201605000-00005.
3. Murphey MD, Vidal JA, Fanburg-Smith JC, et al. Imaging of synovial chondromatosis with radiologic-pathologic correlation. Radiographics 2007;27(5): 1465–88.
4. Gambarotti M, Pacheco M, Ruengwanichayakun P, et al. Synovial chondrosarcoma: a single-institution

experience with molecular investigations and review of the literature. Histopathology 2020;77(3):391–401.

5. Agaram NP, Zhang L, Dickson BC, et al. A molecular study of synovial chondromatosis. Genes Chromosomes Cancer 2020;59(3):144–51.

6. Amary F, Perez-Casanova L, Ye H, et al. Synovial chondromatosis and soft tissue chondroma: extraosseous cartilaginous tumor defined by FN1 gene rearrangement. Mod Pathol 2019;32(12):1762–71.

7. Amary F, Bacsi K, Maggiani F, et al. IDH1 and IDH2 mutations are frequent events in central chondrosarcoma and central and periosteal chondromas but not in other mesenchymal tumours. J Pathol 2011;224(3):334–43.

8. Panagopoulos I, Gorunova L, Lund-Iversen M, et al. Recurrent fusion of the genes FN1 and ALK in gastrointestinal leiomyomas. Mod Pathol 2016;29(11):1415–23.

9. Puls F, Hofvander J, Magnusson L, et al. FN1-EGF gene fusions are recurrent in calcifying aponeurotic fibroma. J Pathol 2016;238(4):502–7.

10. Bertoni F, Unni KK, Beabout JW, et al. Chondrosarcomas of the synovium. Cancer 1991;67(1):155–62.

11. Campanacci DA, Matera D, Franchi A, et al. Synovial chondrosarcoma of the hip: report of two cases and literature review. Chir Organi Mov 2008;92(3):139–44.

12. Evans S, Boffano M, Chaudhry S, et al. Synovial chondrosarcoma arising in synovial chondromatosis. Sarcoma 2014;1-4:647939.

13. McCarthy C, Anderson WJ, Vlychou M, et al. Primary synovial chondromatosis: a reassessment of malignant potential in 155 cases. Skeletal Radiol 2016;45(6):755–62.

14. Muramatsu K, Miyoshi T, Moriya A, et al. Extremely rare synovial chondrosarcoma arising from the elbow joint: case report and review of the literature. J Shoulder Elbow Surg 2012;21(2):e7–11.

15. Zamora EE, Mansor A, Vanel D, et al. Synovial chondrosarcoma: report of two cases and literature review. Eur J Radiol 2009;72(1):38–43.

16. Jonckheere J, Shahabpour M, Willekens I, et al. Rapid malignant transformation of primary synovial chondromatosis into chondrosarcoma. JBR-BTR 2014;97(5):303–7.

17. Anract P, Katabi M, Forest M, et al. Synovial chondromatosis and chondrosarcoma: a study of the relationship between these two diseases. Rev Chir Orthop Reparatrice Appar Mot 1996;82(3):216–24.

18. Ichikawa T, Miyauchi M, Nikai H, et al. Synovial chondrosarcoma arising in the temporomandibular joint. J Oral Maxillofac Surg 1998;56:890–4.

19. Totoki Y, Yoshida A, Hosoda F, et al. Unique mutation portraits and frequent COL2A1 gene alteration in chondrosarcoma. Genome Res 2014;24(9):1411–20.

20. Perez-Casanova L, Ye H, Strobl AC, et al. Recurrent FN1 and/or ACVR2A fusion genes are implicated in

the pathogenesis of synovial chondromatosis, chondrosarcoma secondary to synovial chondromatosis, and soft tissue chondroma. J Pathol 2018;246(S1). Abstract 019.

21. Gouin F, Noailles T. Localized and diffuse forms of tenosynovial giant cell tumor (formerly giant cell tumor of the tendon sheath and pigmented villonodular synovitis). Orthop Traumatol Surg Res 2017;103(1S):S91–7.

22. Monaghan H, Salter DM, Al-Nafussi A. Giant cell tumour of tendon sheath (localised nodular tenosynovitis): clinicopathological features of 71 cases. J Clin Pathol 2001;54(5):404–7.

23. Jones FE, Soule EH, Coventry MB. Fibrous xanthoma of synovium (giant-cell tumor of tendon sheath, pigmented nodular synovitis). A study of one hundred and eighteen cases. J Bone Joint Surg Am 1969;51(1):76–86.

24. Ushijima M, Hashimoto H, Tsuneyoshi M, et al. Giant cell tumor of the tendon sheath (nodular tenosynovitis). A study of 207 cases to compare the large joint group with the common digit group. Cancer 1986;57(4):875–84.

25. Ottaviani S, Ayral X, Dougados M, et al. Pigmented villonodular synovitis: a retrospective single-center study of 122 cases and review of the literature. Semin Arthritis Rheum 2011;40(6):539–46.

26. Myers BW, Masi AT. Pigmented villonodular synovitis and tenosynovitis: a clinical epidemiologic study of 166 cases and literature review. Medicine (Baltimore) 1980;59(3):223–38.

27. Somerhausen NS, Fletcher CD. Diffuse-type giant cell tumor: clinicopathologic and immunohistochemical analysis of 50 cases with extraarticular disease. Am J Surg Pathol 2000;24(4):479–92.

28. Murphey MD, Rhee JH, Lewis RB, et al. Pigmented villonodular synovitis: radiologic-pathologic correlation. Radiographics 2008;28(5):1493–518.

29. Mastboom MJL, Hoek DM, Bovée JVMG, et al. Does CSF1 overexpression or rearrangement influence biological behaviour in tenosynovial giant cell tumours of the knee? Histopathology 2019;74(2):332–40.

30. West RB, Rubin BP, Miller MA, et al. A landscape effect in tenosynovial giant-cell tumor from activation of CSF1 expression by a translocation in a minority of tumor cells. Proc Natl Acad Sci U S A 2006;103(3):690–5.

31. Al-Ibraheemi A, Ahrens WA, Fritchie K, et al. Malignant tenosynovial giant cell tumor: the true "Synovial Sarcoma?" A clinicopathologic, immunohistochemical, and molecular cytogenetic study of 10 cases, supporting origin from synoviocytes. Mod Pathol 2019;32(2):242–51.

32. Bertoni F, Unni KK, Beabout JW, et al. Malignant giant cell tumor of the tendon sheaths and joints (malignant pigmented villonodular synovitis). Am J Surg Pathol 1997;21(2):153–63.

33. Nakayama R, Jagannathan JP, Ramaiya N, et al. Clinical characteristics and treatment outcomes in

six cases of malignant tenosynovial giant cell tumor: initial experience of molecularly targeted therapy. BMC Cancer 2018;18(1):1296.

34. Righi A, Gambarotti M, Sbaraglia M, et al. Metastasizing tenosynovial giant cell tumour, diffuse type/pigmented villonodular synovitis. Clin Sarcoma Res 2015;5:15.

35. Li CF, Wang JW, Huang WW, et al. Malignant diffuse-type tenosynovial giant cell tumors: a series of 7 cases comparing with 24 benign lesions with review of the literature. Am J Surg Pathol 2008;32(4):587–99.

36. Mastboom MJL, Verspoor FGM, Verschoor AJ, et al. Higher incidence rates than previously known in tenosynovial giant cell tumors. Acta Orthop 2017; 88(6):688–94.

37. Mastboom MJL, Palmerini E, Verspoor FGM, et al. Surgical outcomes of patients with diffuse-type tenosynovial giant-cell tumours: an international, retrospective, cohort study. Lancet Oncol 2019;20(6):877–86.

38. Chen EL, de Castro CM, Hendzel KD, et al. Histologically benign metastasizing tenosynovial giant cell tumor mimicking metastatic malignancy: a case report and review of literature. Radiol Case Rep 2019;14(8):934–40.

39. Blay JY, El Sayadi H, Thiesse P, et al. Complete response to imatinib in relapsing pigmented villonodular synovitis/tenosynovial giant cell tumor (PVNS/TGCT). Ann Oncol 2008;19(4):821–2.

40. Cassier PA, Gelderblom H, Stacchiotti S, et al. Efficacy of imatinib mesylate for the treatment of locally advanced and/or metastatic tenosynovial giant cell tumor/pigmented villonodular synovitis. Cancer 2012;118(6):1649–55.

41. Cassier PA, Italiano A, Gomez-Roca CA, et al. CSF1R inhibition with emactuzumab in locally advanced diffuse-type tenosynovial giant cell tumours of the soft tissue: a dose-escalation and dose-expansion phase 1 study. Lancet Oncol 2015;16(8):949–56.

42. Tap WD, Gelderblom H, Palmerini E, et al. Pexidartinib versus placebo for advanced tenosynovial giant cell tumour (ENLIVEN): a randomised phase 3 trial. Lancet 2019;394(10197):478–87.

Undifferentiated Small Round Cell Sarcomas of Bone

Brendan C. Dickson, BA, BSc, MD, MSc, FRCPC[a,b,]*

KEYWORDS

- Ewing family tumor • CIC-associated sarcoma • BCOR-associated sarcoma • FET • ETS
- Undifferentiated round cell sarcoma

Key points

- Undifferentiated small round cell sarcomas represent a heterogeneous group of neoplasms of uncertain origin.
- Ewing family tumors are currently defined as having fusion between a FET RNA-binding protein and ETS transcription factor.
- A subset of genetically distinct undifferentiated round cell sarcomas lacks FET and ETS fusion products, including *CIC*-associated and *BCOR*-associated sarcomas.
- *EWSR1/FUS* may fuse with non-ETS partners to yield additional permutations of genetically distinct neoplasms.
- This is currently an area of active discovery. The nomenclature and classification of these, and related, neoplasms is actively evolving.

ABSTRACT

U ndifferentiated small round cell sarcomas represent a heterogeneous group of mesenchymal neoplasms. While imprecise, this term nevertheless provides a useful framework for conceptualizing these tumors. This article highlights current trends in their classification based on morphology, immunohistochemistry, and advanced molecular techniques. As next-generation sequencing becomes commonplace in diagnostic laboratories pathologists can expect to differentiate these tumors with increasing confidence, and actively contribute to related discoveries. Ultimately, when synthesized with rigorous clinical outcome data and other investigative techniques, a more robust landscape for the molecular diagnosis and classification of undifferentiated small round cell sarcomas is expected to emerge in the future.

INTRODUCTION

Tumors lacking objective evidence in support of a line of differentiation, or cell of origin, are considered undifferentiated; they can be further, admittedly arbitrarily, subcategorized based on their predominant cell shape (ie, round cell, spindle cell, pleomorphic).[1] Undifferentiated small round cell sarcomas arising in bone frequently overlap with those occurring elsewhere (eg, soft tissue

---

[a] Department of Pathology and Laboratory Medicine, Mount Sinai Hospital, 600 University Avenue, Toronto, Ontario M5G 1X5, Canada; [b] Department of Laboratory Medicine and Pathobiology, University of Toronto, Toronto, Ontario, Canada
* Department of Pathology and Laboratory Medicine, Mount Sinai Hospital, 600 University Avenue, Toronto, Ontario M5G 1X5, Canada.
E-mail address: Brendan.Dickson@sinaihealth.ca

Surgical Pathology 14 (2021) 679–694
https://doi.org/10.1016/j.path.2021.06.009

and viscera). Historically, many of these tumors were classified as Ewing sarcoma; however, with the advent of next-generation sequencing, new, and genetically distinct, entities are increasingly recognized. This is an area undergoing significant evolution, and, like other subspecialties, the classification of these tumors is trending toward their underlying molecular attributes—given overlapping and nonspecific morphologies and immunophenotypes. Naturally, the rarity of these tumors adds additional complexity to their study, and this is particularly acute when it comes to understanding their behavior and developing successful therapies.

The classification of these tumors is actively evolving and anticipated to change in the future as next-generation sequencing, expression profiling, and epigenetic characterization, among other methodologies, refines our understanding of the breadth and interrelations of these neoplasms. At present, they can be envisaged, based on the current World Health Organization (WHO) classification, as forming 3 broad categories: (1) FET-ETS-associated sarcomas (ie, Ewing family tumors), (2) non-FET-non-ETS-associated sarcomas (eg, BCOR- and CIC [capicua transcriptional repressor]-associated sarcoma), and (3) FET-non-ETS-associated sarcomas (eg, EWSR1/FUS-NFATC2, and EWSR1-PATZ1). What follows is an overview of undifferentiated small round cell sarcomas of bone based on this nascent molecular classification.

FET-ETS-ASSOCIATED SARCOMA (EWING FAMILY TUMOR)

James Ewing, in 1921, first reported a series of tumors composed of sheets of small polyhedral cells arising in the bones of adolescents.[2] Related neoplasms were subsequently reported, including Askin tumor and primitive neuroectodermal tumor/peripheral neuroepithelioma; however, it was not until the identification of a common cytogenetic event, t(11;22)(q24;q12),[3,4] that these entities could be consolidated under the rubric of Ewing family tumors (EFTs).

EFTs are clinically aggressive neoplasms that predominate in children and young adults,[5,6] and rarely older adults.[7] Although they most frequently arise in bone, about 20% are extraosseous, occurring in the soft tissues and viscera, an event that is more common in adults.[5] A slight male predilection has been reported, and individuals of European ancestry tend to be affected more than others.[6] Presenting symptoms often include pain, mass, fever, and/or pathologic fracture.

Ewing sarcoma is currently defined as neoplasm involving fusion of a FET (FUS, EWSR1, and TAF15) RNA-binding protein to an ETS (E26 transforming sequence [E-twenty-six-specific sequence]) transcription factor (eg, FLI1, ERG, ETV1, ETV4, FEV) (Fig. 1).[1,6,8] Although TAF15 is a FET family member (it can be associated with fusions in other sarcomas, such as TAF15-NR4A3 in extraskeletal myxoid chondrosarcoma),[9] fusions involving this gene and ETS members have not, to date, been reported in sarcoma. Similarly, there are many additional ETS family members, but these have yet to be reported as partnering with FET members.

Gross Features

Samples that have not underdone neoadjuvant therapy tend to be white-gray, soft, and friable and show variable hemorrhage and necrosis. The margins are usually infiltrative. Reported sizes range from less than 1 cm to greater than 20 cm.

Microscopic Features

Tumors tend to show a limited range of morphologies. Architecturally most cases are arranged in sheets and lobules (classic variant) (Fig. 2), but a subset contains rosettes/primitive neuroectodermal tumor (PNET) (Fig. 3).[10] The cells are typically small and round-polyhedral, but rarely they may be large (the so-called atypical variant).[10] Epithelial differentiation (adamantinoma-like variant), most commonly in the head and neck region, is also possible (see Fig. 3).[11]

Except for the atypical variant, the cytoplasm is usually scant and the cell borders are indistinct. The cells range from eosinophilic-amphophilic and often contain clear intracytoplasmic glycogen (this can readily be illustrated using the periodic acid-Schiff method, with and without diastase (Fig. 4). The nuclei are round-ovoid, with minimal atypia and variable mitotic activity. Tumors are typically supported by a delicate thin-walled vasculature. Rarely there may be prominent hyalinized stroma.[10] Necrosis is often present and ranges from scattered degenerating cells to broad swaths with a so-called geographic pattern.

There is no specific immunohistochemical marker for EFTs. Most cases show diffuse membranous staining with CD99 (MIC2) and nuclear immunoreactivity with NKX2.2.[12] Depending on their underlying fusion event, tumors may also show FLI1 or ERG expression. Keratin staining may be identified in up to 20% to 30% of cases, although this is usually only focal to patchy.[13,14] A minority of cases have staining for other routine markers, such as synaptophysin and S100 (see Fig. 4.)

Fig. 1. Circos plot demonstrating the chromosomes involved in the various fusion events in Ewing family tumors.[68] Tumors are defined by fusion of a member of the FET family of RNA-binding proteins (*EWSR1, FUS, TAF15*) to a member of the ETS family of transcription factors (*ERG, ETV1, ETV4, FEV, FLI1*). Note: hashed lines represent theoretic possibilities; likewise, fusions involving *TAF15* and ETS members have not been reported.

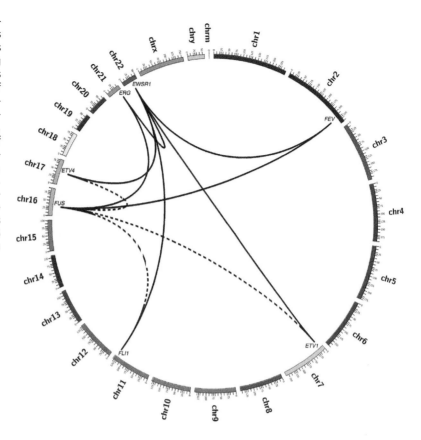

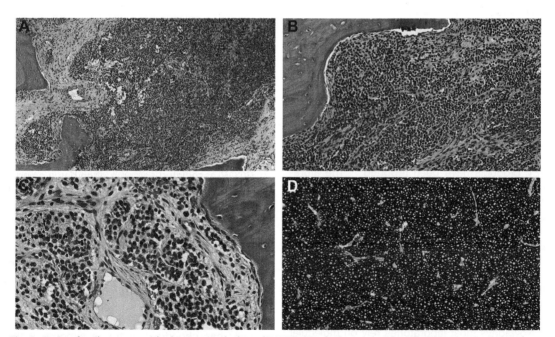

Fig. 2. Ewing family tumor with classic morphology (*EWSR1-FLI1* fusion gene identified by RNA-Seq). (*A*) Sheets and lobules of small round cells with scant eosinophilic cytoplasm. (*B*) The tumor permeates native bone trabecular; it contains a delicate thin-walled vasculature. (*C*) The nuclei are round and monomorphic, with small nucleoli; mitotic activity is not conspicuous. (*D*) There is diffuse membranous immunostaining with CD99.

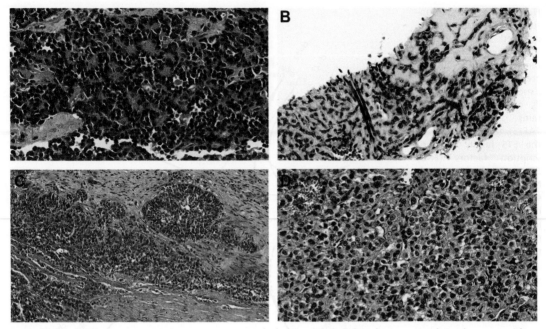

Fig. 3. Ewing family tumors with less common morphologies. (*A*) Peripheral neuroectodermal tumor with rosettes (*EWSR1-FLI1* fusion gene) [Original magnification 400X]. (*B*) Ewing family tumor with abundant hyaline stroma (*EWSR1-ERG* fusion gene) [Original magnification 400X] (*C*) Adamantinomalike Ewing sarcoma, with epithelial differentiation (*EWSR1-FLI1* fusion gene [case previously published[69]]) [Original magnification 200X]. (*D*) Atypical Ewing sarcoma with large cells, abundant pale cytoplasm, and prominent nucleoli (*EWSR1-ERG* fusion gene) [Original magnification 400X].

Molecular Features

Approximately 85% of cases contain a *EWSR1-FLI1* fusion gene, which is the result of t(11;22)(q24;q12).[6] The next most common fusion product, representing about 10% of cases, is the *EWSR1-ERG* fusion gene arising from t(21;22)(q22;q12).[6] Rarely, other ETS member genes have reported to partner with *EWSR1*, including *ETV1*, *ETV4*, and *FEV* (see **Fig. 1**).[15] *FUS* can serve as a proxy for *EWSR1*, so it is presumed that each of the aforementioned, and perhaps other, ETS members may fuse with *FUS*; however, to date, only *FUS-ERG* and *FUS-FEV* products have been reported.[16] The aforementioned fusion genes are currently considered disease-defining for EFTs; however, next-generation sequencing is revealing molecular pleiotropy among several fusion products (ie, an *EWSR1-ATF1* fusion product is present in several distinct entities, including subsets of clear cell sarcoma, angiomatoid fibrous histiocytoma, mesothelioma, and hyalinizing clear cell carcinoma), and it is possible that this understanding may evolve in the future.

Nowadays most laboratories rely on molecular assays, such as fluorescence in situ hybridization (FISH), reverse-transcriptase polymerase chain reaction (RT-PCR), and next-generation sequencing, for the diagnosis of EFTs. The large number of potential fusion genes, as well as breakpoints, makes techniques such as RNA sequencing (RNA-Seq) particularly appealing in this regard.

Differential Diagnosis

There is a relatively broad differential diagnosis for EFTs; however, in primary tumors of bone this is largely restricted to other undifferentiated round cell sarcomas (eg, *BCOR*-associated sarcoma), small cell osteosarcoma, mesenchymal chondrosarcoma, and hematolymphoid neoplasms.

BCOR-associated sarcoma often has a spindle and/or myxoid component, which may offer a morphologic clue to the diagnosis. These tumors have variable staining for CD99, but, in contrast to EFTs, they are usually positive for SATB2. Molecular testing can be used to confirm the presence of *BCOR* rearrangement. Small cell osteosarcoma may disclose osteoid matrix as a morphologic clue. These tumors are positive for SATB2, but usually have no more than focal staining for CD99.[17] Mesenchymal chondrosarcoma usually has chondroid matrix in support of the diagnosis. Immunohistochemistry is of limited value because tumors sometimes express both CD99 and SATB2. Molecular testing is valuable because it can be used to confirm the presence of NCOA2 rearrangement.[18] Although many lymphomas express CD99 (eg, anaplastic large cell, acute lymphoblastic, and acute myelogenous), a broad hematolymphoid panel usually allows appropriate differentiation. In some instances, molecular testing may be useful for establishing the diagnosis in a subset of these neoplasms (eg, ALK rearrangement).

Diagnosis

Although not imperative,[1] confirmation of a disease-defining fusion product is the current gold standard for the diagnosis of an EFT. Owing to the plethora of neoplasms associated with EWSR1 and FUS rearrangement, caution must be used when relying on a fluorescence in situ break-apart probe alone in the diagnosis of EFTs. More specific techniques, such as RT-PCR and RNA-Seq, are preferable.

Prognosis

Metastasis at diagnosis is the most important prognostic indicator, followed by tumor location (in the absence of metastasis, proximal tumors are associated with a worse outcome than distal).[5] Other clinical factors associated with worse outcome include large tumor size and age at diagnosis (>18 years).[5] Localized tumors are managed with a multimodal approach involving a combination of chemotherapy, and surgery and/or radiation therapy. The 5-year survival for localized disease is 65% to 75%, and much less with metastases.[19] There is currently no consensus for the management of recurrent disease.[20]

△△ **Differential Diagnosis**

- BCOR-associated sarcoma
- CIC-associated sarcoma
- Small cell osteosarcoma
- Mesenchymal chondrosarcoma
- Hematolymphoid neoplasm

Non–FET–Non-ETS-ASSOCIATED SARCOMA

EFTs are associated with FET-ETS fusions, whereas other undifferentiated small round cell sarcomas may lack one (eg, EWSR1-non-ETS), or both, of these family members. Historically such neoplasms were known as Ewing-like

sarcoma, a term that is no longer recommended.[1] Many genetically distinct entities fall within this category when this broad molecular definition is applied. A subset have known genetic drivers, whereas others remain to be characterized (unclassified). Applying the existing WHO classification framework, this subsection will be restricted to discussion of recognized entities within this category, namely, BCOR- and CIC-associated sarcomas.[1] That being said, this broad molecular definition could conceivably be applied to other round cell sarcomas of bone, such as mesenchymal chondrosarcoma (genetic drivers include HEY1-NCOA2 and IRF2BP2-CDX1 fusion products). Moreover, many other such examples exist in the soft tissues (eg, undifferentiated small round cell sarcoma with CRTC1-SS18).[21]

BCOR (BCL6 Corepressor)-Associated Sarcoma

Pierron and colleagues,[22] in 2012, applied RNA-Seq to a cohort of undifferentiated small round cell sarcoma of bone and soft tissue lacking canonical FET-ETS fusions—this led to the identification of a novel BCOR-CCNB3 fusion gene that, on expression profiling, was confirmed to be distinct from EFTs. These tumors are very rare. These tumors most often occur in children and adolescents,[22,23] although older adults may be affected.[24] Tumors markedly predominate in males.[22,23,25] Although they often arise in bone, an origin from the soft tissue and viscera is likewise possible.[22,25,26] Presenting symptoms most often include pain, swelling, limp, and fever; bone involvement may be associated with pathologic fracture.[23]

Gross Features

Samples that have not underdone neoadjuvant therapy are white-tan.[27] The margins are usually circumscribed,[28] and bone involvement is frequently accompanied by soft tissue extension.[23] Reported sizes range from 2.5 to greater than 20 cm.[26,29]

Microscopic Features

A spectrum of morphologies is possible (**Figs. 5** and **6**). Architecturally most cases consist of sheets and fascicles of cells with scant-moderate eosinophilic cytoplasm.[25] The cell shape ranges from round to ovoid-spindled, with some tumors containing an admixture of both.[22,23,30] The nuclei are round-ovoid-angulated and lack significant atypia; mitotic activity is usually conspicuous.[22] In less cellular areas the stroma may be myxoid-edematous or even collagenous.[25] Necrosis is frequently present.

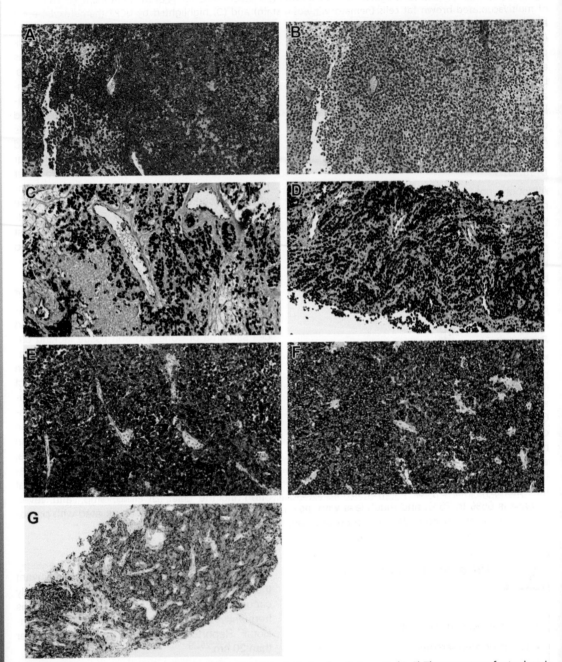

Fig. 4. Ancillary special stains and immunohistochemistry in Ewing family tumors. (*A, B*) The presence of cytoplasmic glycogen is demonstrated by periodic acid-Schiff staining with, and without, diastase [Original magnification 200X]. (*C*) Tumors with *FLI1* fusion partners express FLI1 (*EWSR1-FLI1* fusion gene) [Original magnification 200X]. (*D*) Tumors with *ERG* fusion partners express ERG (*FUS-ERG* fusion gene). On occasion tumors may show significant staining for [Original magnification 200X] (*E*) S100 (*EWSR1-FLI1* fusion gene), (*F*) synaptophysin (*EWSR1-FEV* fusion gene) [Original magnification 200X], and (*G*) keratin (*EWSR1-ERG* fusion gene) [Original magnification 200X].

There is no specific immunohistochemical marker for *BCOR*-associated sarcoma. Tumors are generally positive for BCOR,[31] cyclin D1,[29,32] SATB2,[31] and TLE1[33]; CD99 expression occurs in about half of the cases, and several patterns are possible, including, membranous, cytoplasmic, and dotlike staining.[23] Variable expression of pan-TRK,[34] BCL-2,[27] and CD117[27] has been reported. Cases containing *BCOR-CCNB3* fusions are associated with cyclin B3 expression.[23,25] These neoplasms are usually negative for desmin, S100, keratins, and WT1[26] (**Fig. 7**).

Molecular Features

The most common fusion product in *BCOR*-associated sarcomas is the *BCOR-CCNB3* fusion gene, resulting from an X chromosome paracentric inversion.[22] Less common fusion partners include *BCOR-MAML3*,[26] and *BCOR-CHD9*,[34] as well as *CIITA-BCOR*,[24] *KMT2D-BCOR*,[34] and *ZC3H7B-BCOR*.[26] (The significance of having *BCOR* at the 5′, or 3′ area of the fusion product remains to be clarified.) Another form of *BCOR* genetic alteration, *BCOR* internal tandem duplication, has also be described in undifferentiated round cell sarcomas, and a subset of these tumors are presumed to be related.[29,35] Many of these *BCOR* events are pleiotropic and may be found in other tumors (eg, endometrial stromal sarcoma, ossifying fibromyxoid tumor, clear cell sarcoma of kidney).[36–40]

Differential Diagnosis

BCOR-associated tumors with round cell morphology have a differential diagnosis that overlaps with EFTs (please see earlier discussion). Tumors that additionally contain a spindle cell component may raise the prospect of synovial sarcoma; in such cases, immunohistochemistry for CD99 and TLE1 is unhelpful, and definitive classification may require molecular confirmation.

Diagnosis

Although not imperative,[1] molecular illustration of a fusion product, or *BCOR* ITDs, is the current gold standard in the diagnosis of *BCOR*-associated tumors.

Prognosis

Limited outcome data exist for these tumors due to their rarity, but early indicators suggest a prognosis that is roughly similar to EFTs.[41] The 5-year survival is approximately 75% to 80%.[23,27] Most patients receive multimodal therapy similar to those diagnosed with EFTs. A significant number of patients present with metastases[27]; despite treatment, this tumor is associated with a high rate of local recurrence.[25]

Pathologic Key Features

- Tumors are generally circumscribed. Bone involvement is often associated with soft tissue extension.

- A spectrum of morphologies is possible. Architecturally most cases consist of sheets and fascicles of round to ovoid-spindled cells with no more than mild atypia. Myxoid-edematous stroma is often present.

- Immunohistochemistry is typically positive for BCOR, SATB2, and TLE1. CD99 expression is variable, with membranous, cytoplasmic, and/or dotlike patterns.

- Diverse molecular alterations are possible; these include multiple potential *BCOR* fusion partners; *BCOR* placement at either the 5′ (head), or 3′ (tail), of the fusion gene; and BCOR internal tandem duplication.

CIC-ASSOCIATED SARCOMA

Richkind and colleagues,[42] in 1996, provided the first detailed description of an undifferentiated small round cell sarcoma with a t(4;19)(q35;q13.1) event. Subsequent publications demonstrated that this cytogenetic event resulted in a *CIC-DUX4* fusion gene product.[43] Expression profiling confirms these tumors to be genetically distinct from other small round cell sarcomas, including EFTs and *BCOR*-associated sarcoma.[30,44,45] These neoplasms are rare; they most often occur in young adults, but occurrence ranges from childhood to the elderly.[46,47] Tumors seem to occur slightly more often in males.[47] To date few, if any, details have been reported on the presenting symptoms associated with these neoplasms. Although they most often arise in soft tissue, an origin from bone and viscera is also possible.[46–48]

Gross Features

Samples that have not undergone neoadjuvant therapy are white-gray and frequently necrotic.[48,49] The margins are usually circumscribed.[28,49] Reported sizes range from 0.7 to greater than 20 cm.[47]

Microscopic Features

Architecturally most cases are arranged in sheets and lobules, and less commonly cords, reticular, and/or pseudoalveolar patterns.[47,49,50] (Fig. 8). The cells may be round, epithelioid, and/or spindled in shape. The cytoplasm ranges from scant to moderately abundant, and eosinophilic to amphiphilic with occasional clear vacuoles.[47,49] The nuclei are round-ovoid and often contain mild random pleomorphism; small nucleoli are often present; and mitotic activity is typically brisk.[46,47,49,50] The intervening stroma is usually scant but may be desmoplastic, myxoid, or sclerotic.[48,49] Necrosis is often present.[47–49]

There is no specific immunohistochemical marker for *CIC*-associated sarcoma. Most cases

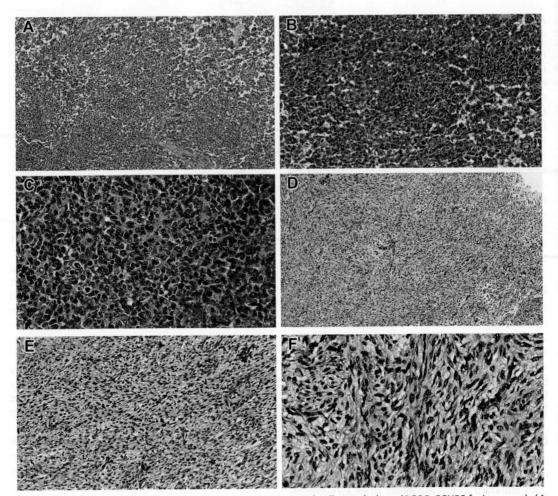

Fig. 5. *BCOR*-associated sarcoma showing a predominant round cell morphology (*BCOR-CCNB3* fusion gene). (*A–C*) Round-epithelioid cells arranged in sheets and lobules [A, (Original magnification 100X), B, [Original magnification 200X], C, [Original magnification 400X], D, [Original magnification 100X], E [Original magnification 200X], F, [Original magnification 400X]). There is scant-medium eosinophilic cytoplasm. The nuclei are round with mild atypia and conspicuous mitotic activity. *BCOR*-associated sarcoma showing a predominant spindle cell morphology (*BCOR-CCNB3* fusion gene). (*D-F*) Spindle cells with a short fascicular to storiform pattern. The cytoplasm is pale and amphophilic. The nuclei are ovoid and monomorphic. Interspersed between cells there is delicate fibrous stroma and myxocollagenous stroma.

are positive for WT1, ETV4, and FLI-1, with variable immunoreactivity for CD99.[44,49–51] Focal staining for S100, keratins, and epithelial membrane antigen may be present.[44,46,48,49,52] Desmin and myogenin give negative results (**Fig. 9**).

Molecular Features

Most tumors have a *CIC* paired with *DUX4* corresponding to t(4;19)(q35;q13), or its paralog *DUX4L*.[43,45,46] Other *CIC* partners include *FOXO4*, and *NUTM1*.[51,53] False-negative results have been reported in a minority of cases using both FISH[54] and RNA-Seq.[55] This risk can be mitigated on next-generation sequencing platforms by limiting automatic filtering of these events and applying the "grep" command in suspicious cases.[56]

Differential Diagnosis

The differential diagnosis for *CIC*-associated sarcomas overlaps with EFT and *BCOR*-rearranged sarcoma (please see earlier discussion). Desmoplastic small round cell tumors may also enter the differential but can readily be excluded based on the characteristic clinical presentation, desmoplastic stroma, polyphenotypic immunoprofile, and presence of an *EWSR1-WT1* fusion product.

Diagnosis

Although not imperative,[1] molecular confirmation of *CIC* rearrangement is the current gold standard in the diagnosis of *BCOR*-associated tumors.

Prognosis

This neoplasm is highly aggressive, and roughly half of the patients are found to have metastatic spread on presentation.[46] The 5-year overall survival is 49% in patients presenting with localized disease, and it is worse in those with metastatic spread.[47] Most patients currently receive multimodal EFT therapy, although the prognosis seems to be worse than both EFTs and *BCOR*-associated sarcoma.[41,57]

Pitfalls

! These tumors often morphologically resemble EFTs; however, the presence of mild random pleomorphism is sometimes a giveaway.

! The intervening stroma may be desmoplastic, resembling desmoplastic small round cell tumor. Potential confusion may be exacerbated by the frequent presence of WT1 staining

! Similar to EFTs, a subset of cases may show diffuse membranous CD99 staining.

! In addition to DUX4, CIC may pair with multiple potential fusion partners (eg, *DUX4L, FOXO4, NUTM1*), so care is necessary in selecting and interpreting a diagnostic assay.

! There is a potential risk of false-negative testing using both FISH and RNA-Seq assays.

FET–NON–ETS–ASSOCIATED SARCOMA

In contrast to EFTs, this recently recognized category encompasses round and spindle cell sarcomas with fusions between a FET RNA-binding protein (*EWSR1, FUS*, or *TAF15*) and a gene unrelated to the ETS transcription factor family. The current WHO classification specifically lists *EWSR1/FUS-NFATC2* (nuclear factor of activated T-cells, cytoplasmic, calcineurin-dependent 2) and *EWSR1-PATZ1* (POZ/BTB and AT hook containing zinc finger 1) as falling under this rubric.[1] Countless other round-spindle cell sarcomas of bone and soft tissue fulfill this admittedly broad molecular definition, such as epithelioid-spindle cell rhabdomyosarcoma, which has a strong predilection for bone (*EWSR1/FUS-TFCP2* fusion gene),[58] and extraskeletal myxoid chondrosarcoma, which, paradoxically, can rarely occur as a primary bone sarcoma (*EWSR1/TAF15/TCF12/ TFG-NR4A3*).[59] Extraskeletal myxoid chondrosarcoma is particularly illustrative, and potentially

exculpatory for this simplified approach to genetic categorization, because it is able to partner either FET or non-FET genes with *NR4A3*, thus potentially undermining this early form of classification (ie, *EWSR1*-non-ETS). It is therefore conceivable that this, and related, molecular classification systems will continue to evolve over time. As such, this section is limited to *EWSR1/FUS-NFATC2*-associated tumors.

Sarcomas with *EWSR1/FUS-NFATC2* fusion genes are rare. They predominate in young adults, but range from childhood to the elderly.[16,60–63] There is a strong predilection for males.[62,63] Presenting symptoms include pain, burning, and mass.[63–65] Although they most often arise in bone, these tumors may also occur in the soft tissue.[60–63]

Gross Features

Tumors with *EWSR1/FUS-NFATC2* rearrangement in bone may be circumscribed or ill-defined and associated with soft tissue extension.[62] These tumors are lobulated, gray-white to pink-tan, and fleshy.[62,63] Reported sizes range from 2.0 to greater than 20 cm.[16,60,62,63]

Microscopic Features

Tumors with *EWSR1/FUS-NFATC2* rearrangement exhibit a range in morphologies[60,62] Architecturally most cases are arranged in sheets and lobules, and less commonly pseudoacinar, anastomosing cords, and trabecular patterns.[62,63] The cells are small-medium and round-spindle shaped.[62,63] The cytoplasm is eosinophilic and ranges from scant to moderate.[62,63] The nuclei are round-ovoid with minimal atypia; mitotic activity, although usually low, may be brisk in a subset of cases.[62,63] Many tumors contain abundant stroma that ranges from fibrous to myxoid, and less commonly osteoidlike and chondroid.[62,63] Necrosis may be present[62] (**Fig. 10**).

There is no specific immunohistochemical marker for *EWSR1/FUS-NFATC2*-associated sarcoma. Tumors are positive for AGGRECAN, and CD99 expression is present in most cases and several patterns are possible, including membranous, cytoplasmic, and dotlike.[62,63] A subset of cases may show focal or dotlike keratin and/or epithelial membrane antigen staining.[63] These cases are typically negative for desmin, smooth muscle actin, S100, WT1, and SATB2.[60,62,63]

Molecular Features

NFATC2 is much more frequently partnered with *EWSR1* than *FUS*. It should be emphasized that there is molecular pleiotropy with the *EWSR1/*

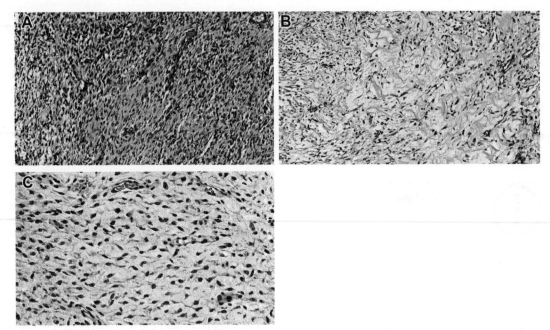

Fig. 6. *BCOR*-associated sarcomas showing different stromal patterns (*BCOR-CCNB3* fusion gene). (*A*) Delicate bands of "wiry" collagen reminiscent of that seen in synovial sarcoma [Original magnification 200X]. (*B*) Abundant edematous stroma with irregular bands of hyalinized collagen [Original magnification 200X]. (*C*) Abundant myxoid stroma, with occasional clear extracellular vacuoles [Original magnification 400X].

FUS-NFATC2 fusion genes, which was recently identified in simple bone cysts[66,67]; the relationship, if any, between these neoplasms is currently unclear.

Differential Diagnosis

The differential diagnosis of *EWSR1/FUS-NFATC2*-associated tumors includes EFTs (please see earlier discussion), myoepithelial tumors,

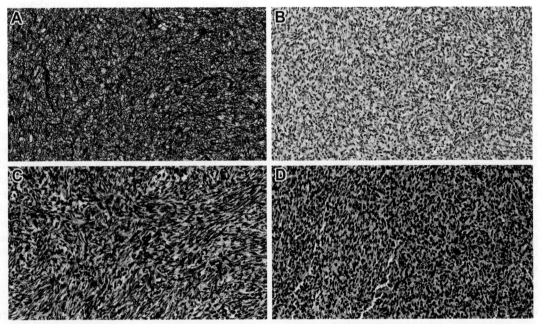

Fig. 7. Immunohistochemistry of *BCOR*-associated sarcoma showing (*A*) CD99, (*B*) SATB2, (*C*) BCL-2, and (*D*) cyclin D1. (*A-D,* Original magnification 200X)

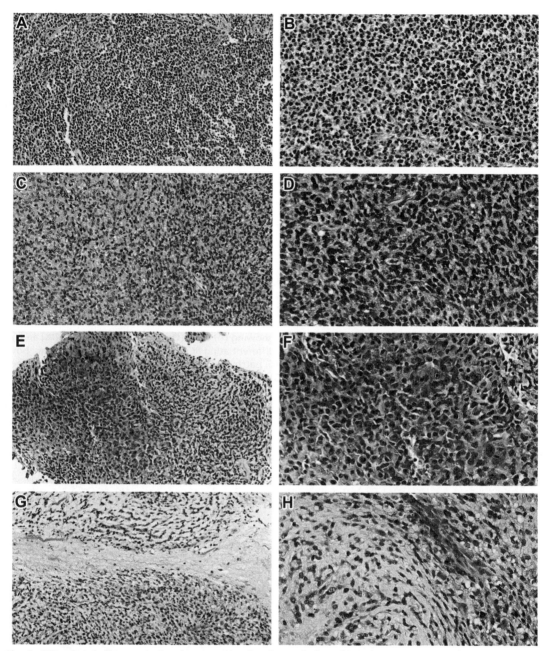

Fig. 8. *CIC*-associated sarcoma showing a conventional morphology (*CIC* rearrangement confirmed by fluorescence in situ hybridization). (*A*) Sheets of small round cells with scant eosinophilic cytoplasm and occasional thin fibrous septa [Original magnification 100X]. (*B*) The nuclei are round, with minimal atypia. Another case of *CIC*-associated sarcoma, this one showing a syncytial morphology (*CIC* rearrangement confirmed by fluorescence in situ hybridization) [Original magnification 200X]. (*C*) Irregular fascicles of ovoid cells [Original magnification 200X]. (*D*) The nuclei are round-ovoid with conspicuous mitotic activity. *CIC*-associated sarcoma showing an epithelioid morphology (*CIC-DUX4L* fusion gene) [Original magnification 400X]. (*E*) Sheets of plump epithelioid cells centrally, with smaller spindle shaped cells peripherally [Original magnification 200X]. (*F*) The nuclei are round-ovoid with mild-moderate atypia and conspicuous nucleoli. *CIC*-associated sarcoma showing a predominant spindle cell morphology (*CIC-DUX4L* fusion gene) [Original magnification 400X]. (*G*) Spindle cells arranged in cords and nodules with abundant intervening hyaline stroma [Original magnification 200X]. (*H*) The cells have amphophilic cytoplasm. The nuclei are ovoid with mild atypia and small nucleoli [Original magnification 400X].

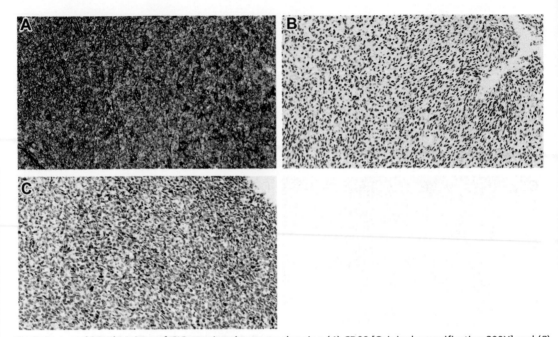

Fig. 9. Immunohistochemistry of *CIC*-associated sarcoma showing (*A*) CD99 [Original magnification 200X] and (*B*) WT1 staining. SATB2 is reported to be a useful marker in differentiating *BCOR*- and *CIC*-associated sarcomas; however, this case contained [Original magnification 200X] (*C*) patchy SATB2 staining, thereby highlighting the need for rigorous molecular confirmation of the diagnosis [Original magnification 200X].

sclerosing epithelioid fibrosarcoma, and small cell osteosarcoma. Immunohistochemistry for MUC4 and molecular testing can be used to exclude the possibility of sclerosing epithelioid fibrosarcoma. Given significant morphologic and immunohistochemical overlap with myoepithelial tumors molecular testing may be necessary to differentiate these entities.

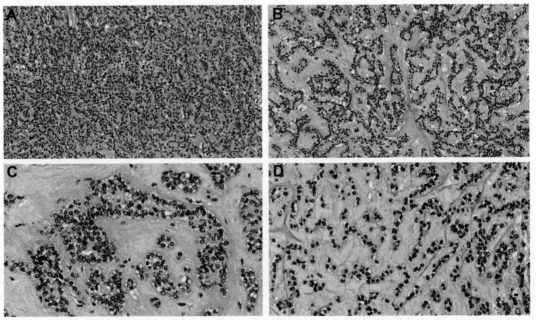

Fig. 10. *EWSR1-NFATC2*-associated sarcoma. (*A–D*) Anastomosing cords of round-polygonal cells, with variable abundance of intervening myxoid stroma. The nuclei are round-ovoid and monomorphic; mitotic activity is inconspicuous. [A, Original magnification 200X]; B, [Original magnification 200X]; C, [Original magnification 400X]; D, [Original magnification 400X]

Diagnosis

Molecular confirmation illustrating either *EWSR1* amplification of the 5' probe, or identification of the fusion product, in the appropriate histopathologic context is essential for this diagnosis.[1]

Prognosis

Limited reports exist on the prognosis of *EWSR1/FUS-NFATC*-associated sarcomas. Many tumors follow an aggressive clinical course, with local recurrence and/or metastasis in approximately 50% of cases.[62] These tumors show a poor response to EFT regimens.[63]

SUMMARY

Although imprecise, the term undifferentiated small round cell sarcoma offers a tentative framework for the classification of these heterogeneous neoplasms. Given tremendous overlap in morphology and immunophenotype, the accurate classification of these tumors can be challenging and often requires advanced molecular techniques (eg, RNA-Seq). These same diagnostic techniques also routinely contribute to the discovery of novel fusion products, underscoring how much remains to be established in our understanding of these neoplasms. Ultimately, the classification of these neoplasms will presumably undergo significant evolution in the decade ahead.

DIAGNOSTIC ALGORITHM BOX

Undifferentiated round cell sarcoma of bone.

1. Assuming this is a primary bone tumor, are there morphologic clues to the diagnosis based on architecture, cytology, and/or extracellular matrix?
2. Perform a broad immunohistochemical screening panel to encompass the aforementioned entities, as well as excluding potential mimics based on the clinical context (including hematolymphoid and epithelial neoplasms).
3. In the absence of a definitive diagnosis based on morphology and immunohistochemistry, and assuming the diagnosis will affect management, application of a targeted next generation sequencing molecular panel should be considered.

ACKNOWLEDGEMENTS

Panov2 research fund, and generous donation from Dr. Martin E. Blackstein patient donation fund.

DISCLOSURE

Not applicable.

REFERENCES

1. Board WCoTE. Soft tissue and bone tumours. France: International Agency for Research on Cancer Lyon; 2020.
2. Ewing J. Classics in oncology. Diffuse endothelioma of bone. James Ewing. Proceedings of the New York Pathological Society, 1921. CA Cancer J Clin 1972;22(2):95–8.
3. Turc-Carel C, Philip I, Berger MP, et al. Chromosomal translocation (11; 22) in cell lines of Ewing's sarcoma. C R Seances Acad Sci III 1983;296(23):1101–3, [in French].
4. Ewing's sarcoma and its congeners: an interim appraisal. Lancet 1992;339(8785):99–100.
5. Riggi N, Suva ML, Stamenkovic I. Ewing's Sarcoma. N Engl J Med 2021;384(2):154–64.
6. Grunewald TGP, Cidre-Aranaz F, Surdez D, et al. Ewing sarcoma. Nat Rev Dis Primers 2018;4(1):5.
7. Jahanseer K, Folpe AL, Graham RP, et al. Ewing sarcoma in older adults: a clinicopathologic study of 50 cases occurring in patients aged >/=40 years, with emphasis on histologic mimics. Int J Surg Pathol 2020;28(4):352–60.
8. Sizemore GM, Pitarresi JR, Balakrishnan S, et al. The ETS family of oncogenic transcription factors in solid tumours. Nat Rev Cancer 2017;17(6):337–51.
9. Agaram NP, Zhang L, Sung YS, et al. Extraskeletal myxoid chondrosarcoma with non-EWSR1-NR4A3 variant fusions correlate with rhabdoid phenotype and high-grade morphology. Hum Pathol 2014;45(5):1084–91.
10. Folpe AL, Goldblum JR, Rubin BP, et al. Morphologic and immunophenotypic diversity in Ewing family tumors: a study of 66 genetically confirmed cases. Am J Surg Pathol 2005;29(8):1025–33.
11. Bridge JA, Fidler ME, Neff JR, et al. Adamantinoma-like Ewing's sarcoma: genomic confirmation, phenotypic drift. Am J Surg Pathol 1999;23(2):159–65.
12. Yoshida A, Sekine S, Tsuta K, et al. NKX2.2 is a useful immunohistochemical marker for Ewing sarcoma. Am J Surg Pathol 2012;36(7):993–9.
13. Gu M, Antonescu CR, Guiter G, et al. Cytokeratin immunoreactivity in Ewing's sarcoma: prevalence in 50 cases confirmed by molecular diagnostic studies. Am J Surg Pathol 2000;24(3):410–6.
14. Collini P, Sampietro G, Bertulli R, et al. Cytokeratin immunoreactivity in 41 cases of ES/PNET confirmed by molecular diagnostic studies. Am J Surg Pathol 2001;25(2):273–4.
15. Wang L, Bhargava R, Zheng T, et al. Undifferentiated small round cell sarcomas with rare EWS gene fusions: identification of a novel EWS-SP3 fusion and of additional cases with the EWS-ETV1 and EWS-FEV fusions. J Mol Diagn 2007;9(4):498–509.

16. Tsuda Y, Zhang L, Meyers P, et al. The clinical heterogeneity of round cell sarcomas with EWSR1/FUS gene fusions: impact of gene fusion type on clinical features and outcome. Genes Chromosomes Cancer 2020;59(9):525–34.

17. Righi A, Gambarotti M, Longo S, et al. Small cell osteosarcoma: clinicopathologic, immunohistochemical, and molecular analysis of 36 cases. Am J Surg Pathol 2015;39(5):691–9.

18. Wang L, Motoi T, Khanin R, et al. Identification of a novel, recurrent HEY1-NCOA2 fusion in mesenchymal chondrosarcoma based on a genome-wide screen of exon-level expression data. Genes Chromosomes Cancer 2012;51(2):127–39.

19. Gaspar N, Hawkins DS, Dirksen U, et al. Ewing sarcoma: current management and future approaches through collaboration. J Clin Oncol 2015;33(27):3036–46.

20. Italiano A, Mir O, Mathoulin-Pelissier S, et al. Cabozantinib in patients with advanced Ewing sarcoma or osteosarcoma (CABONE): a multicentre, single-arm, phase 2 trial. Lancet Oncol 2020;21(3):446–55.

21. Alholle A, Karanian M, Brini AT, et al. Genetic analyses of undifferentiated small round cell sarcoma identifies a novel sarcoma subtype with a recurrent CRTC1-SS18 gene fusion. J Pathol 2018;245(2):186–96.

22. Pierron G, Tirode F, Lucchesi C, et al. A new subtype of bone sarcoma defined by BCOR-CCNB3 gene fusion. Nat Genet 2012;44(4):461–6.

23. Cohen-Gogo S, Cellier C, Coindre JM, et al. Ewing-like sarcomas with BCOR-CCNB3 fusion transcript: a clinical, radiological and pathological retrospective study from the Societe Francaise des Cancers de L'Enfant. Pediatr Blood Cancer 2014;61(12):2191–8.

24. Yoshida A, Arai Y, Hama N, et al. Expanding the clinicopathologic and molecular spectrum of BCOR-associated sarcomas in adults. Histopathology 2020;76(4):509–20.

25. Peters TL, Kumar V, Polikepahad S, et al. BCOR-CCNB3 fusions are frequent in undifferentiated sarcomas of male children. Mod Pathol 2015;28(4):575–86.

26. Specht K, Zhang L, Sung YS, et al. Novel BCOR-MAML3 and ZC3H7B-BCOR gene fusions in undifferentiated small blue round cell sarcomas. Am J Surg Pathol 2016;40(4):433–42.

27. Puls F, Niblett A, Marland G, et al. BCOR-CCNB3 (Ewing-like) sarcoma: a clinicopathologic analysis of 10 cases, in comparison with conventional Ewing sarcoma. Am J Surg Pathol 2014;38(10):1307–18.

28. Brady EJ, Hameed M, Tap WD, et al. Imaging features and clinical course of undifferentiated round cell sarcomas with CIC-DUX4 and BCOR-CCNB3 translocations. Skeletal Radiol 2021;50(3):521–9.

29. Antonescu CR, Kao YC, Xu B, et al. Undifferentiated round cell sarcoma with BCOR internal tandem duplications (ITD) or YWHAE fusions: a clinicopathologic and molecular study. Mod Pathol 2020;33(9):1669–77.

30. Kao YC, Owosho AA, Sung YS, et al. BCOR-CCNB3 fusion positive sarcomas: a clinicopathologic and molecular analysis of 36 cases with comparison to morphologic spectrum and clinical behavior of other round cell sarcomas. Am J Surg Pathol 2018;42(5):604–15.

31. Kao YC, Sung YS, Zhang L, et al. BCOR overexpression is a highly sensitive marker in round cell sarcomas with BCOR genetic abnormalities. Am J Surg Pathol 2016;40(12):1670–8.

32. Matsuyama A, Shiba E, Umekita Y, et al. Clinicopathologic diversity of undifferentiated sarcoma with BCOR-CCNB3 fusion: analysis of 11 cases with a reappraisal of the utility of immunohistochemistry for BCOR and CCNB3. Am J Surg Pathol 2017;41(12):1713–21.

33. Li WS, Liao IC, Wen MC, et al. BCOR-CCNB3-positive soft tissue sarcoma with round-cell and spindle-cell histology: a series of four cases highlighting the pitfall of mimicking poorly differentiated synovial sarcoma. Histopathology 2016;69(5):792–801.

34. Kao YC, Sung YS, Argani P, et al. NTRK3 overexpression in undifferentiated sarcomas with YWHAE and BCOR genetic alterations. Mod Pathol 2020;33(7):1341–9.

35. Malik F, Zreik RT, Hedges DJ, et al. Primary bone sarcoma with BCOR internal tandem duplication. Virchows Arch 2020;476(6):915–20.

36. Panagopoulos I, Thorsen J, Gorunova L, et al. Fusion of the ZC3H7B and BCOR genes in endometrial stromal sarcomas carrying an X;22-translocation. Genes Chromosomes Cancer 2013;52(7):610–8.

37. Marino-Enriquez A, Lauria A, Przybyl J, et al. BCOR internal tandem duplication in high-grade uterine sarcomas. Am J Surg Pathol 2018;42(3):335–41.

38. Antonescu CR, Sung YS, Chen CL, et al. Novel ZC3H7B-BCOR, MEAF6-PHF1, and EPC1-PHF1 fusions in ossifying fibromyxoid tumors–molecular characterization shows genetic overlap with endometrial stromal sarcoma. Genes Chromosomes Cancer 2014;53(2):183–93.

39. Roy A, Kumar V, Zorman B, et al. Recurrent internal tandem duplications of BCOR in clear cell sarcoma of the kidney. Nat Commun 2015;6:8891.

40. Argani P, Kao YC, Zhang L, et al. Primary renal sarcomas with BCOR-CCNB3 gene fusion: a report of 2

cases showing histologic overlap with clear cell sarcoma of kidney, suggesting further link between BCOR-related sarcomas of the kidney and soft tissues. Am J Surg Pathol 2017;41(12):1702–12.

41. Davis JL, Rudzinski ER. Small round blue cell sarcoma other than ewing sarcoma: what should an oncologist know? Curr Treat Options Oncol 2020; 21(11):90.

42. Richkind KE, Romansky SG, Finklestein JZ. t(4;19)(q35;q13.1): a recurrent change in primitive mesenchymal tumors? Cancer Genet Cytogenet 1996;87(1):71–4.

43. Kawamura-Saito M, Yamazaki Y, Kaneko K, et al. Fusion between CIC and DUX4 up-regulates PEA3 family genes in Ewing-like sarcomas with t(4;19)(q35;q13) translocation. Hum Mol Genet 2006;15(13):2125–37.

44. Specht K, Sung YS, Zhang L, et al. Distinct transcriptional signature and immunoprofile of CIC-DUX4 fusion-positive round cell tumors compared to EWSR1-rearranged Ewing sarcomas: further evidence toward distinct pathologic entities. Genes Chromosomes Cancer 2014;53(7):622–33.

45. Watson S, Perrin V, Guillemot D, et al. Transcriptomic definition of molecular subgroups of small round cell sarcomas. J Pathol 2018;245(1):29–40.

46. Italiano A, Sung YS, Zhang L, et al. High prevalence of CIC fusion with double-homeobox (DUX4) transcription factors in EWSR1-negative undifferentiated small blue round cell sarcomas. Genes Chromosomes Cancer 2012;51(3):207–18.

47. Antonescu CR, Owosho AA, Zhang L, et al. Sarcomas with CIC-rearrangements are a distinct pathologic entity with aggressive outcome: a clinicopathologic and molecular study of 115 cases. Am J Surg Pathol 2017;41(7):941–9.

48. Choi EY, Thomas DG, McHugh JB, et al. Undifferentiated small round cell sarcoma with t(4;19)(q35;q13.1) CIC-DUX4 fusion: a novel highly aggressive soft tissue tumor with distinctive histopathology. Am J Surg Pathol 2013;37(9):1379–86.

49. Yoshida A, Goto K, Kodaira M, et al. CIC-rearranged sarcomas: a study of 20 cases and comparisons with Ewing sarcomas. Am J Surg Pathol 2016; 40(3):313–23.

50. Hung YP, Fletcher CD, Hornick JL. Evaluation of ETV4 and WT1 expression in CIC-rearranged sarcomas and histologic mimics. Mod Pathol 2016; 29(11):1324–34.

51. Le Loarer F, Pissaloux D, Watson S, et al. Clinicopathologic features of CIC-NUTM1 sarcomas, a new molecular variant of the family of CIC-fused sarcomas. Am J Surg Pathol 2019;43(2):268–76.

52. Graham C, Chilton-MacNeill S, Zielenska M, et al. The CIC-DUX4 fusion transcript is present in a subgroup of pediatric primitive round cell sarcomas. Hum Pathol 2012;43(2):180–9.

53. Sugita S, Arai Y, Tonooka A, et al. A novel CIC-FOXO4 gene fusion in undifferentiated small round cell sarcoma: a genetically distinct variant of Ewing-like sarcoma. Am J Surg Pathol 2014; 38(11):1571–6.

54. Yoshida A, Arai Y, Kobayashi E, et al. CIC break-apart fluorescence in-situ hybridization misses a subset of CIC-DUX4 sarcomas: a clinicopathological and molecular study. Histopathology 2017;71(3):461–9.

55. Kao YC, Sung YS, Chen CL, et al. ETV transcriptional upregulation is more reliable than RNA sequencing algorithms and FISH in diagnosing round cell sarcomas with CIC gene rearrangements. Genes Chromosomes Cancer 2017;56(6):501–10.

56. Panagopoulos I, Gorunova L, Bjerkehagen B, et al. The "grep" command but not FusionMap, FusionFinder or ChimeraScan captures the CIC-DUX4 fusion gene from whole transcriptome sequencing data on a small round cell tumor with t(4;19)(q35;q13). PLoS One 2014;9(6):e99439.

57. Pappo AS, Dirksen U. Rhabdomyosarcoma, Ewing sarcoma, and other round cell sarcomas. J Clin Oncol 2018;36(2):168–79.

58. Agaram NP, Zhang L, Sung YS, et al. Expanding the spectrum of intraosseous rhabdomyosarcoma: correlation between 2 distinct gene fusions and phenotype. Am J Surg Pathol 2019;43(5):695–702.

59. Finos L, Righi A, Frisoni T, et al. Primary extraskeletal myxoid chondrosarcoma of bone: report of three cases and review of the literature. Pathol Res Pract 2017;213(5):461–6.

60. Wang GY, Thomas DG, Davis JL, et al. EWSR1-NFATC2 translocation-associated sarcoma clinicopathologic findings in a rare aggressive primary bone or soft tissue tumor. Am J Surg Pathol 2019; 43(8):1112–22.

61. Yoshida KI, Machado I, Motoi T, et al. NKX3-1 is a useful immunohistochemical marker of EWSR1-NFATC2 sarcoma and mesenchymal chondrosarcoma. Am J Surg Pathol 2020;44(6):719–28.

62. Perret R, Escuriol J, Velasco V, et al. NFATc2-rearranged sarcomas: clinicopathologic, molecular, and cytogenetic study of 7 cases with evidence of AGGRECAN as a novel diagnostic marker. Mod Pathol 2020;33(10):1930–44.

63. Diaz-Perez JA, Nielsen GP, Antonescu C, et al. EWSR1/FUS-NFATc2 rearranged round cell sarcoma: clinicopathological series of 4 cases and literature review. Hum Pathol 2019;90:45–53.

64. Sadri N, Barroeta J, Pack SD, et al. Malignant round cell tumor of bone with EWSR1-NFATC2 gene fusion. Virchows Arch 2014;465(2):233–9.

65. Cohen JN, Sabnis AJ, Krings G, et al. EWSR1-NFATC2 gene fusion in a soft tissue tumor with

epithelioid round cell morphology and abundant stroma: a case report and review of the literature. Hum Pathol 2018;81:281–90.

66. Hung YP, Fisch AS, Diaz-Perez JA, et al. Identification of EWSR1-NFATC2 fusion in simple bone cysts. Histopathology 2021;78(6):849–56.

67. Pizem J, Sekoranja D, Zupan A, et al. FUS-NFATC2 or EWSR1-NFATC2 fusions are present in a large proportion of simple bone cysts. Am J Surg Pathol 2020;44(12):1623–34.

68. Panigrahi P, Jere A, Anamika K. FusionHub: a unified web platform for annotation and visualization of gene fusion events in human cancer. PLoS One 2018;13(5):e0196588.

69. Weinreb I, Goldstein D, Perez-Ordonez B. Primary extraskeletal Ewing family tumor with complex epithelial differentiation: a unique case arising in the lateral neck presenting with Horner syndrome. Am J Surg Pathol 2008;32(11):1742–8.

Giant Cell-Rich Tumors of Bone

Wolfgang Hartmann, MD[a], Dorothee Harder, MD[b], Daniel Baumhoer, MD[c],*

KEYWORDS

- Giant cell tumor • Giant cell granuloma • Non-ossifying fibroma • Aneurysmal bone cyst
- USP6-rearranged lesions

Key points

- Multinucleated giant cells can be found in a distinct group of bone tumors and generally represent bystanders of the actual neoplastic population

- Most giant cell-rich bone tumors show characteristic molecular alterations that can aid in the differential diagnosis and primarily involve mutations of the *H3.3, KRAS,* and *FGFR1* genes as well as rearrangements of the *USP6* gene

- Benign fibrous histiocytoma (BFH) is no longer listed as a separate entity in the latest WHO classification and believed to represent giant cell tumor with regressive changes

- Giant cell lesion of the small tubular bones has also been eliminated as a distinct entity in the latest WHO classification and thought to represent solid aneurysmal bone cyst

- Rearrangements of the USP6 gene are not limited to classical aneurysmal bone cysts but occur in a variety of formerly "difficult to classify" lesions

ABSTRACT

The term *giant cell-rich tumors of bone* refers to a shared morphologic pattern in a group of different osseous lesions, that is, the abundance of osteoclastlike giant cells. Fitting with a broad spectrum of clinical presentations and biological behavior, the recent detection of characteristic molecular alterations in giant cell tumor of bone (*H3-3*), nonossifying fibroma (*KRAS, FGFR1*), giant cell granuloma of the jaws (*KRAS, FGFR1, TRPV4*), and aneurysmal bone cyst (*USP6*) have contributed significantly to the biological understanding of these morphologically related but clinically distinct lesions and their systematic classification, highlighting differences and pathogenic relationships.

GIANT CELL TUMOR OF BONE

INTRODUCTION

Conventional giant cell tumor constitutes 4% to 5% of all primary bone tumors. This tumor is considered a locally aggressive and rarely metastasizing neoplasm that can undergo malignant transformation into a high-grade sarcoma.[1] Giant cell tumor of bone (GCT) predominantly develops in the epiphyseal/metaphyseal region of long tubular bones after skeletal maturity (>20 years). In less than 10% of cases, tumors occur while the growth plates are still open and are then centered more proximally in the metaphyses.[2] Most commonly involved sites include the distal femur, the proximal tibia, and the distal radius. In

[a] Division of Translational Pathology, Gerhard-Domagk-Institut of Pathology, University Hospital Münster, Albert-Schweitzer-Campus 1, Münster 48149, Germany; [b] Department of Radiology, University Hospital Basel, University of Basel, Petersgraben 4, Basel 4031, Switzerland; [c] Bone Tumor Reference Center, Institute of Medical Genetics and Pathology, University Hospital Basel, University of Basel, Schoenbeinstrasse 40, Basel 4031, Switzerland
* Corresponding author.
E-mail address: daniel.baumhoer@usb.ch

Surgical Pathology 14 (2021) 695–706
https://doi.org/10.1016/j.path.2021.06.010

the spine, the vertebral bodies are affected. GCT is exceptionally rare in the craniofacial bones.

IMAGING FEATURES

As GCTs lack formation of mineralized matrix, they appear purely lytic in radiographs and computed tomographic (CT) scans without sclerotic margins. GCTs are usually large, intramedullary, eccentrically located, and well defined (**Fig. 1**A). Cortical scalloping and penetration can occur in advanced lesions, but aggressive periosteal reactions are usually absent. MRI of GCT shows nonspecific, usually heterogeneous signal intensity on T1-weighted images before and after contrast administration; T2-weighted images are also nonspecific but can demonstrate (pseudo-)cystic change (fluid-fluid levels, see **Fig. 1**C).

GROSS AND MICROSCOPIC FEATURES

Tumors are mostly solid and consist of friable brown tissue with varying amounts of hemorrhage, cystic change, and necrosis. Tumors usually measure 5 to 15 cm in diameter.

Microscopically, abundant and remarkably large multinucleated giant cells are the hallmark of the disease. Although intermingled smaller giant cells can occur in a variety of different lesions, the amount and size of giant cells demonstrating more than 50 nuclei per tissue section is typical for GCT (**Fig. 1**B). The neoplastic cell population, however, is composed of mostly monomorphic oval or polygonal cells arranged in a haphazard manner; it shows ill-defined cell borders and a slightly eosinophilic cytoplasm. Nuclei tend to appear round to ovoid with vesicular chromatin and central nucleoli; they are practically identical to the nuclei of the giant cell component. Mitotic activity, mild to moderate cytologic atypia, and areas of necrosis can be observed, as well as vascular invasion. GCT can undergo regressive changes with prominent accumulation of siderophages and foam cells; other secondary changes include (pseudo-)cystic change and reactive new bone formation.

Following antiresorptive therapy (eg, with denosumab), the microscopic appearance markedly changes. The multinucleated giant cells disappear, and the lesional mononuclear cells decrease and partly transform into osteoblasts forming varying amounts of immature woven bone trabeculae.[3,4] This observation is in line with gene expression profiles of the mononuclear component of GCT that

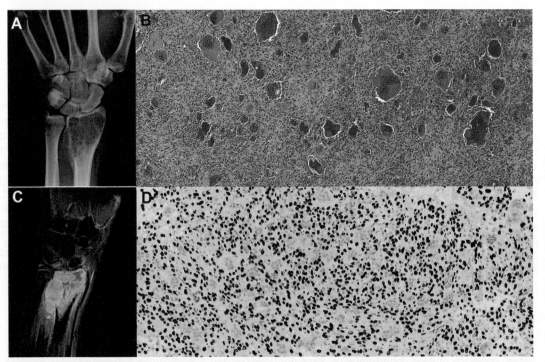

Fig. 1. GCT in the distal radius of a 17-year old boy. The conventional radiograph shows a well-demarcated, slightly expansile lytic lesion extending to the subchondral bone (*A*) with heterogeneous enhancement in a T1-weighted, fat-saturated MRI sequence after contrast administration (*C*). Microscopically, multiple (nonneoplastic) large giant cells are embedded in a background of monomorphic mononuclear spindle cells arranged in a haphazard manner (*B*) [hematoxylin-eosin, original magnification, 50x]. H3.3 G34W immunoreactivity can be observed in the mononuclear spindle cells (*D*) [original magnification, 100x].

resemble those of cells with early osteoblastic differentiation.[5] In some cases, reactive atypia can be striking and mimic malignant transformation.[3]

Malignant GCT can show different kinds of presentation. Typically, parts of a regular GCT can be found adjacent to a high-grade sarcoma, similar to dedifferentiated liposarcoma or chondrosarcoma. The characteristic histone H3.3 mutation of GCT usually remains detectable in the sarcomatous component, and malignant transformation can occur in the primary manifestation or after local recurrences of the GCT. Osteosarcoma (OS) or undifferentiated pleomorphic sarcoma (UPS) comprise the most common histologic patterns found in malignant GCT. OS or UPS without a detectable GCT component but revealing an H3.3 mutation most likely also represent malignant GCT. Genetically, malignant GCT resembles OS and UPS and shows a high degree of aneuploidy.[6]

IMMUNOPHENOTYPE AND MOLECULAR PATHOLOGY FEATURES

Virtually all GCTs (96%) harbor mutations in the *H3-3A* gene specifically involving Glycine 34, with G34W (p.Gly34Trp) accounting for 90% of cases and G34L (p.Gly34Lys) for a smaller minority.[7–9] The G34W mutation can be detected reliably by immunohistochemistry showing nuclear positivity in the mononuclear cell population only (**Fig. 1D**). The functional impact is still largely unknown so far, but recent studies point to a massive effect on the global epigenetic landscape that seems to impair normal osteogenic differentiation.[10] Apart from this driver mutation, GCTs show a relatively low mutation burden and a flat copy number profile.

DIFFERENTIAL DIAGNOSIS

The histology in the typical clinical and imaging context is fairly diagnostic for GCT without additional analyses, whereas H3.3 testing confirmed that *giant cell granulomas of the jaws*, *aneurysmal bone cyst (ABC)*, *giant cell lesions of the small tubular bone,* and *non-ossifying fibroma* are not related to GCT. On the other hand, lesions formerly classified as *BFH*, histologically resembling non-ossifying fibroma but mainly occurring later in life and centered in the epiphyses of long tubular bones, turned out to represent giant cell tumors with marked regressive changes and are no longer listed as a separate entity in the current World Health Organization (WHO) classification (**Fig. 2**). In case of doubt, immunohistochemical testing for the G34W mutation is usually sufficient to

confirm GCT. The detection of rarer mutations still requires sequencing.[11]

SUMMARY AND PROGNOSIS

Conventional GCT recurs locally following curettage in 15% to 50%, usually within 2 years. Tumors can occasionally metastasize to the lungs, which is believed to result from embolization of intravascular growth. Metastases occur in 3% to 7% of cases, often following local recurrence; show limited growth dynamics; and can regress spontaneously. The prognosis of malignant GCT is similar to those of other high-grade sarcomas of bone.

CLINICS CARE POINTS

- Most cases present as lytic mass lesions in the epiphyseal region of long tubular bone in patients older than 20 years
- Abundant large multinucleated giant cells distributed evenly among mononuclear spindle cells are characteristic; H3.3 testing can confirm the diagnosis
- Regressive changes, either following denosumab or without prior treatment (formerly known as BFH), can significantly alter the histologic and radiologic appearance of GCT
- Metastases can occur but often follow an indolent clinical course; primary/secondary malignant GCTs represent high-grade bone sarcomas requiring a multidisciplinary treatment approach

NON-OSSIFYING FIBROMA OF BONE (NOF)

INTRODUCTION

NOF is the most common benign tumor of bone.[12] As it usually follows an asymptomatic course and undergoes spontaneous resolution, most cases are clinically not recognized, which is why the actual incidence of NOF is difficult to determine. It has been estimated, however, that 30% to 40% of children develop one or even multiple occult lesions during skeletal growth.[13] The first edition of the WHO classification of bone tumors published in 1972 described NOF as a nonneoplastic bone lesion of "obscure etiology"; the second edition from 1993 continued to recognize NOF as a tumorlike lesion, probably representing a developmental anomaly.[14,15] In 2002 the third edition of the WHO classification was published and did not list NOF as a separate bone tumor entity; in the fourth edition from 2013 NOF was described together with benign fibrous histiocytoma as a fibrohistiocytic lesion.[16] After recurrent pathogenic

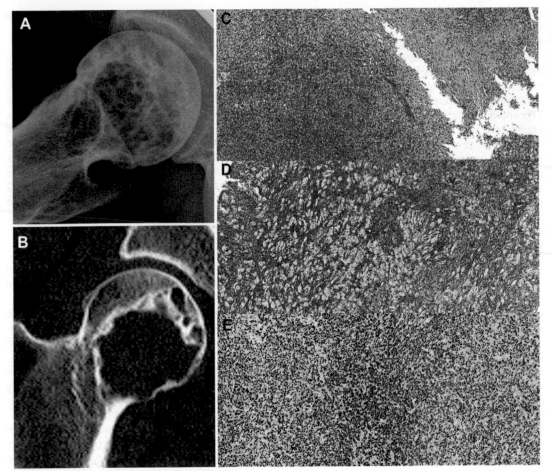

Fig. 2. GCT with regressive changes (former BFH). Conventional radiographs (*A*) and coronal CT reconstruction (*B*) of the proximal femur of a 33-year old woman show a well-demarcated osteolysis of the femoral head with a peripheral sclerotic rim. Microscopically, a dense spindle cell proliferation with only few intermingled multinucleated giant cells (*C*) and extensive foam cell change [hematoxylin-eosin, original magnification, 50x] (*D*) is visible, resembling non-ossifying fibroma (NOF) of bone [hematoxylin-eosin, original magnification, 50x]. (*E*) The tumor cells are consistently positive for H3-3A (G34W mutation 50x).

mutations in the mitogen-activated protein (MAP) kinase signaling pathway were identified recently, NOF was finally recognized as a benign neoplasm and is now listed under the osteoclastic giant cell-rich tumors in the current and fifth edition of the WHO blue book.

NOF exclusively develops in the first 2 decades of life and generally affects the metaphyses of long tubular bones, mainly around the knee and in the distal tibia. Multiple lesions can occur sporadically and also in distinct syndromes, mostly belonging to the spectrum of RASopathies and including neurofibromatosis type 1 (NF1) and Jaffe-Campanacci syndrome.

IMAGING FEATURES

The presentation of NOF on plain radiographs is usually so characteristic that no biopsy confirmation is required. Lesions appear well defined, polylobulated (grapelike), and lytic. Lesions are centered in the cortex and show sclerotic and scalloped borders (**Fig. 3**A, B). Remarkably, (residual) NOF is only rarely encountered in adults, which is probably caused by spontaneous regression and resolution over time.

GROSS AND MICROSCOPIC FEATURES

Most NOFs consist of solid brown tissue with variable amounts of hemorrhage and (pseudo-) cystic change. Necrosis is usually only present after a prior pathologic fracture.

Histologically, the tumors are composed of histiocytelike spindle cells arranged in storiform patterns. Mitoses can be found but are usually scant. There is no significant cytologic atypia. Throughout the lesion, intermingled

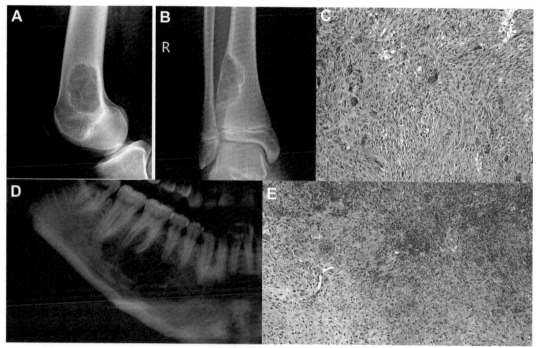

Fig. 3. Plain radiographs of non-ossifying fibroma in the distal femur of a 16-year old girl (*A*) and in the distal tibia of a 14-year old boy (*B*) displaying well-defined, eccentric, and lobulated radiolucent lesions with sclerotic borders. Microscopically, histiocytelike spindle cells are arranged in storiform patterns with intermingled osteoclastlike giant cells (*C*) [hematoxylin-eosin, original magnification, 50x]. (*D*) Mandibular central giant cell granuloma in a 28-year old woman presenting as a well-circumscribed lytic lesion. Microscopically, monomorphic mononuclear spindle cells and scattered multinucleated giant cells can be observed in association with areas of hemorrhage (*E*) [hematoxylin-eosin, original magnification, 50x].

multinucleated giant cells can be observed that appear rather small (>10 nuclei per tissue section) and cluster around areas of hemorrhage (**Fig.** 3C). Aggregations of siderophages and foam cells are other typical findings, the background can be rich in collagen fibers. Reactive new bone formation is rare (*non-ossifying* fibroma) but can be seen following a fracture. The histology of NOF strongly resembles that of giant cell granuloma of the jaws.

IMMUNOPHENOTYPE AND MOLECULAR PATHOLOGY FEATURES

In the vast majority of cases, NOF can be reliably diagnosed without additional analysis but requires radiologic correlation. The immunophenotype is nonspecific and highlights the histiocytic differentiation of the lesional cells. Sequencing revealed mutually exclusive hotspot mutations affecting *KRAS* and *FGFR1* in greater than 80% of cases, which strongly argues for a neoplastic nature.[11] The reason why NOF ceases to grow at some point and completely resolves over time without leaving a trace remains unclear. A similar

mechanism like in fibrous dysplasia in which the lesional cells carrying the *GNAS* mutation get diminished over time by undergoing apoptosis might be a possible explanation.[17]

DIFFERENTIAL DIAGNOSIS

In the appropriate clinical and imaging context, the diagnosis of NOF is usually straightforward. A nearly identical morphology in the jaws can be found in *giant cell granuloma (GCG)*, which is outlined in more detail later discussion. Solid parts of *ABC* can appear similar microscopically but lack the typical radiologic appearance of NOF. In case of doubt, a fluorescence in situ hybridization (FISH) analysis of the *USP6* gene is helpful to support the diagnosis of ABC. Another histologic mimic is GCT with regressive changes, which was formerly believed to represent a distinct lesion designated as *benign fibrous histiocytoma (BFH)*. The histology can appear identical to NOF, but age and the involved sites mirror the distribution of GCT. Immunohistochemical detection of the *H3.3* mutation is an easy way to diagnose or rule out GCT with regressive changes.

SUMMARY AND PROGNOSIS

Surgical pathologists only infrequently encounter NOF in their daily routine because it is only biopsied or curetted in case of (imminent) fracture. The prognosis is excellent, and local recurrences are rare. Malignant transformation has not been described so far. As the *KRAS* and *FGFR1* mutations found in NOF are virtually absent in conventional OS, a relationship between these 2 lesions seems highly unlikely.

CLINICS CARE POINTS

- Most common benign tumor of bone
- Pathognomonic presentation on plain radiographs showing a well-defined, grapelike osteolysis with a sclerotic rim centered in the cortex of the metaphysis of long tubular bones
- Mutations in the MAP kinase signaling pathway drive NOF
- Histologic mimics can be easily ruled out by radiologic correlation and few molecular tests (H3.3, USP6)

GIANT CELL GRANULOMA OF THE JAWS (GCG)

INTRODUCTION

Giant cell granuloma is a benign and sometimes locally aggressive tumor of the jaws; it can develop inside the bone (central giant cell granuloma of the jaws [GCG]) or in the gingival/alveolar mucosa (peripheral GCG). Central GCG most commonly affects patients in the first 2 decades of life and accounts for 10% of all benign tumors of the jaws. The anterior aspects of the mandible (and maxilla) are most frequently involved.[18] Peripheral GCG (synonym giant cell epulis) usually occurs later in life (fifth and sixth decades) and most commonly develops in the mandible.[19]

GCG has long been considered to be of reactive nature, and central GCG has also been referred to as reparative GCG. In the current WHO classification of head and neck tumors published in early 2017, central GCG is defined as a benign "lesion" and peripheral GCG is described to result from chronic irritation. In 2018, Gomes and colleagues,[20] however, discovered recurrent mutations in the MAP kinase signaling pathway in both central and peripheral GCG, strongly arguing in favor of a neoplastic origin.

Imaging Features

Central GCG typically presents as a slowly growing, well-delineated, and expansile osteolysis with cortical thinning (**Fig. 3**D). If large, a multilobulated and/or soap bubble appearance can be

observed. Locally aggressive lesions show cortical penetration and soft tissue infiltration. Tooth resorption or displacements are sometimes evident. Peripheral GCG can erode the underlying bone, which can be visible on radiographs or sectional images.

GROSS AND MICROSCOPIC FEATURES

GCGs have a similar morphology independent of their site of origin. The tissue is brittle and brown with varying amounts of hemorrhage and (pseudo-)cystic change.

Microscopically, GCGs consist of monomorphic and histiocytelike spindle cells arranged in haphazard lobules. Multinucleated giant cells are usually abundant and unevenly distributed throughout the tumor. These cells are rather small (<10 nuclei per tissue section) and cluster around areas of hemorrhage (**Fig. 3**E). The tumor is incompletely subdivided by fibrous septa containing woven bone trabeculae. Secondary changes include accumulation of siderophages, and a thin peripheral rim of reactive new bone formation may be present. Mitotic activity can vary but is usually low. Significant cytologic atypia is not a typical feature of GCG. With the exception of the fibrous septa, the histology is very similar to non-ossifying fibroma (NOF) of the peripheral skeleton.

IMMUNOPHENOTYPE AND MOLECULAR PATHOLOGY FEATURES

Immunohistochemistry is unspecific and not useful. The mononuclear cells express histiocytic markers including CD68 and CD163. Sequencing analyses have revealed recurrent *KRAS* and *FGFR1* mutations, similar to non-ossifying fibroma of bone, in both central and peripheral GCG. In addition, *TRPV4* mutations have been exclusively detected in central GCG (and neither in peripheral GCG nor in NOF so far).[20] This finding is in line with the fact that GCGs can develop in several syndromes, all belonging to the spectrum of RASopathies, including NF1 as well as Noonan, LEOPARD, and Jaffe-Campanacci syndromes. Notably, some patients develop both GCG and NOF. Multiple GCGs point to a syndrome-related pathogenesis.

DIFFERENTIAL DIAGNOSIS

Brown tumors caused by hyperparathyroidism are rare in the Western population but can appear histologically identical to GCGs.

Syndrome-related GCGs are also virtually indistinguishable from sporadic cases and can be the initial presenting symptom. Even in the absence of more specific signs of Noonan syndrome or

NF1, a thorough clinical examination or screening for the relevant germline alterations should be considered, particularly in patients with multiple GCGs. Histologically, some cases show a more prominent spindle cell component with lesser giant cells and a notably storiform pattern of growth without being specific. Lesions tend to reach a considerable size and behave locally aggressive.[21]

Cherubism is a rare benign disease characterized by symmetric enlargement of all 4 quadrants of the jaws. Cherubism is caused by a mutation of the SH3BP2 gene with approximately 50% being inherited in an autosomal dominant trait and 50% arising as de novo mutations. The disease manifests before the age of 6 years and is usually easy to diagnose in the appropriate clinical and imaging contexts. Histologically, however, cherubism appears similar to (syndrome-related) GCG.

ABC is generally characterized by a multicystic architecture composed of blood-filled spaces subdivided by fibrous septa containing multinucleated giant cells. Imaging shows expansile lesions with fluid-fluid levels in MRI. Some ABCs, however, lack the defining cystic appearance and strongly resemble GCGs microscopically; they are referred to as solid ABCs. If this differential diagnosis is considered, USP6 FISH analysis might be helpful to substantiate it.

Conventional GCT practically does not exist in the jaws. Histologically, it shows a higher number and more evenly distributed giant cells that contain more than 50 nuclei per tissue section. *H3-3A* mutations are absent in GCG.

SUMMARY AND PROGNOSIS

Peripheral GCGs are usually excised and recur only infrequently, particularly if the underlying periosteum is included in the excision. Central GCGs are frequently treated by curettage. Recurrence rates differ depending on the aggressiveness of individual lesions.

CLINICS CARE POINTS

- Benign tumors exclusively occurring in the craniofacial skeleton and can be clinically classified as nonaggressive and locally aggressive types
- Sporadic cases are usually solitary and commonly affect the anterior mandible; multiple lesions point to a syndrome-related cause
- Mutations in the MAP kinase signaling cascade drive GCG (*KRAS, FGFR1, TRPV4*)
- Histologic mimics can be ruled out by thorough clinical/imaging correlation and

laboratory tests (parathormone). Molecular tests are rarely needed (*USP6* FISH)

ANEURYSMAL BONE CYST

INTRODUCTION

ABC is another lesion of bone that has originally been assumed to be of reactive nature. In the first 2 editions of the WHO classification, it was listed under the tumorlike lesions; in the third and fourth editions it was listed under the category of tumors of undefined neoplastic nature. The first evidence of underlying genetic rearrangements involving the USP6 gene date back to 1991 and have been described in the WHO blue book since its third edition.[22] However, it is only since the fourth edition published in 2013 that ABC has been defined as a true neoplasm and regarded to be of intermediate biological potential (locally aggressive). In the current and fifth edition, ABC is listed under the osteoclastic giant cell-rich tumors; disputably the editors have revised the biological behavior from locally aggressive to benign.[23]

ABC usually affects children and adolescents; 80% of cases occur in the first 2 decades of life. Typically, the metaphyses of long tubular bones and the posterior elements of the vertebrae are involved; patients present with pain and swellings.

IMAGING FEATURES

Radiologically, ABCs appear expansile, lytic, and eccentric with well-defined margins and commonly a thin shell of reactive bone. Highly aggressive features and periosteal reactions are not typical for ABC, but ill-defined margins, penetration of the cortex, and an extraosseous extension are also possible. MRI highlights fluid-fluid levels that are highly characteristic (**Fig. 4**A); contrast administration primarily shows septal enhancement. Solid components can be present but are usually not predominating and should raise suspicion of other differential diagnoses, including telangiectatic osteosarcoma (TAEOS).

GROSS AND MICROSCOPIC FEATURES

The multicystic architecture of ABC shows blood-filled spaces of varying size that are separated by thin, tan-white septa. Solid areas appear brown and fragile.

Microscopically, the cyst walls are composed of monomorphic and fibroblastlike spindle cells and scattered multinucleated giant cells. Mitotic activity can be brisk, but high-grade atypia and atypical mitoses do not occur in ABC. Both giant cells and mononuclear spindle cells form smooth and

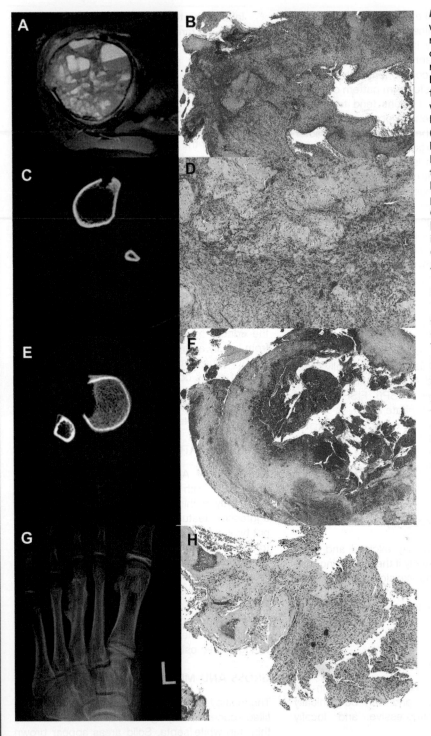

Fig. 4. Different tumors with USP6 rearrangement. Conventional ABC of the right proximal humerus of a 10-year-old boy showing multiple fluid-fluid levels on T2-weighted MRI (A). Histologically, solid and (pseudo-)cystic areas can be distinguished. The lesion contains an immature and reactive new bone formation that appears partly basophilic (so-called blue bone) (B) [hematoxylin-eosin, original magnification, 25x]. CT scans of intracortical ABC in the left tibia of a 19-year-old man (C) and in the right tibia of a 13-year old girl (E) appear lytic and locally aggressive but show a typical morphology of partly solid ABC (D, F) [hematoxylin-eosin, original magnification, 50x]. Juxtacortical ABC in the third metatarsal bone of a 13-year old boy presenting with a broad ossification (G, radiograph). Histologically, only minor parts of the lesion resemble ABC adjacent to abundant and reactive new bone formation (H) [hematoxylin-eosin, original magnification, 50x].

continuous flattened layers that line the (pseudo-) cystic spaces filled by blood and serous fluid (Fig. 4B). Siderophages can be numerous, and reactive new bone formation is another common finding. In at least a third of cases, the woven bone is mineralized in an irregular fashion and appears bluish (so-called blue bone, see Fig. 4B). This peculiar matrix is not specific but a highly characteristic feature of ABC. Necrosis is uncommon if not secondary to pathologic fracture. Solid components show a similar cellular composition.

IMMUNOPHENOTYPE AND MOLECULAR PATHOLOGY FEATURES

Immunohistochemistry of ABC is nonspecific and generally not helpful in the diagnosis. Approximately 70% of ABCs show rearrangements of the *USP6* gene that fuses with various partner genes including *CDH11* (most common, 30% of cases), *THRAP3*, *CNBP*, *OMD*, *COL1A1*, *CTNNB1*, *STAT3*, *FOSL2*, *EIF1*, *SPARC*, *PAFAH1B1*, *USP9X*, and *RUNX2*.[23] The translocations result in upregulation of *USP6* transcription and are only present in the mononuclear spindle cell component. So far individual rearrangements have not been associated with a distinct clinical behavior. Notably, *USP6* rearrangements have not been reported in malignant tumors so far.

DIFFERENTIAL DIAGNOSIS

Various soft tissue, bone, and gnathic tumors can show secondary changes that mimic ABC. This phenomenon has formerly been referred to as *secondary ABC* and is not associated with USP6 rearrangements. As it only represents reactive and nonspecific changes and not a separate entity or a collision tumor, the WHO recommends using the term *ABC-like changes.*

TAEOS is an important differential diagnosis that can mimic ABC. However, in TAEOS there is frank high-grade atypia with pleomorphic high-grade nuclei and usually abundant atypical mitoses. Imaging usually shows more aggressive features and a greater amount of solid areas, but there is an overlap in imaging features with those of ABC. TAEOS does not show *USP6* rearrangements.

In the jaws, solid ABC can virtually be indistinguishable from *GCG*. However, ABC is rather rare in the jaws and usually shows the classic (pseudo-)cystic presentation. Testing for *USP6* rearrangements can help in ambiguous cases.

In the small tubular bones, lesions with a similar histology like GCGs have formerly been classified as *giant cell lesions of the small bones*.[24] As most of those tumors were shown to harbor USP6 rearrangements they are no longer listed in the current WHO classification as a separate entity but considered to constitute solid ABC[25] (**Fig. 5**).

SUMMARY AND PROGNOSIS

ABC is a benign bone tumor usually occurring in children and adolescents. Recurrence rates vary significantly in the literature but probably range between 15% and 30%. Malignant transformation has been described but most likely represented unusual TAEOS; so far, no convincing case of malignant transformation and underlying *USP6* rearrangement has been reported.

CLINICS CARE POINTS

- Benign, expansile, and eccentrically located bone tumor developing in the metaphyses of long tubular bones and the posterior elements of the vertebrae
- Usually well defined and lytic on imaging; can show an (incomplete) sclerotic rim; aggressive imaging features are not typical, but possible; primarily cystic appearance on MRI with characteristic fluid-fluid levels
- *USP6* rearrangements in 70% of cases

OTHER TUMORS OF BONE WITH USP6 REARRANGEMENTS

INTRODUCTION

With increasing molecular testing more and more soft tissue and bone lesions that have formerly been regarded as reactive pseudotumors or tumorlike lesions were shown to harbor recurrent genetic alterations and are now considered true neoplasms. Highly specific findings such as *H3.3* mutations in GCT and chondroblastoma can be extremely helpful in routine diagnostics and often warrant a reliable diagnosis even in smaller core needle biopsies. Other genes are involved in a variety of neoplasms so a mutation or rearrangement itself limits the spectrum of differential diagnoses but is not specific for a distinct lesion per se. Remarkably, several mutations that have been considered the driver genes of highly malignant tumors have recently been shown to also drive benign and sometimes even self-limiting lesions including pathogenic *KRAS* hotspot mutations in non-ossifying fibroma (NOF) and *EWSR1* rearrangements in simple bone cyst.[11,26]

USP6 rearrangements are one prominent example of highly promiscuous alterations occurring in several but so far unequivocally benign neoplasms. The consecutive discovery in distinct lesions caused confusion in the nomenclature prompting the question if a shared molecular alteration is sufficient to assume a direct relation between lesions that otherwise appear distinct from each other. As the first cases of myositis ossificans (MO) were reported to harbor *USP6* rearrangements, those lesions were temporarily suggested to represent *soft tissue variants of ABC,* although clinical and microscopic features were distinct from ABC. In the meantime, it has been increasingly accepted that MO as well as fibro-osseous pseudotumor of digits both belong to the

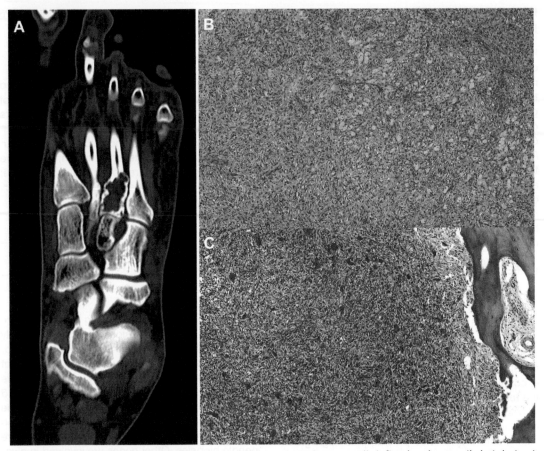

Fig. 5. Solid ABC (former giant cell lesion of the small bones). CT shows a well-defined and expansile lytic lesion in the third right metatarsal of a 29-year-old woman (*A*). Microscopically, the tumor presents uniformly solid with foam cell changes (*B*) [hematoxylin-eosin, original magnification, 50x] and areas resembling giant cell granuloma of the jaws (*C*) [hematoxylin-eosin, original magnification, 50x].

spectrum of *USP6*-related neoplasms.[27,28] The term *solid ABC* is somehow contradictory in itself (as is giant cell tumor without giant cells) but now introduced in the WHO classification to designate lesions in the small tubular bones formerly classified as a separate entity (giant cell lesions of the small bones). ABC can also develop inside and on the surface of cortical bone, which both can appear highly unusual on imaging. USP6-rearranged juxtacortical lesions can cause massive new bone formation and have been designated as *periostitis ossificans*, *periosteal fasciitis*, *juxtacortical ABC*, and *cranial fasciitis*, all with markedly distinct clinical presentation and behavior.[29,30]

IMAGING FEATURES

Intracortical ABCs are usually lytic and well defined but can extend into the adjacent soft tissues (**Fig. 4**C, E). Periosteal reactions sometimes appear aggressive, indicating rapid growth; still,

tumors usually present thin shells of reactive woven bone at their periphery. Solid tumors often reveal homogeneous contrast enhancement prompting a broad spectrum of differential diagnoses. The presentation of lesions developing on the surface of tubular bones varies but can be characterized by abundant new bone formation (**Fig. 4**G, H).

GROSS, MICROSCOPIC, AND MOLECULAR PATHOLOGY FEATURES

The macroscopic and microscopic aspects of USP6-related lesions are mostly similar to ABC or nodular fasciitis. However, secondary changes can predominate and obscure the more characteristic findings. Searching for an *USP6* rearrangement by FISH or RNA sequencing should be considered in unusual intracortical and juxtacortical bone tumors that at least have some resemblance to conventional ABC or nodular fasciitis (**Fig. 4**).

SUMMARY AND PROGNOSIS

The spectrum of USP6-related tumors is increasing and includes rare manifestations at unusual sites. If any peculiar lesion of bone with an underlying *USP6* fusion transcript should be classified as (intracortical, juxtacortical, or solid) ABC will need to be decided as soon as larger series become available and potentially highlight differences in presentation and clinical behavior; currently, only few case reports have been published. In any case, the identification of *USP6* rearrangements appears particularly important because, at least so far, they do not seem to occur in malignant tumors.

CLINICS CARE POINTS

- *USP6*-related neoplasms can show unusual presentation in bone and include solid, intracortical, and surface-related manifestations
- *USP6* rearrangements have not been described in malignant tumors so far
- *USP6* testing is advocated in any lesion of bone that shows at least some morphologic similarity to conventional ABC or nodular fasciitis

ACKNOWLEDGEMENTS

Dr DB was supported by the Swiss National Science Foundation, the Foundation of the Bone Tumor Reference Center, the Gertrude von Meissner Stiftung and the Stiftung für krebskranke Kinder, Regio Basiliensis.

DISCLOSURE

The authors have nothing to disclose.

REFERENCES

1. Flanagan AM, Larousserie F, O'Donnell PG, et al. Giant cell tumour of bone. In: Board WCoTE, editor. WHO classification of tumours, soft tissue and bone tumours. 5th edition. France: IARC Press; 2020. p. 440–6.
2. Al-Ibraheemi A, Inwards CY, Zreik RT, et al. Histologic spectrum of giant cell tumor (GCT) of bone in patients 18 years of age and below: a study of 63 patients. Am J Surg Pathol 2016;40(12):1702–12.
3. Kerr DA, Brcic I, Diaz-Perez JA, et al. Immunohistochemical characterization of giant cell tumor of bone treated with denosumab: support for osteoblastic differentiation. Am J Surg Pathol 2021;45(1):93–100.
4. Treffel M, Lardenois E, Larousserie F, et al. Denosumab-treated giant cell tumors of bone: a clinicopathologic analysis of 35 cases from the French group of bone pathology. Am J Surg Pathol 2020;44(1):1–10.
5. Jain SU, Khazaei S, Marchione DM, et al. Histone H3.3 G34 mutations promote aberrant PRC2 activity and drive tumor progression. Proc Natl Acad Sci U S A 2020;117(44):27354–64.
6. Fittall MW, Lyskjaer I, Ellery P, et al. Drivers underpinning the malignant transformation of giant cell tumour of bone. J Pathol 2020;252(4):433–40.
7. Amary F, Berisha F, Ye H, et al. H3F3A (Histone 3.3) G34W immunohistochemistry: a reliable marker defining benign and malignant giant cell tumor of bone. Am J Surg Pathol 2017;41(8):1059–68.
8. Behjati S, Tarpey PS, Presneau N, et al. Distinct H3F3A and H3F3B driver mutations define chondroblastoma and giant cell tumor of bone. Nat Genet Dec 2013;45(12):1479–82.
9. Presneau N, Baumhoer D, Behjati S, et al. Diagnostic value of H3F3A mutations in giant cell tumour of bone compared to osteoclast-rich mimics. J Pathol Clin Res 2015;1(2):113–23.
10. Lutsik P, Baude A, Mancarella D, et al. Globally altered epigenetic landscape and delayed osteogenic differentiation in H3.3-G34W-mutant giant cell tumor of bone. Nat Commun 2020;11(1): 5414.
11. Baumhoer D, Kovac M, Sperveslage J, et al. Activating mutations in the MAP-kinase pathway define non-ossifying fibroma of bone. J Pathol May 2019; 248(1):116–22.
12. Baumhoer D, Rogozhin DV. Non-ossifying fibroma. In: Board WCoTE, editor. WHO classification of tumours, soft tissue and bone tumours. 5th edition. France: IARC Press; 2020. p. 447–8.
13. Mallet JF, Rigault P, Padovani JP, et al. Non-ossifying fibroma in children: a surgical condition? Chir Pediatr 1980;21(3):179–89. Le fibrome non ossifiant chez l'enfant: une affection chirurgicale?
14. Schajowicz F, Ackerman LV, Sissons HA. Histologic typing of bone tumours. 1st edition WHO international histological classification of tumours. World Health Organization. Berlin: Springer; 1972.
15. Schajowicz F. Histologic typing of bone tumours. 2nd edition WHO international histological classification of tumours. World Health Organization. Berlin: Springer; 1993.
16. Nielsen GP, Kyriakos M. Non-ossifying fibroma/ benign fibrous histiocytoma of bone. In: Fletcher CDM, Bridge J, Hogendoorn PCW, et al, editors. WHO classification of tumours of soft tissue and bone. 4th edition. Lyon, France: IARC Press; 2013. p. 302–4.
17. Kuznetsov SA, Cherman N, Riminucci M, et al. Age-dependent demise of GNAS-mutated skeletal stem cells and "normalization" of fibrous dysplasia of bone. J Bone Miner Res 2008;23(11):1731–40.

18. Raubenheimer E, Jordan RC. Central giant cell granuloma. In: El-Naggar AK, Chan JKC, Grandis JR, et al, editors. WHO classification of head and neck tumours. Lyon, France: IARC Press; 2017. p. 256–7.

19. Raubenheimer E, Jordan RC. Peripheral giant cell granuloma. In: El-Naggar AK, Chan JKC, Grandis JR, et al, editors. WHO classification of head and neck tumours. Lyon, France: IARC Press; 2017. p. 257.

20. Gomes CC, Gayden T, Bajic A, et al. TRPV4 and KRAS and FGFR1 gain-of-function mutations drive giant cell lesions of the jaw. Nat Commun 2018; 9(1):4572.

21. Flanagan AM, Speight PM. Giant cell lesions of the craniofacial bones. Head Neck Pathol 2014;8(4): 445–53.

22. Pfeifer FM, Bridge JA, Neff JR, et al. Cytogenetic findings in aneurysmal bone cysts. Genes Chromosomes Cancer 1991;3(6):416–9.

23. Agaram NP, Bredella MA. Aneurysmal bone cyst. In: Board WCoTE, editor. WHO classification of tumours, soft tissue and bone tumours. 5th edition. Lyon, France: IARC Press; 2020. p. 437–9.

24. Forsyth R, Jundt G. Giant cell lesion of the small bones. In: Fletcher CDM, Bridge J, Hogendoorn PCW, et al, editors. WHO classification of tumours of soft tissue and bone. 4th edition. Lyon, France: IARC Press; 2013. p. 320.

25. Agaram NP, LeLoarer FV, Zhang L, et al. USP6 gene rearrangements occur preferentially in giant cell reparative granulomas of the hands and feet but not in gnathic location. Hum Pathol 2014;45(6): 1147–52.

26. Pizem J, Sekoranja D, Zupan A, et al. FUS-NFATC2 or EWSR1-NFATC2 fusions are present in a large proportion of simple bone cysts. Am J Surg Pathol 2020. https://doi.org/10.1097/PAS.000000000000 1584.

27. Flucke U, Shepard SJ, Bekers EM, et al. Fibro-osseous pseudotumor of digits - Expanding the spectrum of clonal transient neoplasms harboring USP6 rearrangement. Ann Diagn Pathol 2018;35: 53–5.

28. Bekers EM, Eijkelenboom A, Grunberg K, et al. Myositis ossificans - Another condition with USP6 rearrangement, providing evidence of a relationship with nodular fasciitis and aneurysmal bone cyst. Ann Diagn Pathol 2018;34:56–9.

29. Paulson VA, Stojanov IA, Wasman JK, et al. Recurrent and novel USP6 fusions in cranial fasciitis identified by targeted RNA sequencing. Mod Pathol 2020;33(5):775–80.

30. Laaveri M, Heikinheimo K, Baumhoer D, et al. Periosteal fasciitis in a 7-year old girl: a diagnostic dilemma. Int J Oral Maxillofac Surg 2017;46(7): 883–5.

Fibrous and Fibro-Osseous Lesions of Bone

Ivan Chebib, MD[a],*, Connie Y. Chang, MD[b], Santiago Lozano-Calderon, MD, PhD[c]

KEYWORDS

• Fibrous • Fibro-osseous • Fibrous dysplasia • Ossifying fibroma • Desmoplastic fibroma

Key points

- Desmoplastic fibromas are rare tumors comprising bland-appearing fibroblasts without bone formation, morphologically resembling fibromatosis.
- Fibrous dysplasia may involve one (monostotic) or multiple (polyostotic) bones.
- Fibrous dysplasia shows a characteristic mixture of cellular fibroblastic proliferation surrounding woven bone without prominent osteoblasts.
- Cemento-ossifying fibromas are well-circumscribed tumors of the jaw arising from molar or premolar teeth.

ABSTRACT

Fibrous and fibro-osseous tumors are some of the most common benign lesions involving bones. Although many of the histomorphologic features of these tumors overlap significantly, an interdisciplinary approach helps to consolidate the classification of these tumors. Herein, the clinical, radiologic, and pathologic features of lesions within these categories are described.

FIBROUS TUMORS OF BONE

DESMOPLASTIC FIBROMA

Introduction

Desmoplastic fibroma is an uncommon tumor of bone that is morphologically comparable to fibromatosis.[1–4] It is a locally aggressive tumor with a wide age range at presentation but most commonly affects those in the second and third decade. There is no gender predilection. Desmoplastic fibroma most commonly affects the craniofacial skeleton, especially the mandible and long bones. In long bones, they arise in the metaphysis with extension into the diaphysis and less commonly involve the epiphysis as well. Patients typically present with a mass lesion, swelling, deformity, or associated pain secondary to a pathologic fracture.

Radiologic Features

By imaging, desmoplastic fibromas typically show an expansile and osteolytic but well-defined tumor[5–7] (**Fig. 1**). The margins are often nonsclerotic, with the expansion of the native bone by periosteal new bone formation. There is no evidence of a mineralized matrix, but tumors can show thick internal pseudotrabeculae. Cross-sectional imaging may show extension into surrounding soft tissue. By T1-weighted MRI, the tumor shows low signal intensity, with T2-weighted images showing variably increased signal.

Microscopic Features

There are 2 distinctive morphologies that have been classified as desmoplastic fibroma. Those

[a] James Homer Wright Pathology Laboratories, Harvard Medical School, Massachusetts General Hospital, 55 Fruit Street, Boston, MA 02114, USA; [b] Division of Musculoskeletal Imaging, Department of Radiology, Harvard Medical School, Massachusetts General Hospital, 55 Fruit Street, Boston, MA 02114, USA; [c] Department of Orthopaedic Oncology, Harvard Medical School, Massachusetts General Hospital, 55 Fruit Street, Boston, MA 02114, USA
* Corresponding author.
E-mail address: ichebib@mgh.harvard.edu

Surgical Pathology 14 (2021) 707–721
https://doi.org/10.1016/j.path.2021.06.011

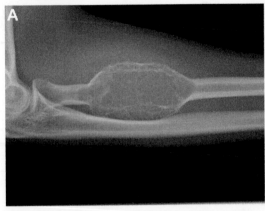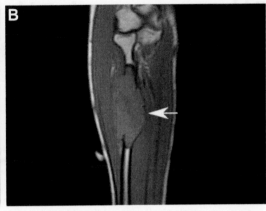

Fig. 1. Desmoplastic fibroma. (*A*) Radiograph of the proximal radius shows a large and expansile mass. (*B*) MRI of the proximal radius shows an expansile mass (*arrow*) with extension into soft tissue.

that show long fascicles of fibroblastic spindle cells have significant morphologic overlap with fibromatosis. However, most desmoplastic fibromas show the haphazard distribution of bland-appearing fibroblasts/myofibroblasts embedded within an abundant collagenous stroma but without a fascicular distribution (**Figs. 2** and **3**). Cellularity may be variable, with areas showing hypercellularity and rare mitotic figures. There is usually no evidence of bone formation except secondarily in tumors with secondary fracture.

Molecular Features

Unlike soft tissue (desmoid-type) fibromatosis, desmoplastic fibromas are only rarely associated with *CTNNB1* (beta-catenin) or *APC* mutations.[8–10] Recurrent amplifications were identified in *COL1A1* and *FGFR2*.[10] Some cases that were

negative for beta-catenin mutations have been shown to express nuclear positivity for beta-catenin by immunohistochemistry (IHC).[8]

Differential Diagnosis

There can be significant overlap between desmoplastic fibroma and low-grade osteosarcoma, which may be dominated by the fibrous stromal component, especially on small biopsy.[11] Significant infiltration of bone or soft tissue is diagnostic of malignancy. Low-grade surface and intramedullary osteosarcomas may harbor *MDM2* amplification that can be identified by fluorescence in situ hybridization and screened for by MDM2 IHC.[12] Soft tissue fibromatosis with the involvement of bone will be nearly impossible to differentiate from desmoplastic fibroma by light microscopy alone. The distinction is clear, however, by reviewing clinical and radiologic features. Fibrous

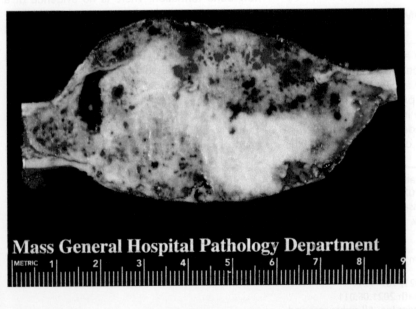

Fig. 2. Desmoplastic fibroma. Gross image shows a white to tan solid expansile mass with thinning and loss of surrounding cortex and areas of hemorrhage.

Mass General Hospital Pathology Department

METRIC   1   2   3   4   5   6   7   8   9

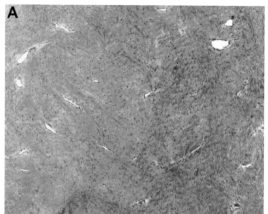 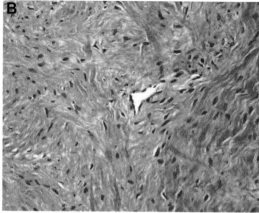

Fig. 3. Desmoplastic fibroma. (*A*) Low-power image shows a fibroblastic proliferation with collagenous matrix and without bone formation (hematoxylin and eosin, original magnification ×100). (*B*) High-power image shows bland spindle cells within densely fibrous stroma (hematoxylin and eosin, original magnification ×400).

dysplasia (FD) may also be difficult to differentiate, especially on small biopsies that fail to capture woven bone deposition. Again, clinical and radiologic features will help differentiate these tumors, as FD typically shows mineralization on imaging and may be polyostotic. Molecular pathology may assist in identifying *GNAS* mutations, characteristic of FD, which is not seen in desmoplastic fibroma. Care must be taken to not overinterpret bone at the edge of desmoplastic fibroma as a fibro-osseous tumor.

Prognosis

Desmoplastic fibroma is a locally aggressive tumor that may recur with incomplete resection or curettage. Wide resection is curative.

Summary

Desmoplastic fibroma is a locally aggressive tumor. By light microscopy, it shows a fibroblastic/myofibroblastic proliferation of spindle cells in a fascicular pattern, with collagenous background and without osteoid matrix production, resembling soft tissue fibromatosis.

Clinics Care Points

- Desmoplastic fibroma is a locally aggressive tumor.
- Two distinct morphologies: those resembling fibromatosis show fascicular fibroblastic/myofibroblastic proliferation; however, most cases show a haphazard population of spindle cells within abundant collagenous stroma without a specific pattern of growth.
- These tumors rarely harbor *CTNNB1* mutations but may express beta-catenin IHC.
- Recently, recurrent amplification of *COL1A1* and *FGFR2* has been described.

FIBRO-OSSEOUS TUMORS OF BONE

FIBROUS DYSPLASIA

Introduction

FD is the prototypical fibro-osseous lesion[13–15] and can either involve a single bone (monostotic) or multiple bones (polyostotic). Sporadic monostotic FD presents equally in men and women and often occurs in pediatric or adolescent patients (10–15 years) but has a wide age range, especially tumors arising proximal to the extremities.[16–18] The most common locations are the long bones, craniofacial skeleton, and ribs. Although many asymptomatic cases are identified incidentally on imaging, most symptomatic patients present with limping, pain, or swelling of the affected extremity, or rarely, pathologic fracture.[17,18]

Polyostotic FD most commonly affects the long bones of the lower extremities, pelvis, and craniofacial bones but is not uncommonly found in the small bones of the hands and feet and rarely the vertebral body.[17] Polyostotic FD involving the proximal femur causes foreshortening secondary to microfractures in the area of the compression zone of the femoral neck, resulting in leg length discrepancy, bowing abnormality, and varus angulation (shepherd's crook deformity)[17] (**Fig. 4**). Craniofacial polyostotic FD is common and associated with facial asymmetry, swelling, and displacement of the orbit.[17] Although polyostotic FD typically follows a benign clinical course, the progression of polyostotic FD may be severely debilitating (**Fig. 5**) and very rarely undergoes malignant transformation to high-grade sarcoma.[17]

There are 2 syndromes associated with polyostotic FD: McCune-Albright syndrome[19,20] and Mazabraud (Henschen-Mazabraud) syndrome.[21,22]

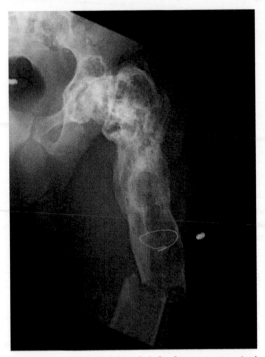

Fig. 4. FD. Radiograph of left femur extensively involved and deformed by FD (shepherd crook deformity) with distal fracture.

McCune-Albright syndrome is associated with mosaic postzygotic somatic activating mutations in *GNAS*.[23] Patients with McCune-Albright syndrome show mucocutaneous pigmentation (café-au-lait spots with irregular borders resembling the "coast of Maine"), endocrine abnormalities (sexual precocity, short stature, goiter, pituitary adenomas, rarely somatotroph [growth hormone producing] pituitary adenoma leading to acromegaly) in association with polyostotic FD.[24,25] Patients with Mazabraud syndrome typically show polyostotic FD and multiple soft tissue myxomas.[26] It is associated with activating *GNAS* mutations as it has sporadic intramuscular myxomas.[27] Tumors arise in older patients, with FD and myxomas identified synchronously or myxomas occurring decades after the initial FD diagnosis (**Fig. 6**).

Radiologic Features

On radiograph and computed tomography (CT) scan, FD appears as circumscribed, intramedullary lesions with radiolucent to ground-glass appearance, smooth borders, and cortical thinning[17,28–34] (**Fig. 7**). There is no periosteal reaction, except in association with pathologic fracture.

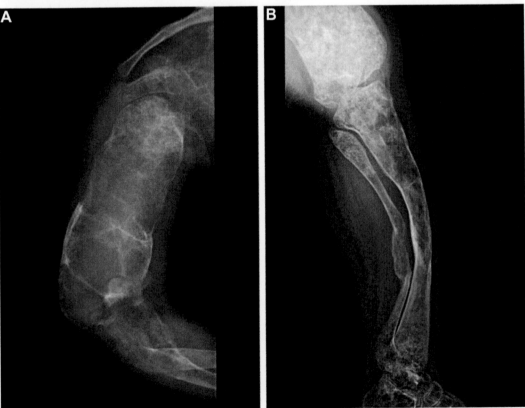

Fig. 5. Polyostotic FD. Extensive involvement and deformity of (*A*) humerus, radius, and ulna as well as (*B*) distal femur, tibia, and fibula.

Fig. 6. Mazabraud syndrome. Patient with intramuscular myxoma involving the right buttock (*white arrow*) and polyostotic FD involving ilium and proximal femur (*black arrows*).

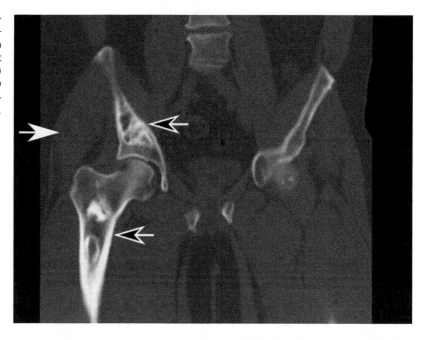

Rarely, tumors may undergo cyst formation. MRI may be more variable with low to intermediate intensity signal on T1-weighted sequences and intermediate to high signal on T2-weighted images, dependent on the extent of ossification. On bone scan, tumors may show increased uptake of radioisotope.[35,36]

Microscopic Features

By light microscopy, FD is composed of uniform, variably cellular, stellate spindle cells arranged in whorling fascicles with intermixed, often interconnected meshwork of woven bone[14–17,37,38] (**Fig. 8**). The spindle cell component resembles fibroblasts/myofibroblasts and lacks atypia and necrosis. Mitoses are rare and never atypical. The amount of bone formation in FD can vary: some tumors are dominated by bone formation, imparting an osteoma-like appearance, whereas others are bone-poor, dominated by the fibrous component. The bone is classically described as curvilinear but may have variable appearance, with areas

Fig. 7. FD. CT chest scan shows polyostotic FD involving the left rib (*white arrow*) and transverse process (*black arrow*).

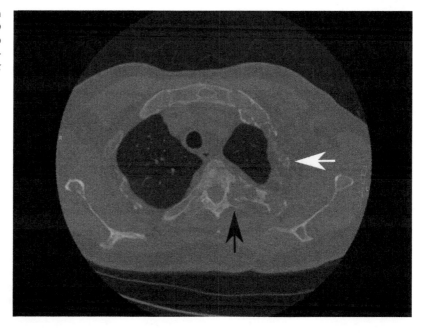

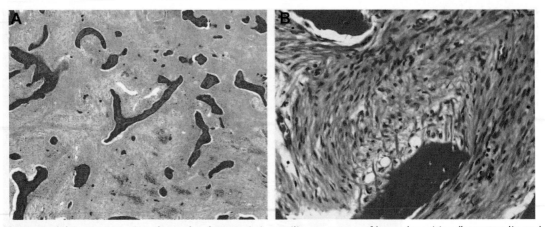

Fig. 8. FD. (*A*) Low-power view shows the characteristic curvilinear pattern of bone deposition (hematoxylin and eosin, original magnification ×100). (*B*) High-power image shows bland proliferation of fibroblastic spindle cells and Sharpey-like fibers. (hematoxylin and eosin, original magnification ×400).

resembling psammomatous calcification (cementoid bodies), lamellar linear arrangement mimicking low-grade central osteosarcoma, or thickened woven bone resembling Paget disease of bone (**Fig. 9**). The neoplastic bone is lined by

inconspicuous flattened "resting" osteoblasts; plump plasmacytoid or epithelioid osteoblasts are rarely present but may be seen in reactive bone formation following a fracture. Sharpey-like fibers are often seen merging between bone

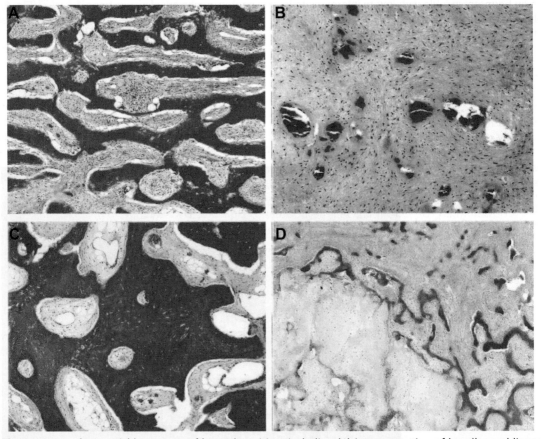

Fig. 9. FD may show variable patterns of bone deposition, including (*A*) interconnection of lamellar and linear bone deposition; (*B*) psammomatoid pattern of bone deposition; (*C*) Pagetoid-pattern of bone deposition; (*D*) FD with chondroid differentiation.

formation and fibrous tissue (**Fig. 10**). Foamy macrophages are present, and rare foci of cartilaginous or fatty differentiation may be found. Secondary aneurysmal bone cystlike changes may be seen.

Malignant transformation occurs in less than 1% of cases[39–42] (**Fig. 11**). The morphology is typically an undifferentiated spindle to pleomorphic sarcoma, with rare transdifferentiation to osteosarcoma, chondrosarcoma, or angiosarcoma.[43,44] These high-grade sarcomas typically arise in patients with severe polyostotic disease or prior exposure to radiation and occur in younger patients than monostotic FD.

Molecular Pathology Features

Originally identified in McCune-Albright syndrome,[45,46] both monostotic and polyostotic syndrome-associated FD have been associated with activating mutations of *GNAS* R201 or, rarely, Q227 (**Fig. 12**).

Differential Diagnosis

Differential diagnoses include other fibro-osseous lesions: ossifying fibromas of the craniofacial bones (**Fig. 13**), osteofibrous dysplasia, or well-differentiated (osteofibrous dysplasia-like) adamantinoma, and low-grade central osteosarcoma. Clinically, the most relevant distinction to make is with well-differentiated osteosarcoma, which typically arises in the distal femur or proximal tibia; histologically, it shows parallel orientation of woven

bone with some cytologic atypia. Identification of tumor infiltration around preexisting trabecular bone is diagnostic of malignancy but unlikely to be present on small biopsies. Therefore, molecular testing has become important to distinguish these entities: FD contains *GNAS* mutations, while low-grade osteosarcoma harbors *MDM2* amplification in most cases.[44–50] Osteofibrous dysplasia and well-differentiated adamantinoma arise in the cortex of the tibia or fibula in children; histologically, there are plump osteoblasts surrounding woven bone. Single or small clusters of keratin-positive spindle cells also help in differentiating these tumors from FD.

Prognosis

FD is a benign tumor and can be followed clinically with serial radiographs to show maturation and ossification. However, if there is an atypical presentation or atypical radiologic features, a biopsy might be necessary to confirm the diagnosis. In cases of mechanical pain secondary to impending or complete pathologic fracture, curettage with allograft packing plus mechanical stabilization with plate and screws or intramedullary rods may be performed. Sarcomas arising in the background of FD are treated as de novo primary bone sarcomas in which resection with negative margins is the primary oncologic goal along with reconstruction with either an allograft, a metallic endoprosthesis, or a combination of the two (alloprosthesis) to restore function. Polyostotic FD and

Fig. 10. FD shows prominent Sharpey-like fibers (*arrow*) (hematoxylin and eosin, original magnification ×400).

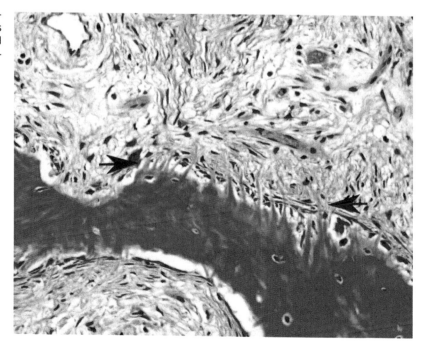

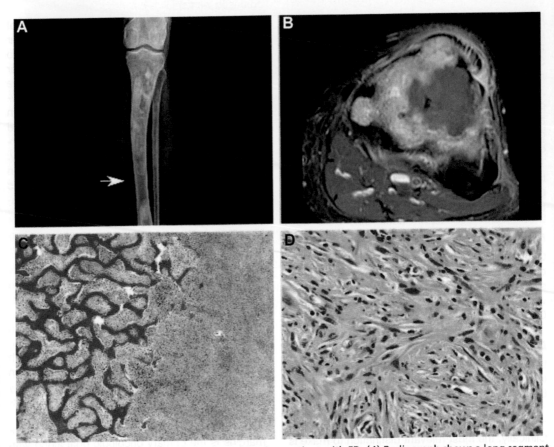

Fig. 11. High-grade undifferentiated sarcoma arising in a patient with FD. (*A*) Radiograph shows a long segment of radius involved by FD with an area of relative lucency (*arrow*). (*B*) MRI shows large mass involving distal tibia with extension into soft tissue. (*C*) Low-power image shows apposition of FD (*left*) and high-grade sarcoma without bone formation (*right*). (*D*) High-power image shows pleomorphic spindle cells without differentiation (hematoxylin and eosin, original magnification ×400).

related syndromes may be locally aggressive, causing structural deformity, fractures, or obstruction of sinonasal or oropharyngeal airways.

Summary

FD is a common tumor of bone with characteristic clinical, radiologic, and pathologic features. It is the quintessential fibro-osseous tumor showing bland spindle cell proliferation surrounding woven bone formation lacking plump osteoblasts. Polyostotic tumors are associated with clinical syndromes: McCune-Albright and Mazabraud syndrome.

Clinics Care Points

- Fibrous dysplasia is a common fibro-osseous tumor of bone.
- Fibrous dysplasia may be mono-ostotic or polyostotic.
- Tumors are composed of cellular but bland-appearing spindle cells surrounding woven bone formation that lacks osteoblastic lining.
- Fibrous dysplasia are associated with *GNAS* mutations.
- McCune-Albright syndrome: FD and endocrinopathies.

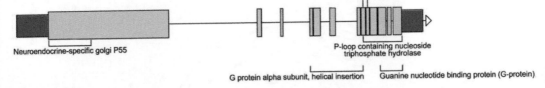

Fig. 12. *GNAS* gene. Most common sites of activating mutations: R201, and less commonly, Q227.

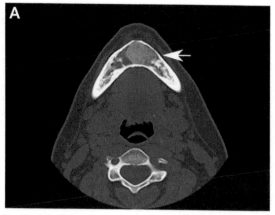

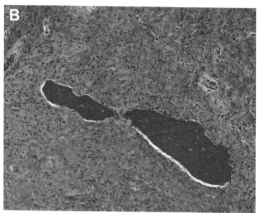

Fig. 13. (*A*) CT face scan shows FD involving the anterior mandible (*arrow*). (*B*) Histologic section of FD involving the mandible. This tumor was originally interpreted as cemento-ossifying fibroma, but on recurrence, it was found to harbor *GNAS* mutation.

- Mazabraud syndrome: FD and intramuscular myxoma.

PROTUBERANT FIBRO-OSSEOUS LESION OF CRANIAL BONES (BULLOUGH LESION)

INTRODUCTION

Protuberant fibro-osseous lesion of the temporal bone is a recently described entity,[51] with only small series and case reports published.[49,50,52–55] They present as protuberant surface lesions, originally described in temporal bone and more recently the occipital bone.[52] The age distribution is wide (18–71 years), and the published reports have predominantly been of female patients.

RADIOLOGIC FEATURES

On imaging, these lesions show a heterogeneously ossified mass protruding from the outer cortex without the involvement of the medullary cavity.

MICROSCOPIC FEATURES

Histologically, this lesion is composed of hypocellular dense fibrous tissue with discrete ovoid islands of lamellar or woven bone, which may show osteoblastic rimming (**Fig. 14**). There is often Sharpey fiber-like extension of collagen fibers from the osseous component.

DIFFERENTIAL DIAGNOSIS

Differential diagnosis may include low-grade parosteal (surface) osteosarcoma, FD, and osteoma. Low-grade parosteal osteosarcoma only exceptionally affects the craniofacial bones and shows a hypercellular stromal component with cytologic atypia of tumor cells and deposition neoplastic

bone often in a layered pattern. They are MDM2 positive by IHC and show *MDM2* amplification. FD is an intramedullary expansile mass and has only rarely been described to expand beyond the cortical surface (FD protuberans).[56] Osteoma typically shows dense bone deposition with only scant loose fibrovascular tissue.

PROGNOSIS

Protuberant fibro-osseous lesions of cranial bones are benign.

SUMMARY

Protuberant fibro-osseous lesions of the cranial bones are rare fibro-osseous tumors comprising hypocellular fibrous tissue and islands of lamellar and woven bone, most often arising from the temporal bone.

CLINICS CARE POINTS

- Protuberant fibro-osseous lesions of the cranial bones are rare fibro-osseous tumors that arise on the temporal or occipital bones.
- Tumors are composed of a hypocellular population of spindle cells and islands of lamellar or woven bone.

FIBRO-OSSEOUS LESIONS OF THE ODONTOGENIC/GNATHIC AND CRANIOFACIAL SKELETON

CEMENTO-OSSIFYING FIBROMA

Introduction

Cemento-ossifying fibroma (ossifying fibroma) occurs in the third and fourth decade of life.[57–59] It

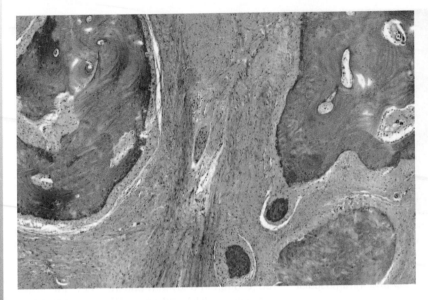

Fig. 14. Protuberant fibro-osseous lesion of the cranial bones. Histologic section shows moderately cellular stroma with variably rounded bone deposition (hematoxylin and eosin, original magnification ×100).

occurs most commonly in the mandible and is associated with the molar or premolar teeth, likely arising from the periodontal ligament of the mandible.

Radiologic Features

By imaging, it is a circumscribed unilocular or multilocular radiolucent lesion (**Fig. 15**).

Gross Features

The tumors lack infiltration and can often be shelled out entirely as a single fragment.

Microscopic Features

By histology, it is composed of bland fibroblast-like spindle cells within a fibrous stroma in association with woven bone, lamellar bone, or spheroid/rounded (cementoid) bone deposition (**Fig. 16**). Similar to FD, thick bony trabeculae may resemble Paget disease of bone. The bony component shows a rim of plump osteoblasts in less than 50% of the cases.

Differential Diagnosis

The main differential diagnosis is craniofacial FD; the presence of plump osteoblasts lining woven

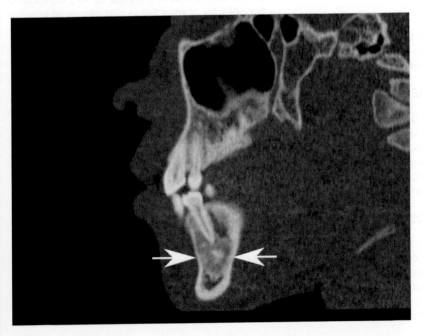

Fig. 15. Cemento-ossifying fibroma. Sagittal CT scan shows a well-circumscribed lesion (*arrow*) of the mandible arising at the root of premolar tooth.

Fig. 16. Cemento-ossifying fibroma. Histologically tumor is composed of bland-appearing spindle cells and woven bone deposition with prominent osteoblasts (hematoxylin and eosin, original magnification ×200).

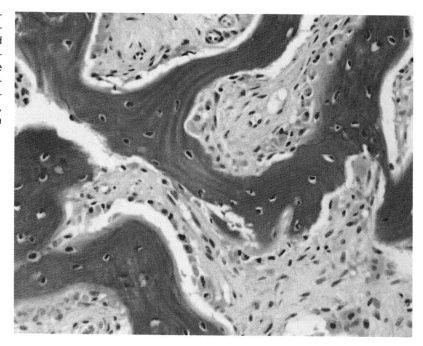

bone and a circumscribed tumor at the base of molar or premolar teeth is characteristic of cemento-ossifying fibroma. Cases can have significant morphologic overlap, and the presence of *GNAS* mutation or extragnathic polyostotic involvement helps confirm FD.

Prognosis

They may recur, however, in up to 30% of patients.

Summary

Cemento-ossifying fibromas are benign fibro-osseous tumors arising most commonly in the mandible, associated with the molar or premolar teeth. They show variably cellular spindle cells surrounding bone formation with prominent osteoblastic rimming.

Clinics Care Points

- Cemento-ossifying fibroma is a fibro-osseous tumor arising in the maxilla or mandible, associated with molar or premolar teeth.
- They most commonly arise in the third and fourth decade.
- Tumors are often circumscribed and shelled out in a single fragment/piece.
- Histology shows variably cellular spindle cells and woven bone formation, sometimes showing plump osteoblastic rimming.

JUVENILE OSSIFYING FIBROMA

Introduction

There are 2 distinct subtypes of juvenile ossifying fibroma: trabecular and psammomatoid subtypes.

Trabecular juvenile ossifying fibroma (TJOF) is an expansile tumor of bone of the facial skeleton that can sometimes undergo rapid and aggressive growth.[60–63] It occurs in variable locations, including molar/premolar mandible/maxilla, maxillary sinus, and less commonly, within the nasal cavity. It occurs most commonly in pediatric and adolescent age groups. Often asymptomatic, its locally aggressive growth may lead to sinonasal obstruction or deformity.

Psammomatoid juvenile ossifying fibroma (PJOF) typically occurs in the first 2 decades of life but has a wide age range.[60,63–65] It arises most commonly in the orbital and sinonasal bones, and less commonly in the maxilla, mandible, and the calvarium. Patients typically present with a painless mass lesion or sinonasal obstruction.

Radiologic Features

By imaging, TJOF has well-defined margins showing mixed radiolucent areas and foci of mineralization, with unilocular or multilocular architecture. Radiologically, PJOF tumors can have a variable appearance from radiolucent to radiodense areas, including some with ground-glass appearance resembling FD (**Fig. 17**).

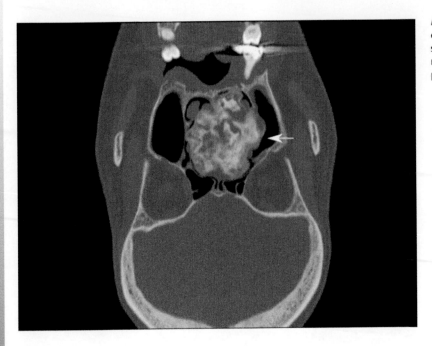

Fig.   17. Psammomatoid ossifying fibroma. CT head scan shows a large sino-nasal mass (*arrow*) with prominent mineralization.

Microscopic Features

Histologically, TJOF is circumscribed and unen-capsulated, composed of cellular proliferation of fibroblast-like spindle cells with scant collagen deposition. There is a prominent deposition of woven bone in an anastomosing trabeculae pattern. Some have suggested that there may be focal infiltration at the periphery of the tumor,[63] but care should be taken to rule out low-grade os-teosarcoma. Multinucleated osteoclast-like giant cells are common.

PJOF shows proliferation of spherical osteoid and woven bone with a cellular spindle cell stroma (**Fig. 18**). Larger cystic areas with hemorrhage and osteoclast-like giant cells may be present, resem-bling aneurysmal bone cyst.

Molecular Pathology Features

Nearly 70% of juvenile ossifying fibroma (trabec-ular and psammomatoid variants) were found to harbor *MDM2* amplification by quantitative poly-merase chain reaction, although none showed MDM2 overexpression by IHC.[66] The degree of *MDM2* amplification (3- to 13-fold) was less than the range seen in low-grade osteosarcoma (3- to 21-fold) and well-dedifferentiated liposarcomas (3- to 40-fold). In fibro-osseous tumors harboring *MDM2*-amplification, this study also identified

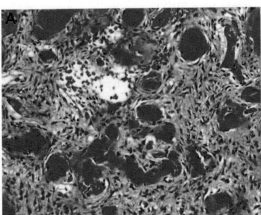
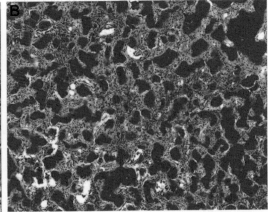

Fig. 18. Psammomatoid ossifying fibroma. Low- (*A*) and high-power (*B*) images show a bland but cellular spindle cell proliferation associated with very characteristic psammomatoid/spherical osteoid deposition.

amplification of *RASAL1*, suggesting relatively large rearrangements of chromosome 12.

Differential Diagnosis

Differentiating TJOF from cemento-ossifying fibroma is usually straightforward as cemento-ossifying fibroma occurs in adult patients, predominantly in the molar/premolar location. Unlike cemento-ossifying fibroma, TJOF cannot be easily shelled out.

Differentiating PJOF from cemento-ossifying fibroma, especially those with spheroid bone deposition, may be difficult. However, an extra-gnathic tumor in a young patient would be characteristic of PJOF. FD not uncommonly affects the craniofacial and sinonasal skeleton and may also have a psammomatoid pattern of bone deposition. In polyostotic cases, FD is favored. In difficult cases, the identification of *GNAS* mutations would be definitive. In tumors involving the calvarium, the differential may include psammomatous meningioma, which is highlighted by epithelial membrane antigen (EMA) and progesterone receptor (PR) IHC.

Prognosis

TJOF and PJOF may locally recur in up to 50% of patients.

Summary

TJOF and PJOF are benign tumors of pediatric patients, although the age range may be wide. PJOF typically arises in extragnathic cranial facial bones, most commonly orbital or sinonasal bones. Histology shows a fibro-osseous lesion composed of fibroblasts and woven bone formation arranged in either trabecular or psammomatoid architecture.

Clinics Care Points

- Trabecular juvenile ossifying fibroma is a locally aggressive fibro-osseous tumor of young patients, most commonly arising in the maxilla and mandible.
- Histomorphology shows a mixture of bland spindle cells and woven bone in an interconnected trabecular pattern.
- Psammomatoid juvenile ossifying fibroma is a locally aggressive fibro-osseous tumor of young patients but with a wide age range, most commonly arising in extragnathic bones, such as orbit and sinonasal.
- Histomorphology shows a mixture of bland spindle cells and woven bone with prominent psammomatoid appearance.

DISCLOSURE

The authors have nothing to disclose.

REFERENCES

1. Rabhan W, Rosai J. Desmoplastic fibroma. Report of ten cases and review of the literature. J Bone Joint Surg 1968;50:487–502.
2. Bertoni F, Calderoni P, Bacchini P, et al. Desmoplastic fibroma of bone. A report of six cases. J Bone Joint Surg Br 1984;66:265–8.
3. Gebhardt M, Campbell C, Schiller A, et al. Desmoplastic fibroma of bone. A report of eight cases and review of the literature. J Bone Joint Surg Am 1985;67:732–47.
4. Inwards CY, Unni KK, Beabout JW, et al. Desmoplastic fibroma of bone. Cancer 1991;68:1978–83.
5. Taconis WK, Schütte HE, van der Heul RO. Desmoplastic fibroma of bone: a report of 18 cases. Skeletal Radiol 1994;23:283–8.
6. Crim JR, Gold RH, Mirra JM, et al. Desmoplastic fibroma of bone: radiographic analysis. Radiology 1989;172:827–32.
7. Frick MA, Sundaram M, Unni KK, et al. Imaging findings in desmoplastic fibroma of bone: distinctive T2 characteristics. AJR Am J Roentgenol 2005;184: 1762–7.
8. Hauben EI, Jundt G, Cleton-Jansen A-M, et al. Desmoplastic fibroma of bone: an immunohistochemical study including β-catenin expression and mutational analysis for β-catenin. Hum Pathol 2005;36:1025–30.
9. Horvai A E, Jordan R C. Fibro-osseous lesions of the craniofacial bones: β-catenin immunohistochemical analysis and CTNNB1 and APC mutation analysis. Head Neck Pathol 2014;8:291–7.
10. Cho S, Bean G, Charville G, et al. Molecular genetics of desmoplastic fibroma of bone. Mod Pathol 2020;33:174–239.
11. Song W, van den Berg E, Kwee TC, et al. Low-grade central fibroblastic osteosarcoma may be differentiated from its mimicker desmoplastic fibroma by genetic analysis. Clin Sarcoma Res 2018;8. https://doi.org/10.1186/s13569-018-0104-z.
12. Habeeb O, Cates J, Kilpatrick S, et al. Molecular and immunohistochemical reappraisal of desmoplastic fibromas reveals a subset of misclassified low-grade central osteosarcomas. Mod Pathol 2020;33: 174–239.
13. WHO Classification of Tumours Editorial Board. WHO classification of tumours of soft tissue and bone. 5th edition. Lyon (France): IARC Press; 2020. Available at: https://publications.iarc.fr/Book-And-Report-Series/Who-Classification-Of-Tumours/Soft-Tissue-And-Bone-Tumours-2020. Accessed June 2, 2020.
14. Lichtenstein L. Polyostotic fibrous dysplasia. Arch Surg 1938;36:874–98.

15. Liechtenstein L, Jaffe H. Fibrous dysplasia of bone: conditions affecting one, several or many bones, graver cases of which may present abnormal pigmentation of skin, premature sexual development, hyperthyroidism, and still other extra-skeletal abnormalities. Arch Patol 1942;33:777–816.

16. Schlumberger HG. Fibrous dysplasia of single bones (monostotic fibrous dysplasia). Mil Surg 1946;99:504–27.

17. Harris W, Dudley H, Barry R. The natural history of fibrous dysplasia: an orthopaedic, pathological, and roentgenographic study. J Bone Joint Surg 1962;44:207–33.

18. Henry A. Monostotic fibrous dysplasia. J Bone Joint Surg Br 1969;51-B:300–6.

19. McCune D. Osteitis fibrosa cystica: the case of a nine year old girl who also exhibits precocious puberty, multiple pigmentation of the skin and hyperthyroidism. Am J Dis Child 1936;52:743–4.

20. Albright F, Butler AM, Hampton AO, et al. Syndrome characterized by osteitis fibrosa disseminata, areas of pigmentation and endocrine dysfunction, with precocious puberty in females. N Engl J Med 1937;216:727–46.

21. Henschen F. Fall von Ostitis fibrosa mit multiplen Tumoren in der umgebenden Muskulatur. Verh Dtsch Ges Pathol 1926;21:93–7.

22. Mazabraud A, Semat P, Roze R. [Apropos of the association of fibromyxomas of the soft tissues with fibrous dysplasia of the bones]. Presse Med 1967; 75:2223–8.

23. McCune-Albright syndrome - conditions - GTR - NCBI. Available at: https://www-ncbi-nlm-nih-gov/gtr/conditions/C0242292/. Accessed April 20, 2020.

24. McCune-Albright syndrome. Genetics home reference. Available at: https://ghr.nlm.nih.gov/condition/mccune-albright-syndrome. Accessed April 20, 2020.

25. Boyce AM, Collins MT. Fibrous dysplasia/McCune-Albright syndrome: a rare, mosaic disease of $G\alpha$ s activation. Endocr Rev 2020;41:345–70.

26. Zoccali C, Teori G, Prencipe U, et al. Mazabraud's syndrome: a new case and review of the literature. Int Orthop 2009;33:605–10.

27. Okamoto S, Hisaoka M, Ushijima M, et al. Activating Gs(alpha) mutation in intramuscular myxomas with and without fibrous dysplasia of bone. Virchows Arch 2000;437:133–7.

28. Gibson MJ, Middlemiss JH. Fibrous dysplasia of bone. Br J Radiol 1971;44:1–13.

29. Utz JA, Kransdorf MJ, Jelinek JS, et al. MR appearance of fibrous dysplasia. J Comput Assist Tomogr 1989;13:845–51.

30. Norris MA, Kaplan PA, Pathria M, et al. Fibrous dysplasia: magnetic resonance imaging appearance at 1.5 Tesla. Clin Imaging 1990;14:211–5.

31. Kransdorf MJ, Moser RP, Gilkey FW. Fibrous dysplasia. RadioGraphics 1990;10:519–37.

32. Jee WH, Choi KH, Choe BY, et al. Fibrous dysplasia: MR imaging characteristics with radiopathologic correlation. AJR Am J Roentgenol 1996;167:1523–7.

33. Bousson V, Rey-Jouvin C, Laredo J-D, et al. Fibrous dysplasia and McCune–Albright syndrome: imaging for positive and differential diagnoses, prognosis, and follow-up guidelines. Eur J Radiol 2014;83: 1828–42.

34. Kinnunen A-R, Sironen R, Sipola P. Magnetic resonance imaging characteristics in patients with histopathologically proven fibrous dysplasia—a systematic review. Skeletal Radiol 2020. https://doi.org/10.1007/s00256-020-03388-x.

35. Machida K, Makita K, Nishikawa J, et al. Scintigraphic manifestation of fibrous dysplasia. Clin Nucl Med 1986;11:426–9.

36. Johns WD, Gupta SM, Kayani N. Scintigraphic evaluation of polyostotic fibrous dysplasia. Clin Nucl Med 1987;12:627–31.

37. Sakamoto A, Oda Y, Iwamoto Y, et al. A comparative study of fibrous dysplasia and osteofibrous dysplasia with regard to expressions of c-fos and c-jun products and bone matrix proteins: a clinicopathologic review and immunohistochemical study of c-fos, c-jun, type I collagen, osteonectin, osteopontin, and osteocalcin. Hum Pathol 1999;30:1418–26.

38. Maki M, Saitoh K, Horiuchi H, et al. Comparative study of fibrous dysplasia and osteofibrous dysplasia: histopathological, immunohistochemical, argyrophilic nucleolar organizer region and DNA ploidy analysis. Pathol Int 2001;51:603–11.

39. Schwartz DTMD, Alpert MMD. The malignant transformation of fibrous dysplasia. J Med Sci 1964; 247:1–20.

40. Huvos AG, Higinbotham NL, Miller TR. Bone sarcomas arising in fibrous dysplasia. J Bone 1972; 54:1047–56.

41. Yabut SM, Kenan S, Sissons HA, et al. Malignant transformation of fibrous dysplasia. A case report and review of the literature. Clin Orthop Relat Res 1988;(228):281–9.

42. Ruggieri P, Sim FH, Bond JR, et al. Malignancies in fibrous dysplasia. Cancer 1994;73:1411–24.

43. Fukuroku J, Kusuzaki K, Murata H, et al. Two cases of secondary angiosarcoma arising from fibrous dysplasia. Anticancer Res 1999;19:4451–7.

44. Eguchi K, Ishi S, Sugiura H, et al. Angiosarcoma of the chest wall in a patient with fibrous dysplasia. Eur J Cardiothorac Surg 2002;22:654–5.

45. Weinstein LS, Shenker A, Gejman PV, et al. Activating mutations of the stimulatory G protein in the McCune-Albright syndrome. N Engl J Med 1991; 325:1688–95.

46. Schwindinger WF, Francomano CA, Levine MA. Identification of a mutation in the gene encoding

the alpha subunit of the stimulatory G protein of adenylyl cyclase in McCune-Albright syndrome. Proc Natl Acad Sci U S A 1992;89:5152–6.

47. Yoshida A, Ushiku T, Motoi T, et al. Immunohistochemical analysis of MDM2 and CDK4 distinguishes low-grade osteosarcoma from benign mimics. Mod Pathol 2010;23:1279–88.

48. Dujardin F, Binh MBN, Bouvier C, et al. MDM2 and CDK4 immunohistochemistry is a valuable tool in the differential diagnosis of low-grade osteosarcomas and other primary fibro-osseous lesions of the bone. Mod Pathol 2011;24:624–37.

49. Sia SF, Fung S, Davidson AS, et al. Protuberant fibro-osseous lesion of the temporal bone: "Bullough lesion. Am J Surg Pathol 2010;34:1217–23.

50. Lee M, Song JS, Chun S-M, et al. Protuberant fibro-osseous lesions of the temporal bone: two additional case reports. Am J Surg Pathol 2014;38:1510–5.

51. Selesnick SH, Desloge RB, Bullough PG. Protuberant fibro-osseous lesions of the temporal bone: a unique clinicopathologic diagnosis. Am J Otol 1999;20:394–6.

52. Sato N, Aoki T, Mukai N, et al. Protuberant fibro-osseous lesion of the skull: two cases with occipital lesions. Virchows Arch 2017;470:717–20.

53. Jiang B, Mushlin H, Zhang L, et al. Bullough's bump: unusual protuberant fibro-osseous tumor of the temporal bone. Case report. J Neurosurg Pediatr 2018;21:107–11.

54. Maroun CA, Khalifeh I, Faddoul DS, et al. A patient with a protuberant fibro-osseous lesion of the temporal bone. J Craniofac Surg 2019;30:e453–4.

55. Sturdà C, Rapisarda A, Gessi M, et al. Bullough's lesion: an unexpected diagnosis after the resection of a slowly growing osseous-like retroauricular bump-case report and review of the literature. World Neurosurg 2019;122:372–5.

56. Dorfman HD, Ishida T, Tsuneyoshi M. Exophytic variant of fibrous dysplasia (fibrous dysplasia protuberans). Hum Pathol 1994;25:1234–7.

57. Hamner JE, Scofield HH, Col JC Lt. Benign fibro-osseous jaw lesions of periodontal membrane origin. An analysis of 249 cases. Cancer 1968;22:861–78.

58. Waldron CA, Giansanti JS. Benign fibro-osseous lesions of the jaws: a clinical-radiologic-histologic review of sixty-five cases: part II. Benign fibro-osseous lesions of periodontal ligament origin. Oral Surg Oral Med Oral Pathol 1973;35:340–50.

59. Eversole LR, Leider AS, Nelson K. Ossifying fibroma: a clinicopathologic study of sixty-four cases. Oral Surg Oral Med Oral Pathol 1985;60:505–11.

60. Makek M. 7. Pathological and clinical characteristics of the proposed new entities. Clin Pathol Fibro Osteo Cemental Lesions Cranio-Facial Jaw Bones 1983;105–211. https://doi.org/10.1159/000185256.

61. Slootweg PJ, Panders AK, Koopmans R, et al. Juvenile ossifying fibroma. An analysis of 33 cases with emphasis on histopathological aspects. J Oral Pathol Med 1994;23:385–8.

62. Williams HK, Mangham C, Speight PM. Juvenile ossifying fibroma. An analysis of eight cases and a comparison with other fibro-osseous lesions. J Oral Pathol Med 2000;29:13–8.

63. El-Mofty S. Psammomatoid and trabecular juvenile ossifying fibroma of the craniofacial skeleton: two distinct clinicopathologic entities. Oral Surg Oral Med Oral Pathol Oral Radiol Endod 2002;93:296–304.

64. Johnson LC, Yousefi M, Vinh TN, et al. Juvenile active ossifying fibroma. Its nature, dynamics and origin. Acta Otolaryngol Suppl 1991;488:1–40.

65. Wenig BM, Vinh TN, Smirniotopoulos JG, et al. Aggressive psammomatoid ossifying fibromas of the sinonasal region: a clinicopathologic study of a distinct group of fibro-osseous lesions. Cancer 1995;76:1155–65.

66. Tabareau-Delalande F, Collin C, Gomez-Brouchet A, et al. Chromosome 12 long arm rearrangement covering MDM2 and RASAL1 is associated with aggressive craniofacial juvenile ossifying fibroma and extracranial psammomatoid fibro-osseous lesions. Mod Pathol 2015;28:48–56.

Osteofibrous Dysplasia and Adamantinoma

Alessandra F. Nascimento, MD[a], Scott E. Kilpatrick, MD[b], John D. Reith, MD[b],*

KEYWORDS

- Osteofibrous dysplasia • Adamantinoma • OFD-like adamantinoma
- Dedifferentiated adamantinoma

Key points

- Osteofibrous dysplasia is a benign fibro-osseous neoplasm easily confused with fibrous dysplasia; careful radiographic correlation is key to separating these entities.
- Osteofibrous dysplasia-like adamantinoma can be difficult to differentiate from osteofibrous dysplasia, particularly when sampling is limited.
- The judicious use of keratin immunostains is often necessary to identify the scattered nests of epithelial cells that characterize osteofibrous dysplasia-like adamantinoma. Treatment for this variant of adamantinoma remains controversial.
- Classic adamantinoma is a biphasic malignant neoplasm with a range of histologic appearances and fully capable of metastasizing.
- The spindled variant may closely resemble synovial sarcoma; indeed, some reported examples of this variant have proven to be intraosseous synovial sarcoma.

ABSTRACT

For decades, the diagnosis, treatment, and even pathogenesis of the osteofibrous dysplasia/osteofibrous dysplasia-like adamantinoma/classic adamantinoma spectrum of neoplasms have been controversial. Herein, we discuss and illustrate the radiographic and histologic spectrum, differential diagnoses, unifying chromosomal and molecular abnormalities, and current controversies and treatment recommendations for each entity.

OSTEOFIBROUS DYSPLASIA

Osteofibrous dysplasia (OFD) is a benign fibro-osseous neoplasm, originally described by Frangenheim in 1921 as congenital osteitis fibrosa.[1] Other names applied to this entity, which are no longer recommended, include congenital fibrous dysplasia (FD) and ossifying fibroma of long bones.[2,3] The term 'osteofibrous dysplasia of the tibia and fibula' was first coined by Campanacci in 1976.[4]

OFD is a disease of young patients, typically arising within the anterior cortex of the diaphyseal region of the tibia and/or fibula.[5,6] Occasionally, lesions also involve the metaphyses of these bones as well.[5] The vast majority of patients diagnosed with OFD are within the first and second decades of life, and males and females seem to be affected equally.[5,6] The most common clinical presentation is pain, reported in 25% to 50% of patients, followed by pathologic fracture and bony (bowing) deformities.[5,6]

RADIOGRAPHIC FEATURES

Radiologically, OFD presents as a single or multiple, variably sized, sharply marginated radiolucencies within the cortex of the tibia and/or

[a] Department of Pathology, University Hospitals Cleveland Medical Center, 11100 Euclid Avenue, Cleveland, OH 44106, USA; [b] Department of Pathology, L25, Cleveland Clinic, 9500 Euclid Avenue, Cleveland, OH 44195, USA
* Corresponding author.
E-mail address: reithj2@ccf.org

Surgical Pathology 14 (2021) 723–735
https://doi.org/10.1016/j.path.2021.06.012

fibula, with a surrounding sclerotic rim (**Fig. 1**). An anterior bowing deformity and/or pathologic fracture may be observed in large, more extensive lesions.[5] However, soft tissue extension is not present, and intramedullary involvement is unusual.[5] Individual lesions often have an internal density similar to FD. A computed tomography scan and MRI are useful for confirming the intracortical location of the lesion. Scintigraphy typically shows intense uptake of radioisotope. There may be considerable overlap in the imaging features between OFD and OFD-like adamantinoma (ADA).

GROSS FEATURES

On macroscopic examination, OFD is an exclusively intracortical lesion with a tan–gray, solid cut surface and a gritty consistency. The periosteum is intact, and the surrounding cortical bone is usually sclerotic and thickened. Intramedullary involvement is not typically seen.

MICROSCOPIC FEATURES

OFD is a well-demarcated, benign fibro-osseous neoplasm characterized by relatively small woven bone trabeculae, often associated with a distinct zoning pattern, with more mature lamellar bone peripherally, all deposited in a loose fibrous stroma (**Fig. 2**A). The lesional spindle cells are arranged in a storiform pattern or short fascicles and show elongated nuclei with tapered ends, vesicular chromatin, inconspicuous nucleoli, and pale eosinophilic cytoplasm with indistinct cell borders (**Fig. 2**B). There is no significant nuclear atypia, necrosis, or mitotic activity. Small immature and irregularly shaped, woven bone trabeculae, rimmed by benign-appearing plump osteoblasts, are distributed haphazardly (**Fig. 2**C). Occasional osteoclast-like giant cells may be present. Secondary aneurysmal bone cyst, intralesional hemorrhage, and hyaline cartilage are not features of this tumor.

Immunohistochemical stains are of little utility for confirming the diagnosis of OFD, but can be useful for excluding other entities in the differential diagnosis (as discussed elsewhere in this article). Scattered individual keratin-positive spindled stromal cells are frequently observed (**Fig. 3**). Pancytokeratins (AE1/AE3) and basal cell type keratins (CK14 and CK19) are more often expressed.[6] Importantly, no keratin-positive cellular nests or clusters should be seen in OFD, helping to separate OFD from ADA.

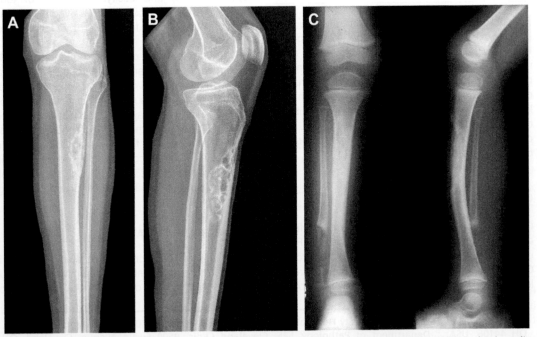

Fig. 1. Radiographic appearance of OFD. (*A, B*) Posteroanterior and lateral radiographs show multiple radiolucent lesions with surrounding sclerotic bone involving the anterolateral tibial cortex of a skeletally mature patient. (*C*) Posteroanterior and lateral radiographs demonstrate concomitant lesions in the tibia and fibula of a skeletally immature patient. The extensive tibial lesion results in an anterior bowing deformity.

Fig. 2. Histologic features of OFD. (*A*) Low power view demonstrating a fibro-osseous lesion merging with the cortex (hematoxylin and eosin stain). (*B*) At medium power, woven bone trabeculae near the cortex demonstrate prominent osteoblastic rimming (hematoxylin and eosin stain).

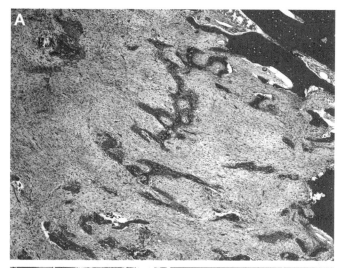

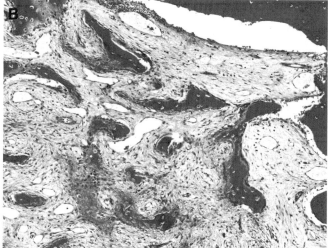

DIFFERENTIAL DIAGNOSIS

The differential diagnosis of OFD is fairly limited and relies heavily on clinical and radiologic findings. The main entities that should be considered in the differential diagnosis include FD, osteoid osteoma and osteoblastoma, and OFD-like ADA. Classic ADA, as discussed elsewhere in this article, is characterized by obvious nests and anastomosing groups of epithelial cells that are easily recognized on conventional hematoxylin and eosin stains; therefore, the distinction between OFD and classic ADA is often straightforward, provided the sample is representative.

FD is also a benign fibro-osseous neoplasm occurring over a wide age range. The femur and craniofacial bones are the most common sites for this tumor; however, any bone can be involved.

In sharp contrast with OFD, FD arises within the medullary canal. Histologically, FD is also composed of a bland fibrous stromal proliferation admixed with randomly distributed woven bone. However, rimming of the bony trabeculae by osteoblasts, a prominent feature in OFD, is less commonly seen in FD, and the keratin–immunoreactive stromal cells of OFD are never observed in FD. Unlike OFD, nodules of benign hyaline cartilage may be present in a subset of FD cases, so-called fibrocartilaginous dysplasia. Finally, FD is characterized at the molecular level by activating missense mutations in *GNAS*, which have not been identified in OFD.[7]

Osteoid osteoma and osteoblastoma are bone-forming neoplasms that often involve the cortex of the long bones of the lower extremity. Other typical

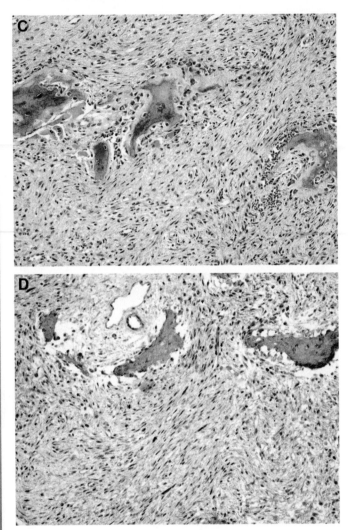

Fig. 2. (*continued*). (*C*) High magnification view shows haphazardly arranged trabeculae of woven bone rimmed by prominent osteoblasts. Osteoclasts and the bland fibrous stroma are evident (hematoxylin and eosin stain). (*D*) An immunostain for cytokeratin AE1/3 is immunoreactive in scattered spindled stromal cells, and no epithelial nests are present.

locations include the femur and spine. Osteoid osteoma and osteoblastoma share nearly identical histologic features, the distinction between them made primarily based on the size of the lesion and more often intramedullary involvement of the latter. Morphologically, both are characterized by an anastomosing proliferation of woven bone rimmed by plump osteoblasts with an intervening paucicellular stroma rich in thin-walled, often dilated blood vessels. These lesions often harbor diagnostic rearrangements involving the *FOS* and less frequently *FOSB* gene loci.[8] Although these bone-forming neoplasms may mimic OFD radiographically, their histologic features are distinguished easily from the fibro-osseous appearance of OFD, and further ancillary studies are not generally required.

OFD and OFD-like ADA have very similar, overlapping clinical, radiographic, and histologic features. Both lesions predominantly occur in patients under the age of 20 years and are intracortical.[6,9,10] Histologically, OFD-like ADA closely resembles OFD, but also contains widely scattered, clearly visible small epithelial nests, as opposed to individual keratin–immunoreactive cells typical of OFD. The isolated nests that define OFD-like ADA may be absent in small biopsy samples and are easily overlooked on routine hematoxylin and eosin–stained biopsies. Therefore, we recommend the routine use of cytokeratin immunostains for any OFD-like lesion.

DIAGNOSIS

In the appropriate clinical and radiologic context, the diagnosis of OFD is usually straightforward, presenting as a well-demarcated intracortical lesion involving the tibia and/or fibula of young

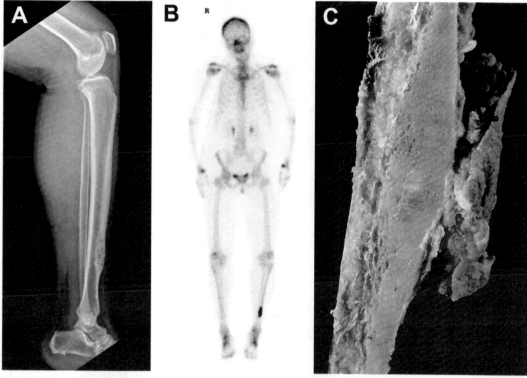

Fig. 3. Radiographic and gross appearance of OFD-like ADA. (*A*) Lateral radiograph showing a fusiform intracortical lesion in the distal tibial diaphysis. The radiolucence in the distal aspect of the lesion is a biopsy tract. (*B*) Scintigraphy demonstrates intense uptake of isotope in the lesion. (*C*) Gross photograph of the resection specimen shows a fusiform, intracortical lesion with a densely ossified cut surface. The oval tan area in the center of the tumor is a cement plug indicating the site of prior biopsy.

patients, showing fibro-osseous morphology with irregular woven bone rimmed by osteoblasts.

PROGNOSIS

The somewhat overlapping clinical, radiologic, and histologic features of OFD, OFD-like ADA, and classic ADA have long raised the possibility of whether these entities belong within a morphologic and clinical continuum, and whether OFD may represent a precursor lesion to ADA.[5,6,9,11–16] This concept has been further questioned because of the documentation of trisomies 7, 8, and 12 in both OFD and ADA.[6,13] However, to date, no confirmed progression from OFD into ADA has been documented persuasively in the literature.[5,6,11,12,15]

OFD lesions may gradually increase in size during the first decade of life. However, the majority ultimately show stabilization or even spontaneous regression around the time of skeletal maturity. Recurrences may be noted after curettage.[15–17] Therefore, surgery should be offered to select symptomatic patients only.[15–17] OFD shows no potential for the development of distant metastases.

SUMMARY

OFD is a benign fibro-osseous neoplasm affecting the anterior cortex of the tibia and/or fibula of young patients. It is a circumscribed lesion characterized by the proliferation of small and irregular trabeculae of woven bone embedded in a bland storiform spindle cell background. Although some features of this lesion may overlap with those of OFD-like ADA, no definitive progression of OFD to ADA has been documented. OFD may spontaneously regress after puberty or develop local nondestructive recurrences, but there is no potential for distant metastases. Symptomatic patients may be treated surgically.

CLINICS CARE POINTS

- OFD is a benign fibro-osseous neoplasm that arises almost exclusively in the anterior cortex of the tibia and/or fibula of children and adolescents.

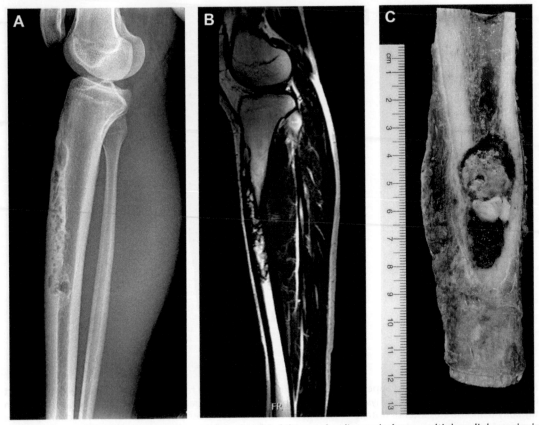

Fig. 4. Radiographic and gross appearance of classic ADA. (*A*) Lateral radiograph shows multiple radiolucencies in the anterior tibial cortex, imparting a "soap bubble" appearance. Medullary cavity invasion is present distally. (*B*) MRI highlights the cortical and medullary cavity involvement of the lesion. (*C*) Grossly, the residual adamantinoma has a fleshy and hemorrhagic cut surface. The white structure in the center of the lesion is a cement plug from a prior biopsy.

- Pain is the most common presenting symptom.
- Morphologically, it is characterized by a benign spindle cell proliferation associated with haphazardly arranged woven bone trabeculae rimmed by osteoblasts.
- Keratin positivity may be noted in rare isolated stromal cells.
- OFD may regress spontaneously, and surgery is reserved for selected symptomatic patients.

ADAMANTINOMA

ADA of the long bones is an extraordinarily rare primary bone neoplasm accounting for approximately 0.5% of all bone malignancies.[18,19] It is regarded in the current World Health Organization Classification of Tumors as a biphasic, locally aggressive or low-grade malignancy.[19] Three major histologic subtypes are recognized: OFD-like ADA (also known as "differentiated" or "juvenile" ADA), classic ADA, and dedifferentiated ADA. Although these subtypes have overlapping clinical

and radiologic features, they differ in their morphologic appearance and outcomes.

Similar to OFD, ADA occurs almost exclusively in the anterior cortex of the diaphysis, and less frequently involves the metaphysis, of the tibia, with a subset of patients also having isolated or concurrent involvement of the fibula.[9,20–32] Rarely, this tumor has reportedly arisen in other bones, such as the humerus, ulna, and radius, among others.[9,20–32] Patients diagnosed with classic ADA are generally within the third and fourth decades of life, whereas those with OFD-like ADA are younger, often within the same age range as patients with OFD.[9] Males are slightly more commonly affected than females.[9,20–32] The clinical presentation is similar to that of OFD, with pain, a palpable mass, and bony deformity as the most commonly reported symptoms. Pathologic fractures may occur.[23] These symptoms may be present for many years before the pathologic diagnosis.[9,20–32]

On conventional radiographs, ADA appears as a well-demarcated, lobulated, radiolucent lesion

Fig. 5. Morphologic spectrum of classic ADA (all medium power, hematoxylin and eosin stain). (A) Tubular architecture. (B) Basaloid appearance with peripheral palisading of cells. (C) Squamous differentiation. (D) Spindled cytomorphology mimicking synovial sarcoma.

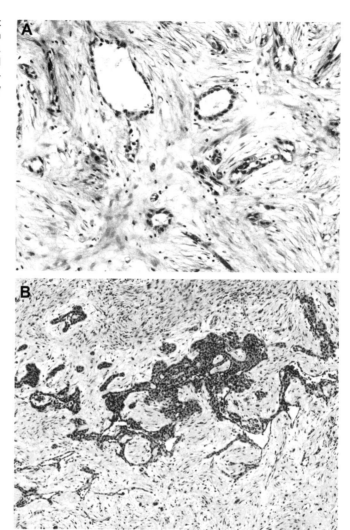

within cortical bone (**Fig. 4**), imparting a "soap bubble" appearance.[23,33] Skip lesions and/or multicentric lesions involving the tibia and/or fibula may be present. Unlike OFD, ADA may breach the cortex, extending into the medullary cavity or adjacent soft tissues. A computed tomography scan and MRI are useful for documenting multifocality, cortical destruction, and soft tissue extension.

GROSS FEATURES

Macroscopically, most examples are solid, well-demarcated, lobulated lesions, with tan–white cut surfaces, although solid and cystic tumors are sometimes noted. Tumors are typically centered within the cortex with variable involvement of the medullary space or extraperiosteal soft tissue. Tumor size varies from less than 1 cm to greater than 10 cm.

MICROSCOPIC FEATURES

Classic ADA is characterized by a predominant epithelial component, embedded in an inconspicuous OFD-like bland spindled or fibro-osseous stroma. The epithelial component forms nests, large anastomosing groups, or sheets of monomorphic cells, displaying tubular or glandular structures (**Fig. 5**A), basaloid architecture with peripheral palisading of neoplastic cells (**Fig. 5**B),

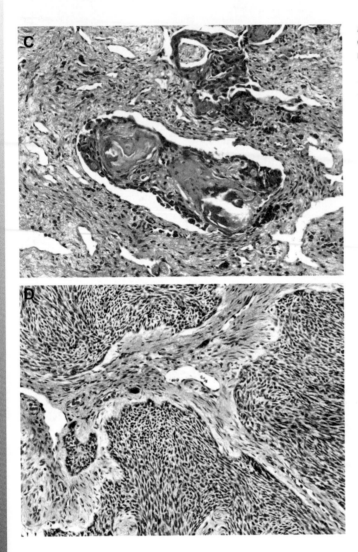

Fig. 5. (*continued*). (*C*) Squamous differentiation. (*D*) Spindled cytomorphology mimicking synovial sarcoma.

squamous differentiation with associated keratinization (**Fig. 5**C), or, least commonly, spindled cytomorphology (**Fig. 5**D) reminiscent of synovial sarcoma. Mitotic activity is usually inconspicuous, and nuclear atypia is not a prominent feature.

As mentioned elsewhere in this article, OFD-like ADA shows considerable morphologic overlap with OFD. Unlike OFD, OFD-like ADA is defined by inconspicuous small nests of epithelial cells embedded in a predominately OFD-like stroma (**Fig. 6**). In most cases, these epithelial nests are not obvious on hematoxylin and eosin–stained sections, may resemble small blood vessels, and are identified only with a keratin immunostain. Therefore, a keratin immunostain should be applied to all OFD-like lesions to aid in distinguishing OFD from OFD-like ADA. The demonstration of

any group or groups of epithelial cells excludes a diagnosis of OFD. Similarly, when an epithelial component is conspicuous at low magnification on hematoxylin and eosin–stained sections, a diagnosis of conventional ADA should be considered.

Dedifferentiated ADA is an extremely rare variant that is defined by the abrupt transition of classic ADA morphology into a less differentiated, usually pleomorphic sarcoma, losing epithelial differentiation and gaining increased mitoses. Osteoid or chondroid matrix may be identified in the dedifferentiated foci.[34]

Immunohistochemical stains for broad spectrum and basal epithelial-type cytokeratins, epithelial membrane antigen, p63, and podoplanin may be used for the diagnosis of ADA.[35,36]

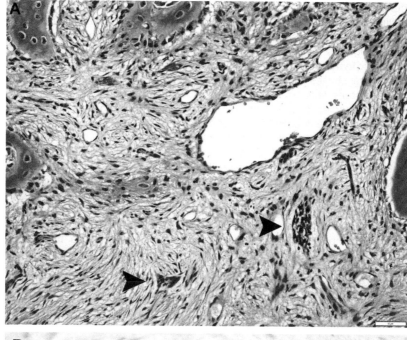

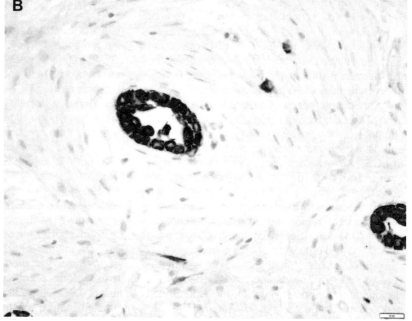

Fig. 6. Histologic features of OFD-like ADA. (*A*) Low magnification shows rare epithelial nests in a predominately OFD-like background (hematoxylin and eosin stain). (*B*) An immunostain for cytokeratin AE1/3 is often necessary to highlight the rare epithelial nests in OFD-like ADA, as seen in this example.

DIFFERENTIAL DIAGNOSIS

The main differential diagnosis of OFD-like ADA is OFD, as discussed elsewhere in this article. Classic ADA should be distinguished from intraosseous synovial sarcoma, ADA-like Ewing sarcoma, and metastatic carcinoma.

Synovial sarcoma is an aggressive sarcoma with a predilection for the soft tissues of the lower extremities of young adults. It harbors the pathognomonic t(X;18) (p11;q11) translocation, resulting in SS18-SSX fusions. Similar to its soft tissue counterpart, rare intraosseous examples of synovial sarcoma are characterized by a monomorphic fascicular proliferation of spindle cells with overlapping oval shaped nuclei, vesicular chromatin, inconspicuous nucleoli, and scant pale eosinophilic cytoplasm. In a recent study, Horvai and colleagues[37] demonstrated a subset of tumors initially diagnosed as spindle cell ADA represent primary intraosseous synovial sarcoma. The differential diagnosis with classic ADA based solely on histologic features may be difficult and immunohistochemical studies using cytokeratins and epithelial membrane antigen are of little use, because these antibodies lack specificity and are also expressed by the neoplastic cells of synovial sarcoma in variable extent. More recently, 2 antibodies, namely, SS18-SSX fusion-specific antibody (E9X9V) and an SSX-specific antibody (E5A2C), have been shown to have more than 95% specificity and sensitivity for the diagnosis of synovial sarcoma in a large cohort of neoplasms.[38] However, the expression of these markers in the epithelial component of ADA is unknown. In difficult cases, fluorescence in situ hybridization using SS18 break apart probes or molecular studies for the SS18–SSX fusion can be performed.

ADA-like Ewing sarcoma is a rare variant of Ewing sarcoma, initially reported in 1975 by van Haelst and de Haas van Dorsser[39] and further characterized by Bridge and colleagues in 1999.[40] Ewing sarcoma is included in the category of aggressive small round cell sarcomas with rearrangements leading to FET–ETS fusion genes in all cases. Although soft tissue examples are seen, this neoplasm affects primarily the long bones, pelvis, and ribs. Classic examples of Ewing sarcoma are characterized by a monotonous proliferation of round cells with inconspicuous intervening stroma. However, several other morphologic variants have been described including, but not limited to, PNET, ADA-like, spindle cell sarcoma-like, sclerosing, and large cell (or "atypical Ewing sarcoma").[41–43] The ADA-like variant of Ewing sarcoma has been described more often in the head and neck region, but may also be encountered in the long bones of the leg, mimicking ADA.[41–45] Histologically, it shows nests or anastomosing trabeculae of epithelial-like cells with peripheral nuclear palisading, embedded in a desmoplastic fibrotic stroma. Overt keratinization and squamous pearls may be present. As expected, this variant displays diffuse and strong membranous expression of CD99, in addition to cytokeratins and p40.[41–45] Given the considerable differences in treatment and prognosis between ADA and Ewing sarcoma, cytogenetic, and/or molecular studies should strongly be considered when the diagnosis is uncertain. Similar to conventional or classic Ewing sarcoma, the ADA-like Ewing sarcoma variant also shows the characteristic EWSR1–FLI1 gene fusion.[41–45]

Finally, classic ADA and its squamous, tubular, or basaloid epithelial elements may be mistaken for metastatic carcinoma. Immunohistochemistry is not useful in distinguishing these lesions; however, careful attention to the cortical location in the tibia (or fibula), younger patient age, and overall histologic features should point to a diagnosis of ADA. In select cases in older individuals, a thorough clinicoradiographic evaluation for a primary neoplasm may be necessary before a diagnosis of classic ADA is rendered.

DIAGNOSIS

The diagnosis of ADA relies on identifying a bland biphasic fibro-osseous low-grade malignant neoplasm arising in the cortex of long bones, almost exclusively involving the tibia and/or fibula, within the appropriate clinicoradiologic setting. Immunohistochemical stains may confirm the epithelial nature of the neoplastic nests of tumor cells. Specific cytogenetic and/or molecular studies may be necessary to rule out other neoplasms, sharing clinical and histologic features.

PROGNOSIS

ADA and its variants are resistant to chemotherapy and radiation therapy; the treatment of choice is surgery. OFD-like ADA shows a local recurrence rate between 14% and 22%, with no propensity to metastasize.[32,46] Therefore, it is probably best considered a locally aggressive disease. Rare cases have been reported to show classic ADA histology in the recurrence, although it is unclear whether this represents true progression from OFD-like ADA or under-recognition (or sampling error) of classic ADA at the initial diagnosis.[47] Because OFD-like ADA is locally aggressive and not known to metastasize, surgical treatment strategies have been controversial. Some authors have advocated for clinical observation of OFD-like ADA in young patients, but en bloc resection for any lesion that progresses.[10,48] However, other investigators recently advocated for wide resection of OFD-like ADA despite the comparatively indolent nature of this lesion compared with classic ADA.[32]

In contrast, patients with a diagnosis of classic ADA show a local recurrence rate of approximately 20% after wide excision, and a metastatic rate of 18%.[23,32,46] The main sites of metastatic disease include the lungs and lymph nodes, and less frequently other bones, the liver, and the central nervous system.[23,32,46] The main factor correlated with increased recurrence or metastatic potential is the presence of contaminated or positive surgical margins.[23,32,46] Other factors associated with increased recurrence or metastatic potential include male sex, female sex associated with young age at presentation, a short duration of symptoms, pain, and lack of squamous differentiation.[19] Classic ADA should be managed with wide resection or amputation for unresectable tumors. Few data are available in the literature regarding the therapy and outcome of dedifferentiated ADA, but it is believed to behave more aggressively.[19,34]

SUMMARY

ADA is a locally aggressive, low-grade malignant neoplasm of the bone, affecting mainly patients in the third to fourth decades of life. Similar to OFD, ADA arises mostly within the anterior cortex of the tibia and/or fibula, with potential extension into the medullary compartment and/or extraosseous soft tissues. Three main histologic variants are recognized: OFD-like ADA, classic ADA, and dedifferentiated ADA. The classic variant is characterized by nests and trabeculae of epithelial cells with a diverse morphologic spectrum: tubular, basaloid, squamous, or spindled. The neoplastic cells forming these nests and trabeculae express cytokeratins, epithelial membrane antigen, p63, and podoplanin. The differential diagnosis includes other sarcomas, such as SS or ADA-like Ewing sarcoma, and metastatic carcinoma. Rarely, the use of cytogenetics and/or molecular studies may be necessary to separate these lesions. Given the potential for local recurrence and metastasis, excision with negative margins represents the gold standard for the treatment of classic ADA.

CLINICS CARE POINTS

- ADA is a rare malignant neoplasm of the bone, occurring almost exclusively in the tibia and/or fibula.

- Classic ADA affects patients within the third and fourth decades of life, whereas patients with OFD-like ADA are typically younger.

- The neoplasm is usually centered in the cortex, within the diaphyseal region, but extension into the medullary cavity and/or soft tissues, with cortical disruption, may be present.

- Three main histologic subtypes are recognized: classic, OFD-like, and dedifferentiated.

- Morphologically, tumors are biphasic and composed of nests and trabeculae of epithelial cells embedded in a variably conspicuous OFD-like stroma.

- Classic ADA may locally recur (20% cases) and less commonly metastasize to the lungs and lymph nodes.

DISCLOSURE

The authors have nothing to disclose.

REFERENCES

1. Frangenheim P. Angeborene Ostitis fibrosa als Ursache einer intrauterinen Unterschenkelfraktur. Arch Klin Chir 1921;117:22–9.
2. Semian DW, Willis JB, Bove KE. Congenital fibrous defect of the tibia mimicking fibrous dysplasia. J Bone Joint Surg Am 1975;57:854–7.
3. Kempson RL. Ossifying fibroma of the long bones. A light and electron microscopic study. Arch Pathol 1966;82:218–33.
4. Campanacci M. Osteofibrous dysplasia of long bone. A new clinical entity. Ital J Orthop Traumatol 1976;2:221–37.
5. Park YK, Unni K, McLeod RA, et al. Osteofibrous dysplasia: clinicopathologic study of 80 cases. Hum Pathol 1993;24:1339–47.
6. Gleason BC, Liegl-Atzwanger B, Kozakewich HP, et al. Osteofibrous dysplasia and adamantinoma in children and adolescents: a clinicopathologic reappraisal. Am J Surg Pathol 2008;32:363–76.
7. Tabareau-Delalande F, Collin C, Gomez-Brouchet A, et al. Diagnostic value of investigating GNAS mutations in fibro-osseous lesions: a retrospective study of 91 cases of fibrous dysplasia and 40 other fibro-osseous lesions. Mod Pathol 2013;26:911–21.
8. Fittall MW, Mifsud W, Pillay N, et al. Recurrent rearrangements of FOS and FOSB define osteoblastoma. Nat Commun 2018;9:2150.
9. Czerniak B, Rojas-Corona RR, Dorfman HD. Morphologic diversity of long bone adamantinoma. The concept of differentiated (regressing) adamantinoma and its relationship to osteofibrous dysplasia. Cancer 1989;64:2319–34.
10. Kuruvilla G, Steiner GC. Osteofibrous dysplasia-like adamantinoma of bone: a report of five cases with immunohistochemical and ultrastructural studies. Hum Pathol 1998;29:809–14.
11. Sweet DE, Vinh TN, Devaney K. Cortical osteofibrous dysplasia of long bone and its relationship to adamantinoma. A clinicopathologic study of 30 cases. Am J Surg Pathol 1992;16:282–90.
12. Ishida T, Iijima T, Kikuchi F, et al. A clinicopathological and immunohistochemical study of osteofibrous dysplasia, differentiated adamantinoma, and adamantinoma of long bones. Skeletal Radiol 1992;21:493–502.
13. Hazelbag HM, Wessels JW, Mollevangers P, et al. Cytogenetic analysis of adamantinoma of long

bones: further indications for a common histogenesis with osteofibrous dysplasia. Cancer Genet Cytogenet 1997;97:5–11.

14. Maki M, Athanasou N. Osteofibrous dysplasia and adamantinoma: correlation of proto-oncogene product and matrix protein expression. Hum Pathol 2004; 35:69–74.

15. Schofield DW, Sadozai Z, Ghali C, et al. Does osteofibrous dysplasia progress to adamantinoma and how should they be treated? Bone Joint J 2017; 99B:409–16.

16. Park JW, Lee C, Han I, et al. Optimal treatment of osteofibrous dysplasia of the tibia. J Pediatr Orthop 2018;38:e404–10.

17. Westacott D, Kannu P, Stimec J, et al. Osteofibrous dysplasia of the tibia in children: outcome without resection. J Pediatr Orthop 2019;39:e614–21.

18. Nielsen GP, Rosenberg AE. Adamantinoma. In: Diagnostic pathology: bone. 2nd edition. Salt Lake City, UT: Elsevier, Inc; 2017. p. 386–91.

19. Nielsen GP, Hogendoorn PCW. Adamantinoma of long bones. In: WHO classification of tumours. Soft tissue and bone tumours. 5th edition. Lyon, France: IARC; 2020. p. 463–6.

20. Huvos AG, Marcove RC. Adamantinoma of long bones. A clinicopathologic study of fourteen cases with vascular origin suggested. J Bone Joint Surg Am 1975;57:148–54.

21. Weiss SW, Dorfman HD. Adamantinoma of long bones. An analysis of nine new cases with emphasis on metastasizing lesions and fibrous dysplasia-like changes. Hum Pathol 1977;8:141–53.

22. Campanacci M, Giunti A, Bertoni F, et al. Adamantinoma of the long bones. The experience at the Instituto Ortopedico Rizzoli. Am J Surg Pathol 1981;5: 533–42.

23. Keeney GL, Unni KK, Beabout JW, et al. Adamantinoma of long bones. A clinicopathologic study of 85 cases. Cancer 1989;64:730–7.

24. Hazelbag HM, Taminiau AH, Fleuren GJ, et al. Adamantinoma of long bones. A clinicopathological study of thirty-two patients with emphasis on histological subtype, precursor lesion, and biological behavior. J Bone Joint Surg Am 1994;76:1482–99.

25. Jundt G, Remberger K, Roessner A, et al. Adamantinoma of long bones. A histopathological and immunohistochemical study of 23 cases. Pathol Res Pract 1995;191:112–20.

26. Desai SS, Jambhekar N, Agarwal M, et al. Adamantinoma of tibia: a study of 12 cases. J Surg Oncol 2006;93:429–33.

27. Van Rijn R, Bras J, Schaap G, et al. Adamantinoma in childhood: report of six cases and review of the literature. Pediatr Radiol 2006;36:1068–74.

28. Szendroi M, Antal I, Arató G. Adamantinoma of long bones: a long-term follow-up study of 11 cases. Pathol Oncol Res 2009;15:209–16.

29. Houdek MT, Sherman CE, Inwards CY, et al. Adamantinoma of bone: long-term follow-up of 46 consecutive patients. J Surg Oncol 2018;118: 1150–4.

30. Aytekin MN, Öztürk R, Amer K. Epidemiological study of adamantinoma from US surveillance, epidemiology, and end results program: III retrospective analysis. J Oncol 2020;8.

31. Schwarzkopf E, Tavarez Y, Healey JH, et al. Adamantinomatous tumors: long-term follow-up study of 20 patients treated at a single institution. J Surg Oncol 2020;122:273–82.

32. Schutgens EM, Picci P, Baumhoer D, et al. Surgical outcome and oncological survival of osteofibrous dysplasia-like and classic adamantinomas: an international multicenter study of 318 cases. J Bone Joint Surg Am 2020;102:1703–13.

33. Khanna M, Delaney D, Tirabosco R, et al. Osteofibrous dysplasia, osteofibrous dysplasia-like adamantinoma and adamantinoma: correlation of radiological imaging features with surgical histology and assessment of the use of radiology in contributing to needle biopsy diagnosis. Skeletal Radiol 2008;37:1077–84.

34. Hazelbag HM, Laforga JB, Roels HJL, et al. Dedifferentiated adamantinoma with revertant mesenchymal phenotype. Am J Surg Pathol 2003;27:1530–7.

35. Kashima TG, Dongre A, Flanagan AM, et al. Podoplanin expression in adamantinoma of long bones and osteofibrous dysplasia. Virchows Arch 2011; 459:416–46.

36. Dickson BG, Gortzak Y, Bell RS, et al. p63 expression in adamantinoma. Virchows Arch 2011;459:109–13.

37. Horvai A, Dashti NK, Rubin BP, et al. Genetic and molecular reappraisal of spindle cell adamantinoma of bone reveals a small subset of misclassified intraosseous synovial sarcoma. Mod Pathol 2019;32:231–41.

38. Baranov E, McBride MJ, Bellizzi AM, et al. A novel SS18-SSX fusion-specific antibody for the diagnosis of synovial sarcoma. Am J Surg Pathol 2020;44: 922–33.

39. van Haelst UJ, de Haas van Dorsser AH. A perplexing malignant bone. Highly malignant so-called adamantinoma or non-typical Ewing's sarcoma. Virchows Arch A Pathol Anat Histol 1975;365:63–74.

40. Bridge JA, Fidler ME, Neff JR, et al. Adamantinoma-like Ewing's sarcoma: genomic confirmation, phenotypic drift. Am J Surg Pathol 1999;23:159–65.

41. Folpe AL, Goldblum JR, Rubin BP, et al. Morphologic and immunophenotypic diversity in Ewing family tumors: a study of 66 genetically confirmed cases. Am J Surg Pathol 2005;29:1025–33.

42. Llombart-Bosch A, Machado I, Navarro S, et al. Histological heterogeneity of Ewing's sarcoma/PNET: an immunohistochemical analysis of 415 genetically confirmed cases with clinical support. Virchows Arch 2009;445:397–411.

43. Rekhi B, Shetty O, Vora T, et al. Clinicopathologic, immunohistochemical, molecular cytogenetic profile with treatment and outcomes of 34 cases of Ewing sarcoma with epithelial differentiation, including 6 cases with "Adamantinoma-like" features, diagnosed at a single institution, India. Ann Diagn Pathol 2020;49: 151625.

44. Bishop JA, Alaggio R, Zhang L, et al. Adamantinoma-like Ewing family tumors of the head and neck: a pitfall in the differential diagnosis of basaloid and myoepithelial carcinomas. Am J Surg Pathol 2015;39:1267–74.

45. Rooper LM, Jo VY, Antonescu CR, et al. Adamantinoma-like Ewing sarcoma of the salivary glands: a newly recognized mimicker of basaloid salivary carcinomas. Am J Surg Pathol 2019;43:187–94.

46. Deng Z, Gong L, Zhang Q, et al. Outcome of osteofibrous dysplasia-like versus classic adamantinoma of long bones: a single-institution experience. J Orthop Surg Res 2020;15:268.

47. Hatori M, Watanabe M, Hosaka M, et al. A classic adamantinoma arising from osteofibrous dysplasia-like adamantinoma in the lower leg: a case report and review of the literature. Tohoku J Exp Med 2006;209:53–9.

48. Springfield D, Rosenberg A, Mankin H, et al. Relationship between osteofibrous dysplasia and adamantinoma. Clin Orthop Rel Res 1994;309:234–44.

Miscellaneous Tumours of Bone

Vaiyapuri P. Sumathi, MD, FRCPath

KEYWORDS

- Intraosseous-schwannoma • Lipoma • Phosphaturic mesenchymal tumor
- Undifferentiated pleomorphic sarcoma of bone

Key points

- Tumours of non-osseous and non-cartilaginous lineage such as neural, adipocytic, smooth muscle can rarely present as primary bone tumours.
- Metastases from other primary sites always needs to excluded.
- Morphologic features are similar to their soft tissue counterparts.

ABSTRACT

There are several tumors that do not easily fit into the specific classifications of primary bone tumors. These tumors include tumors of neural, adipocytic, smooth muscle lineage, and some of uncertain lineage. The pathologic features with recent updates of these tumors are discussed here.

SCHWANNOMA

Schwannoma of bone accounts for less than 0.2% of all primary bone tumors. The most common sites of involvement are the skull, vertebrae, and sacrum. They are usually solitary and sporadic, but a few are associated with type 2 neurofibromatosis.

IMAGING

The tumors appear as large expansile lytic lesions with well-defined sclerotic margins. On a T1-weighted MRI sequence, the lesion appears hypointense or isointense, and on a T2-weighted MRI sequence, the lesion has a heterogenous hyperintense appearance. Cystic changes may be present, which are nonenhancing on T1-weighted postcontrast sequences.[1,2]

GROSS FEATURES

Intraosseous schwannomas are unencapsulated and have a firm, pale tan, cut surface.

MICROSCOPIC FEATURES

Intraosseous schwannoma, similar to its soft tissue counterpart, consists of benign Schwann cells that vary in cellularity. Nuclear palisades, known as Verocay bodies, are present. The tumor cells are strongly positive for S100 and SOX10 (**Fig. 1**).

DIAGNOSTIC CRITERIA

- Expansile lytic lesion that characteristically shows benign, variably cellular spindle cell tumor that expresses S100 and SOX10.

LIPOMATOUS TUMORS AND HIBERNOMA OF BONE

INTRODUCTION

Lipoma and hibernoma of bone are rare primary tumors of the bone that arise within or on the surface of the bone.

Lipoma tumors and hibernoma of bone constitute less than 0.1% of all bone tumors. The age

Department of Musculoskeletal Pathology, The Royal Orthopaedic Hospital, University Hospitals Birmingham, Robert Aitken Institute of Clinical Research, The Medical School, University of Birmingham, Vincent Drive, Birmingham B15 2TT, UK
E-mail address: vaiyapuri.sumathi@nhs.net

Surgical Pathology 14 (2021) 737–750
https://doi.org/10.1016/j.path.2021.06.013

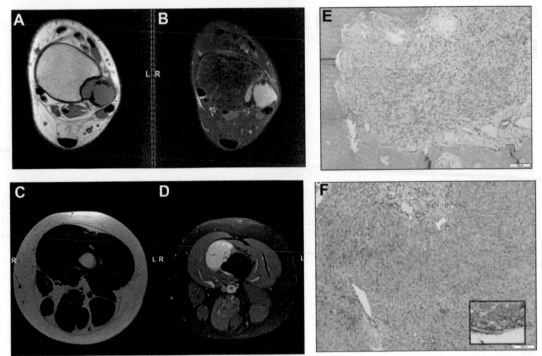

Fig. 1. (*A, B*) Axial T1- and T2-weighted MRIs of an intraosseous schwannoma presenting as a lytic lesion of the distal fibula with cortical breach and extension into soft tissue. (*C, D*) T1-weighted and T2-weighted MRIs of an 8.5-cm periosteal schwannoma arising from the anteromedial aspect of distal femoral diaphysis. (*E, F*) Intraosseous schwannoma of variable cellularity showing nuclear palisades and diffuse S100 positivity (*inset*) [hematoxylin-eosin stain]. L, left; R, right.

range is from the second to the eighth decade, and men are affected more frequently than women. These tumors most commonly occur in the calcaneus and metaphysis of the long bones, particularly of the lower extremities. Parosteal lipoma develops on the diaphysis of the long bones of the extremities. Hibernoma often affects the axial skeleton. They are noted as incidental

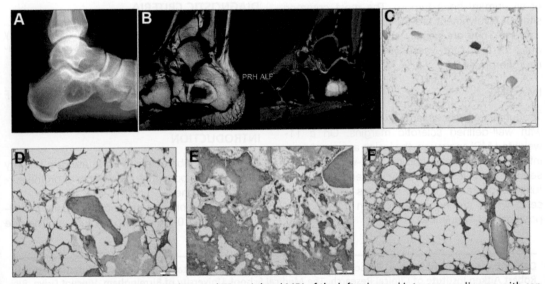

Fig. 2. (*A, B*) Radiograph and sagittal T1- and T2-weighted MRI of the left calcaneal intraosseous lipoma with central nidus like opacity and cystic degeneration. (*C, D*) The lesion consisted of mature adipocytes (hematoxylin-eosin stain)and (*E*) calcified necrotic fat (hematoxylin-eosin stain). (*F*) Areas of degeneration (hematoxylin-eosin stain).

findings on radiographs and are mostly asymptomatic but rarely present with pain.[3-5]

IMAGING

Radiographically, intraosseous lipomas appear of low density on plain radiographs and high signal on T1-weighted MRI with similar intensity to subcutaneous fat. Fat necrosis, cystic degeneration, and calcifications are seen as high density on radiographs and computed tomography (CT) and show signal void on MRI. Hibernoma is characterized by an increased heterogeneous signal on MRI, ill-defined sclerotic appearance on CT, and high uptake of fludeoxyglucose on PET-CT.

GROSS FEATURES

Intraosseous lipomas are well-defined lesions composed of adipose tissue. These tumors are usually less than 5 cm and rarely exceed 10 cm. The bone surrounding the tumor is often sclerotic. An osseous pedicle may be noted in parosteal lipoma.

MICROSCOPIC FEATURES

Intraosseous and parosteal lipoma is composed of lobules of mature adipocytes, which have eccentric nuclei and univacuolated cytoplasm. Foci of fat necrosis with foamy macrophages and dystrophic calcification may be noted (**Fig. 2**). Hibernoma contains brown fat cells, which have multivacuolated and eosinophilic cytoplasm that indents central nuclei. Thin trabecular of woven and lamellar bone may be present within the lesion. Adipocytes are positive for S100, and brown fat is positive for UCP1 (**Fig. 3**).

Liposarcoma of Bone

Primary liposarcoma of bone is extremely rare and has been eliminated for the latest fifth edition of the World Health Organization classification of bone tumors.

Well-differentiated liposarcoma consists of lobules of mature adipocytes with scattered cells with enlarged hyperchromatic and irregular nuclei. Lipoblasts may be present.

Myxoid/round cell liposarcoma consists of mildly atypical ovoid to spindle and round cells

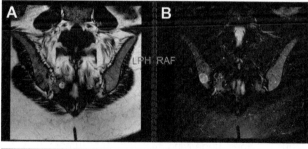
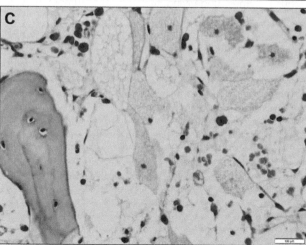
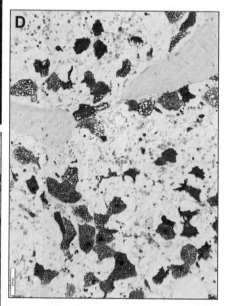

Fig. 3. (*A, B*) Axial T1- and T2-weighted MRIs of 1.5-cm intraosseous hibernoma of the right ilium, (*C*) consisting of multivacuolated brown fat cells (hematoxylin-eosin stain) and (*D*) highlighted by UCP1 (hematoxylin-eosin stain).

with variable numbers of lipoblasts set in a myxoid stroma rich in delicate branching capillary vasculature. Many intraosseous myxoid liposarcomas are metastatic lesions and commonly affect the spinal column[6] (**Fig. 4**). These tumors demonstrate FUS-DDIT3 or EWR1-DDIT3 fusion genes.

Pleomorphic liposarcoma contains a varying proportion of pleomorphic lipoblasts.[7] Very rarely, lipoblastic differentiation may be seen as a component in dedifferentiated chondrosarcoma (**Fig. 5**).

DIFFERENTIAL DIAGNOSIS

Bone infarcts are ill-defined lesions and may have areas of calcifications similar to intraosseous lipoma but can be differentiated by the presence of necrotic host bone.

Parosteal lipoma may mimic osteochondroma radiographically but histologically is distinguishable by the presence of lobules of fat.

ATROPHIC FATTY MARROW CAN RESEMBLE MYXOID LIPOSARCOMA

Diagnostic Criteria

- *Intraosseous lipoma*
    Well-defined tumor consisting of lobules of mature adipocytes
- *Parosteal lipoma*
    Mature adipocytic tumors present on the surface of the bone

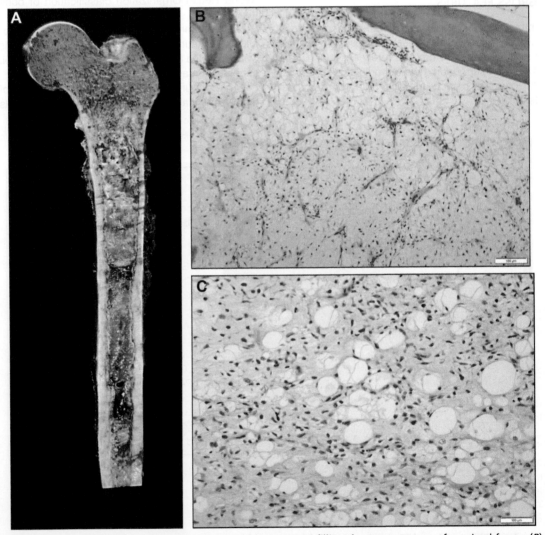

Fig. 4. (*A*) Gross appearance of a metastatic myxoid liposarcoma filling the marrow space of proximal femur. (*B*) Moderately cellular tumor with chicken wire-like arborizing capillary network in a myxoid stroma (hematoxylin-eosin stain). (*C*) Prominent lipoblastic differentiation (hematoxylin-eosin stain).

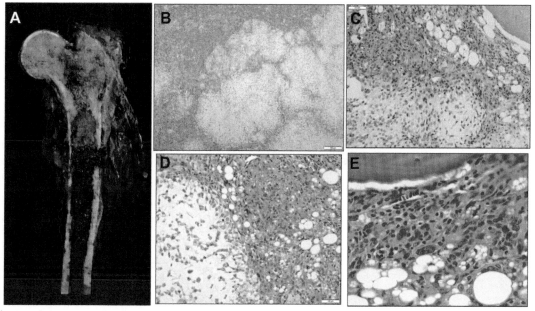

Fig. 5. (A) Gross appearance of proximal femoral dedifferentiated chondrosarcoma with pale yellowish areas. (*B–E*) A biphasic tumor consisting of nodules of grade 2 chondrosarcoma and an abrupt transition to a high-grade pleomorphic liposarcoma with several easily identifiable pleomorphic lipoblasts that contain cytoplasmic lipid droplets that indent the nuclei.

- *Hibernoma*
  Well-defined tumor composed of lobules of brown fat
- *Liposarcoma*
  Most are metastatic and very rarely present as a primary bone tumor

LEIOMYOSARCOMA

INTRODUCTION

Leiomyosarcomas of bone are rare aggressive primary bone sarcomas that show smooth muscle differentiation. Metastases from primary uterine or soft tissue leiomyosarcoma are more common in the bone. These tumors predominantly occur in adults in the third to the fifth decades of life. These tumors usually occur in the long tubular bones of the lower extremities and flat bones of the pelvis and craniofacial skeleton. Pain and pathologic fractures are the most common presenting symptoms.[8–10] Leiomyosarcoma in immunocompromised individuals has been associated with Epstein-Barr virus infection. These tumors have also been associated with familial retinoblastoma syndrome caused by germline mutations of the RB1 gene, and some are related to radiation therapy. Primary leiomyosarcoma of the bone has a high incidence of distant metastases, and 5-year disease-free survival is less than 50%.

IMAGING

Radiographically, these tumors appear as nonspecific lytic, aggressive, and destructive lesions with soft tissue involvement.

GROSS FEATURES

The tumor has a fleshy tan to grayish-white cut surface with areas of necrosis. The margins may be well demarcated but mostly destructive with a soft tissue component.

MICROSCOPIC FEATURES

Similar to leiomyosarcoma of other sites, the lesion is composed of intersecting fascicles of spindle cells that have prominent eosinophilic cytoplasm and elongated blunt-ended nuclei. Nuclear pleomorphism and necrosis are present. Occasionally, osteoclast-like giant cell reaction may be present.

Tumor cells are diffusely and strongly positive with smooth muscle actin (SMA), desmin, and/or h-caldesmon. Focal positivity for keratin is frequently noted (**Fig. 6**).

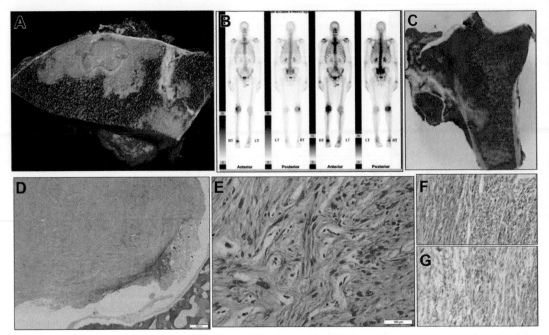

Fig. 6. (*A*) Leiomyosarcoma of ilium adjacent to the sacroiliac joint, which shows a well-circumscribed fibrous tumor. (*B*) Corresponding bone scan, which shows the lesion is solitary. (*C*) Gross appearance of a destructive leiomyosarcoma of the proximal tibia. (*D*, *E*) Interlacing fascicles of atypical smooth muscle cells, which have eosinophilic cytoplasm (hematoxylin-eosin stain). (*F*, *G*) Diffusely positive for smooth muscle actin (SMA) and desmin (hematoxylin-eosin stain).

DIFFERENTIAL DIAGNOSIS

Metastatic leiomyosarcoma is more common than primary leiomyosarcoma of bone, and positivity for estrogen receptor (ER) and progesterone receptor (PR) is strongly suggestive of metastases from a uterine primary.

Primary myofibroblastic sarcoma of bone lacks the characteristic morphologic features of leiomyosarcoma and diffuse strong uniform positivity for smooth muscle immunohistochemical markers.

Metastatic sarcomatoid carcinoma shows strong positivity for epithelial markers.

DIAGNOSTIC CRITERIA

- Exclusion of metastases from other primary sites; characterized by intersecting fascicles of pleomorphic smooth muscle cells; diffuse strong immunoreactivity for SMA, desmin, and/or h-caldesmon.

RHABDOMYOSARCOMA

INTRODUCTION

Primary rhabdomyosarcoma of the bone is extremely rare, and most pediatric cases are metastatic. Rarely, rhabdomyoblastic differentiation may be noted as a divergent differentiation in dedifferentiated chondrosarcoma. Rhabdomyosarcomatous differentiation in osteosarcoma is well recognized.

Embryonal, pleomorphic, and alveolar variants of rhabdomyosarcoma occur in the bone.[11] Radiographically they show lytic destructive features.

MICROSCOPIC FEATURES

Embryonal rhabdomyosarcoma contains primitive mesenchymal cells with a scant amount of amphophilic cytoplasm. Varying stages of muscle differentiation can be seen.

Pleomorphic rhabdomyosarcoma is composed of bizarre, atypical pleomorphic and spindle cells.

The tumor cells typically show diffuse positive immunoreactivity for desmin and variable staining for myogenin and MYOD1 (**Fig. 7**).

MOLECULAR PATHOLOGY

Most alveolar rhabdomyosarcomas harbor PAX3/7-FOXO1. A rare variant of spindle cell rhabdomyosarcoma harbors FUS-TFCP2 (**Fig. 8**).[12]

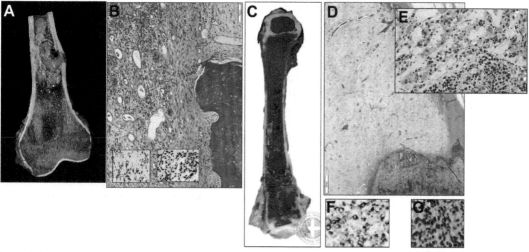

Fig. 7. (*A*) Primary rhabdomyosarcoma of the distal femoral diaphysis, which shows a fleshy tumor. (*B*) Bizarre atypical pleomorphic and spindle cells highlighted with desmin and MYOD1 (*inset*) [hematoxylin-eosin stain]. (*C*) Gross appearance of rhabdomyosarcoma extensively involving the tibia. (*D*) Prominent chemotherapy-induced changes (hematoxylin-eosin stain). (*E*) Varying stages of muscle differentiation are noted (hematoxylin-eosin stain). (*F, G*) Diffusely positive for desmin and MYOD1 (hematoxylin-eosin stain).

DIFFERENTIAL DIAGNOSIS

Rhabdomyosarcomatous differentiation in dedifferentiated chondrosarcoma is well recognized and should be differentiated from primary rhabdomyosarcoma of bone. Mutational analysis for IDH mutation may be helpful to differentiate these entities.

DIAGNOSTIC CRITERIA

- Exclusion of metastases from other primary sites; characterized by primitive mesenchymal cells or pleomorphic cells; diffuse

strong immunoreactivity for desmin, myogenin, and MYOD1.

FIBROCARTILAGINOUS MESENCHYMOMA

INTRODUCTION

Fibrocartilaginous mesenchymoma is a very rare locally aggressive tumor of the bone consisting of mildly atypical cells, nodules of growth platelike cartilage, and bone trabeculae. The tumor usually occurs in the metaphyses of the long bones and rarely involves the pubis, vertebrae, metatarsal

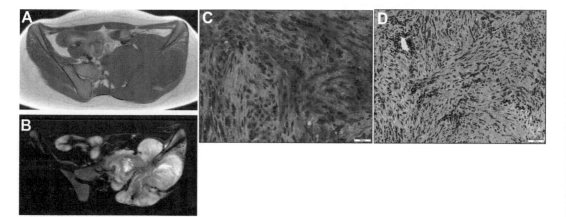

Fig. 8. Axial T1 (*A*) and short tau inversion recovery (*B*) showing large tumor involving the left ilium, crossing the left sacroiliac joint and extending into the left sacral ala and body of the sacrum. (*C, D*) Spindle cell rhabdomyosarcoma of bone showed FUS-TFCP2 gene fusion confirmed by RNA sequencing (hematoxylin-eosin stain).

bones, and ribs.[13] Pain is the most common presenting symptom.

IMAGING

The lesion appears expansile and lytic with foci of calcifications. Cortical destruction is commonly seen. On MRI, the lesion shows low signal intensity on T1-weighted images and high signal intensity on T2-weighted images.

GROSS FEATURES

The tumors have a pale, whitish appearance with glistening bluish-gray areas representing cartilaginous tissue.

MICROSCOPIC FEATURES

Fibrocartilaginous mesenchymoma is composed of fascicles of mildly atypical spindle cells with scattered nodules of hyaline cartilage reminiscent of growth plate, which shows peripheral endochondral ossification. Bony trabeculae of varying sizes are present (**Fig. 9**). The tumor is seen to infiltrate bone and extend into the surrounding soft tissues.

DIFFERENTIAL DIAGNOSIS

Fibrous dysplasia, particularly with cartilaginous nodules, is characterized by curvilinear trabeculae of woven bone surrounded by bland fibroblastic proliferation. Identification of GNAS mutation will help differentiate it from fibrocartilaginous mesenchymoma.

The combination of cartilage and spindle cell components in fibrocartilaginous mesenchymoma may lead to an erroneous diagnosis of dedifferentiated chondrosarcoma, which shows a low-grade cartilaginous tumor with an abrupt transition to high-grade spindle cell sarcoma. Identification of isocitrate dehydrogenase 1 (IDH1) and IDH2 mutation may help differentiate this tumor from fibrocartilaginous mesenchymoma.

The hypercellular fibrous spindle cell component may be mistaken for desmoplastic fibroma, but cartilaginous metaplasia is extremely rare.

DIAGNOSTIC CRITERIA

- Cellular, mildly atypical spindle cells, nodules of growth platelike cartilage, and bone trabeculae.

PHOSPHATURIC MESENCHYMAL TUMOR

INTRODUCTION

Phosphaturic mesenchymal tumors are distinctive neoplasms of the bone that produce FGF23, resulting in tumor-induced osteomalacia. All ages are affected, and any bone may be affected.[14] A germline chromosomal abnormality causing upregulation of α-Klotho may be a predisposing factor.[15] *FN1-FGFR1/FGF1* fusion genes are common in these tumors.

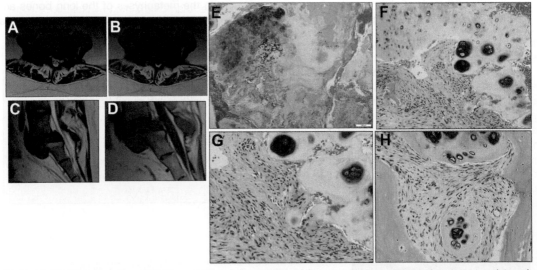

Fig. 9. (*A–D*) Coronal and sagittal T1- and T2-weighted MRIs of fibrocartilaginous mesenchymoma involving the whole vertebral body with soft tissue extension. (*E–H*) Cellular spindle cell proliferation admixed with nodules of growth plate-like hyaline cartilaginous nodules and irregular trabeculae of woven bone (hematoxylin-eosin stain).

Pain may be the presenting symptom, and severe hypophosphatasemia and elevated serum levels of FGF23 are demonstrated.

IMAGING

The tumors appear hyperintense on T2-weighted imaging and show marked homogeneous enhancement on T1-weighted images with contrast on MRI.

GROSS FEATURES

Phosphaturic mesenchymal tumors present as nonspecific masses, and some may contain gritty calcification. Cystic change may be noted.

MICROSCOPIC FEATURES

These tumors are composed of bland spindle cells set in a stroma, which usually contains capillary vessels and larger blood vessels arranged in hemangiopericytoma-like pattern or resembling cavernous hemangioma. The matrix is usually characterized by grungy or flocculent calcification. Occasionally, chondromyxoid stroma resembling chondromyxoid fibroma may be present. Collections of osteoclasts, mature fat, primitive cartilage, or osteoid and cystic change may be noted (Fig. 10).

Malignant phosphaturic mesenchymal tumors show overt features of malignancy, which include marked pleomorphism, necrosis, and brisk mitotic activity resembling fibrosarcoma or undifferentiated pleomorphic sarcoma.

Most tumors express FGF23, FGFR1, and/or SSTR2A.

DIFFERENTIAL DIAGNOSIS

Giant cell tumor of bone contains evenly distributed osteoclast type giant cells, and the mononuclear cells express H3.3pGly34Trp(G34W).

Solitary fibrous tumor with a prominent hemangiopericytoma-like vascular pattern may resemble a phosphaturic mesenchymal tumor. Immunohistochemical expression of STAT6 is helpful to differentiate.

Mesenchymal chondrosarcoma consists of primitive spindle to undifferentiated round cells with chondroid differentiation and hemangiopericytoma-like vascular pattern. Demonstration of HEY1-NCOA2 gene fusion is helpful.

Chondromyxoid fibroma has a lobular architecture and is composed of stellate to round cells with increased cellularity and the presence of multinucleated osteoclast-like giant cells toward the periphery of the lobules. The stroma is myxoid and may contain coarse calcification.

DIAGNOSTIC CRITERIA

- Proliferation of bland spindle cells in a rich vascular stroma with matrix and grungy calcification and clinical evidence of hypophosphatasemia and/or osteomalacia.

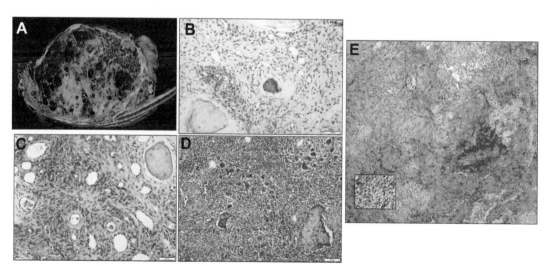

Fig. 10. (A) A large phosphaturic mesenchymal tumor of the rib, which shows solid pale whitish and hemorrhagic cystic areas. (B, C) Bland spindle cell proliferation in a rich vascular network (hematoxylin-eosin stain). (D) Giant cell rich areas (hematoxylin-eosin stain) and (E) large areas of grungy calcification noted; diffuse FGF23 expression (inset) [hematoxylin-eosin stain].

UNDIFFERENTIATED PLEOMORPHIC SARCOMA

INTRODUCTION

Undifferentiated pleomorphic sarcoma of bone is a rare primary bone sarcoma that lacks a specific line of differentiation. These tumors represent less than 2% of all primary malignant bone neoplasms. Tumors commonly arise in the long bones of the lower extremities, particularly the femur, followed by the tibia and humerus.

IMAGING

The tumors appear lytic and have an ill-defined margin and are often associated with cortical destruction and soft tissue extension.

GROSS FEATURES

The cut surface may be grayish-white with a fleshy appearance (**Fig. 11**).

MICROSCOPIC FEATURES

The tumor is composed of fascicles and solid sheets of spindled, epithelioid, and/or large polygonal cells that exhibit marked pleomorphism. Atypical mitoses are readily identified. Multinucleated giant cells, foamy histiocytes, and inflammatory cells are seen admixed with tumor cells. The tumor lacks malignant osteoid or cartilage.

MOLECULAR PATHOLOGY

Somatic gene fusions, CLTC-VMP1 and FARP1-STK24, appear to be recurrent and are characterized by activation of the FGF23 pathway.[16]

DIFFERENTIAL DIAGNOSIS

Dedifferentiated chondrosarcoma is characterized by nodules of hyaline cartilaginous tumor, which shows an abrupt transition to high-grade sarcoma. These tumors may harbor IDH1 or IDH2 mutation.[17]

DIAGNOSTIC CRITERIA

- Fascicles of pleomorphic spindle cells that lack any specific line of differentiation.

MYOEPITHELIOMA

INTRODUCTION

Myoepithelioma of bone is an extremely rare primary bone tumor and has been reported to arise in long bones, pelvis, mandible, vertebra, and small bones of the feet.

GROSS FEATURES

These tumors may have a gelatinous or fleshy appearance. Cortical destruction with soft tissue extension may be noted (**Fig. 12**).

MICROSCOPIC FEATURES

These tumors show varied morphologic features and are often composed of cords, nests, and/or

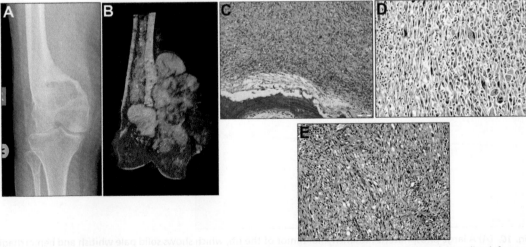

Fig. 11. (*A*) Plain radiograph of a destructive undifferentiated pleomorphic sarcoma involving distal femoral metadiaphysis. (*B*) Gross appearance of the tumor has a lobulated fleshy cut surface with areas of necrosis. (*C–E*) Fascicles and solid sheets of atypical spindled and bizarre tumor cells are noted (hematoxylin-eosin stain).

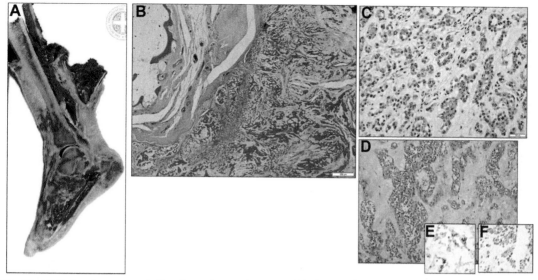

Fig. 12. (*A*) Below knee amputation for a destructive myoepithelioma of the cuboid bone with secondary soft tissue involvement. (*B–D*) Lobules of bland ovoid to epithelioid cells arranged in cords and nests in a prominent myxoid stroma (hematoxylin-eosin stain). (*E*) CAM5.2 (hematoxylin-eosin stain) and (*F*) S100-positive (hematoxylin-eosin stain).

solid sheets of epithelioid to ovoid cells set in a variable amount of myxoid, hyalinized, or sclerotic stroma. Many of the tumors express broad-spectrum keratins and S100, including EMA, GFAP, and SOX10.

MOLECULAR PATHOLOGY

Molecular pathology includes an EWSR1/FUS gene rearrangement involving POU5F1, PBX3, PBX1, ZNF444, KLF15, and KLF17.[18]

DIFFERENTIAL DIAGNOSIS

Metastatic carcinoma lacks positivity for S100 and SOX10.

Chordoma is characterized by large physaliphorous cells, which express brachyury and cytokeratin.

DIAGNOSTIC CRITERIA

- Cords, nests, and/or solid sheets of spindled to epithelioid cells set in a myxoid/hyalinized stroma that expresses keratin and S100, SOX10, or GFAP.

SCLEROSING EPITHELIOID FIBROSARCOMA

INTRODUCTION

Primary sclerosing epithelioid fibrosarcoma of bone is an extremely rare bone tumor and is characterized by cords, nests, or sheets of monotonous epithelioid cells within a dense collagenous background. These tumors may involve any bone and have been described in the long bones, vertebrae, and jaw bones.[19]

IMAGING

These tumors appear as lytic expansile lesions mostly surrounded by sclerotic rims.

GROSS FEATURES

The tumors have a solid, homogeneous, cream- to white-colored cut surface devoid of hemorrhage or necrosis (**Fig. 13**).

MICROSCOPIC FEATURES

These tumors are characterized by solid sheets of monotonous small to medium-sized epithelioid cells with round nuclei and narrow, pale, eosinophilic to clear cytoplasm embedded within a heavily collagenized sclerotic stroma. The tumor cells express MUC4 together with EMA and SMA.

MOLECULAR PATHOLOGY

The tumor cells harbor gene fusion, and the most frequent are EWSR1-CREB3L1. FUS/PAX5 and CREB3L2, CREB3L3, or CREM may be involved.

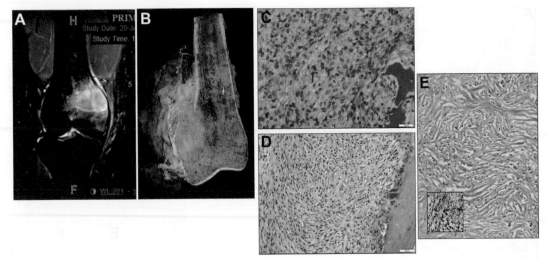

Fig. 13. (*A*) Sagittal T1-weighted MRI of a sclerosing epithelioid fibrosarcoma of the distal femoral metadiaphysis. (*B*) Gross specimen showing a fleshy ill-defined fibrous tumor. (*C, D*) Cords and nests of epithelioid cells with round to oval nuclei set in a densely sclerotic stroma (hematoxylin-eosin stain). (*E*) Hyalinized/sclerotic stroma mimicking osteoid; diffuse strong expression of MUC4 (*inset*) [hematoxylin-eosin stain].

Differential Diagnosis

Osteoblastic osteosarcoma shows significant pleomorphism and lacks MUC4 expression and EWS gene rearrangement.

DIAGNOSTIC CRITERIA

- Densely hyalinized sclerotic tumor, which contains cords and nests of epithelioid fibroblasts; diffuse expression of MUC4.

SOLITARY FIBROUS TUMOR

INTRODUCTION

Solitary fibrous tumors of bone are extremely rare fibroblastic tumors characterized by the presence of staghorn-shaped branching blood vessels. Primary solitary fibrous tumors have been described in the long bones and the vertebrae.[20] Pain and pathologic fracture may be presenting symptoms.

IMAGING

On imaging, the tumor is lytic, and MRI shows variable intensity on T1- and T2-weighted images.

GROSS FEATURES

The tumors have a fleshy tan-colored appearance and may show hemorrhagic and cystic areas (**Fig. 14**).

MICROSCOPIC FEATURES

These tumors consist of haphazardly arranged spindled cells set in a variable collagenous stroma, which contains branching and hyalinized staghorn-shaped blood vessels exhibiting a hemangiopericytomatous pattern. The tumor cells characteristically express CD34 and STAT6.[21]

MOLECULAR PATHOLOGY

NAB2-STAT6 gene fusions are pathognomonic for solitary fibrous tumor.

DIFFERENTIAL DIAGNOSIS

Bone metastases of malignant or meningeal solitary fibrous tumor must be excluded.

The hyalinized stroma in solitary fibrous tumor may mimic osteoid in osteosarcoma. Osteosarcomas lack expression of CD34 and STAT6. NAB2-STAT6 gene fusion is absent in osteosarcoma.

DIAGNOSTIC CRITERIA

- Spindle cells disposed in a random pattern in a variable collagenous stroma; expression of CD34 and/or STAT6. NAB2-STAT6 gene fusion is pathognomonic.

MALIGNANT MESENCHYMOMA

Primary malignant mesenchymoma of bone is an extremely rare malignant tumor that shows 2 or

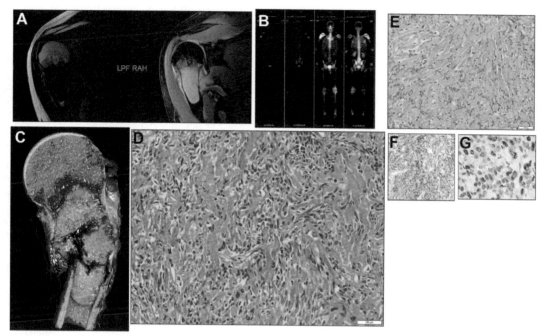

Fig. 14. (*A*) sagittal T1- and T2-weighted MRIs of solitary fibrous tumor of the proximal humerus. (*B*) The lesion is solitary on bone scan. (*C*) Pathologic fracture through a fleshy tumor with hemorrhagic areas. (*D*) Haphazardly arranged ovoid to spindle cells in a collagenous stroma (hematoxylin-eosin stain). (*E*) Extremely collagenous stroma mimicking osteoid (hematoxylin-eosin stain). (*F*) Diffuse expression of CD34 (hematoxylin-eosin stain). (*G*) Nuclear expression of STAT6 (hematoxylin-eosin stain).

more distinct mesenchymal components of divergent differentiation (**Fig. 15**). Tumors that show chondrosarcoma with divergent differentiation are classified as dedifferentiated chondrosarcoma. Osteosarcoma with divergent rhabdomyosarcomatous differentiation is well documented.[22] Some of these tumors have been associated with radiation therapy.

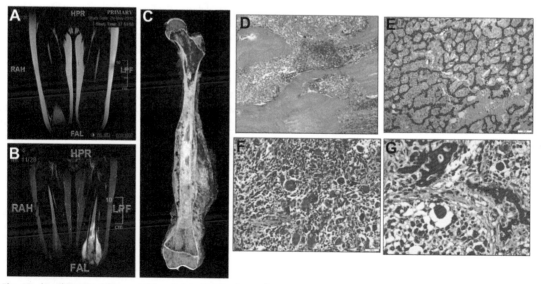

Fig. 15. (*A, B*) Sagittal T1- and T2-weighted MRI of a malignant mesenchymoma involving the entire length of the femur. (*C*) Sagittal section shows an ill-defined pale whitish tumor with a large soft tissue component. (*D–G*) Necrotic permeative tumor with large areas of malignant osteoid production admixed with rhabdomyoblasts (hematoxylin-eosin stain).

DISCLOSURE

The authors have nothing to disclose.

REFERENCES

1. Summers S, Jose J, Barrera CM, et al. Intraosseous schwannomas involving the sacrum: characteristic imaging findings and review of the literature. Neuroradiol J 2018;31(5):531–40.
2. Perera N, de Silva C, Perera V. Large schwannoma of the femur - a common tumor at an unusual site: a case report and review of the literature. J Med Case Rep 2017;11(1):147.
3. Campbell RS, Grainger AJ, Mangham DC, et al. Intraosseous lipoma: report of 35 new cases and a review of the literature. Skeletal Radiol 2003;32(4):209–22.
4. Kang HS, Kim T, Oh S, et al. Intraosseous lipoma: 18 years of experience at a single institution. Clin Orthop Surg 2018;10(2):234–9.
5. Kumar R, Deaver MT, Czerniak BA, et al. Intraosseous hibernoma. Skeletal Radiol 2011;40(5):641–5.
6. Haniball J, Sumathi VP, Kindblom L-G, et al. Prognostic factors and metastatic patterns in primary myxoid/round-cell liposarcoma. Sarcoma 2011; 2011:538085.
7. Torigoe T, Matsumoto T, Terakado A, et al. Primary pleomorphic liposarcoma of bone: MRI findings and review of the literature. Skeletal Radiol 2006;35:536–8.
8. Mori T, Nakayama R, Endo M, et al. Forty-eight cases of leiomyosarcoma of bone in Japan: a multicenter study from the Japanese musculoskeletal oncology group. J Surg Oncol 2016;114(4):495–500.
9. Deyrup, Andrea, Lee VK, et al. Epstein-Barr virus-associated smooth muscle tumors are distinctive mesenchymal tumors reflecting multiple infection events -a clinicopathologic and molecular analysis of 29 tumors from 19 patients. Am J Surg Pathol 2006;30(1):75–82.
10. Brewer P, Sumathi V, Grimer RJ, et al. Primary leiomyosarcoma of bone: analysis of prognosis. Sarcoma 2012;2012:636849.
11. Balogh P, Bánusz R, Csóka M, et al. Primary alveolar rhabdomyosarcoma of the bone: two cases and review of the literature. Diagn Pathol 2016;11(1):99.
12. Dashti NK, Wehrs RN, Thomas BC, et al. Spindle cell rhabdomyosarcoma of bone with FUS-TFCP2 fusion: confirmation of a very recently described rhabdomyosarcoma subtype. Histopathology 2018;73(3): 514–20.
13. Tsuyoshi S, Motoi T, Suehara Y, et al. Fibrocartilaginous mesenchymoma of the tibia with predominant microcystic features: a case report and literature review. Hum Pathol Case Rep 2019;16:100288.
14. Folpe AL. Phosphaturic mesenchymal tumors: a review and update. Semin Diagn Pathol 2019;36(4): 260–8.
15. Lee CH, Su SY, Sittampalam K, et al. Frequent overexpression of klotho in fusion-negative phosphaturic mesenchymal tumors with tumorigenic implications. Mod Pathol 2020;33:858–70.
16. Ali NM, Niada S, Brini AT, et al. Genomic and transcriptomic characterisation of undifferentiated pleomorphic sarcoma of bone. J Pathol 2019;247(2): 166–76.
17. Chen S, Fritchie K, Wei S, et al. Diagnostic utility of IDH1/2 mutations to distinguish dedifferentiated chondrosarcoma from undifferentiated pleomorphic sarcoma of bone. Hum Pathol 2017;65:239–46.
18. Suurmeijer AJH, Dickson BC, Swanson D, et al. A morphologic and molecular reappraisal of myoepithelial tumors of soft tissue, bone, and viscera with EWSR1 and FUS gene rearrangements. Genes Chromosomes Cancer 2020;59(6):348–56.
19. Kosemehmetoglu K, Ardic F, Kilpatrick S, et al. Sclerosing epithelioid fibrosarcoma of bone: morphological, immunophenotypical, and molecular findings of 9 cases. Virchows Arch 2020; 478(4):767–77.
20. Jia C, Crim J, Evenski A, et al. Solitary fibrous tumor of bone developing lung metastases on long-term follow-up. Skeletal Radiol 2020;49:1865–71.
21. Thway K, Ng W, Noujaim J, et al. The current status of solitary fibrous tumor: diagnostic features, variants, and genetics. Int J Surg Pathol 2016;24(4): 281–92.
22. Mrad K, Sassi S, Smida M, et al. Osteosarcoma with rhabdomyosarcomatous component or so-called malignant mesenchymoma of bone. Pathologica 2004;96(6):475–8.

UNITED STATES POSTAL SERVICE ®

Statement of Ownership, Management, and Circulation
(All Periodicals Publications Except Requester Publications)

1. Publication Title	2. Publication Number	3. Filing Date
SURGICAL PATHOLOGY CLINICS	025 – 478	9/18/2021

4. Issue Frequency	5. Number of Issues Published Annually	6. Annual Subscription Price
MAR, JUN, SEP, DEC	4	$228.00

7. Complete Mailing Address of Known Office of Publication (Not printer) (Street, city, county, state, and ZIP+4®)

ELSEVIER INC.
230 Park Avenue, Suite 800
New York, NY 10169

Contact Person
Malathi Samayan
Telephone (Include area code)
215-239-3688

8. Complete Mailing Address of Headquarters or General Business Office of Publisher (Not printer)

ELSEVIER INC.
230 Park Avenue, Suite 800
New York, NY 10169

9. Full Names and Complete Mailing Addresses of Publisher, Editor, and Managing Editor (Do not leave blank)

Publisher (Name and complete mailing address)

DOLORES MELONI, ELSEVIER INC.
1600 JOHN F KENNEDY BLVD. SUITE 1800
PHILADELPHIA, PA 19103-2899

Editor (Name and complete mailing address)

KATERINA HEIDHAUSEN, ELSEVIER INC.
1600 JOHN F KENNEDY BLVD. SUITE 1800
PHILADELPHIA, PA 19103-2899

Managing Editor (Name and complete mailing address)

PATRICK MANLEY, ELSEVIER INC.
1600 JOHN F KENNEDY BLVD. SUITE 1800
PHILADELPHIA, PA 19103-2899

10. Owner (Do not leave blank. If the publication is owned by a corporation, give the name and address of the corporation immediately followed by the names and addresses of all stockholders owning or holding 1 percent or more of the total amount of stock. If not owned by a corporation, give the names and addresses of the individual owners. If owned by a partnership or other unincorporated firm, give its name and address as well as those of each individual owner. If the publication is published by a nonprofit organization, give its name and address.)

Full Name	Complete Mailing Address
WHOLLY OWNED SUBSIDIARY OF REED/ELSEVIER, US HOLDINGS	1600 JOHN F KENNEDY BLVD. SUITE 1800 PHILADELPHIA, PA 19103-2899

11. Known Bondholders, Mortgagees, and Other Security Holders Owning or Holding 1 Percent or More of Total Amount of Bonds, Mortgages, or Other Securities. If none, check box ► ☐ None

Full Name	Complete Mailing Address
N/A	

12. Tax Status (For completion by nonprofit organizations authorized to mail at nonprofit rates) (Check one)
The purpose, function, and nonprofit status of this organization and the exempt status for federal income tax purposes:
☒ Has Not Changed During Preceding 12 Months
☐ Has Changed During Preceding 12 Months (Publisher must submit explanation of change with this statement)

PS Form **3526**, July 2014 [Page 1 of 4 (see instructions page 4)]   PSN: 7530-01-000-9931   PRIVACY NOTICE: See our privacy policy on www.usps.com.

13. Publication Title	14. Issue Date for Circulation Data Below
SURGICAL PATHOLOGY CLINICS	JUNE 2021

15. Extent and Nature of Circulation		Average No. Copies Each Issue During Preceding 12 Months	No. Copies of Single Issue Published Nearest to Filing Date
a. Total Number of Copies (Net press run)		319	306
b. Paid Circulation (By Mail and Outside the Mail)	(1) Mailed Outside-County Paid Subscriptions Stated on PS Form 3541 (Include paid distribution above nominal rate, advertiser's proof copies, and exchange copies)	238	226
	(2) Mailed In-County Paid Subscriptions Stated on PS Form 3541 (Include paid distribution above nominal rate, advertiser's proof copies, and exchange copies)	0	0
	(3) Paid Distribution Outside the Mails Including Sales Through Dealers and Carriers, Street Vendors, Counter Sales, and Other Paid Distribution Outside USPS®	68	67
	(4) Paid Distribution by Other Classes of Mail Through the USPS (e.g., First-Class Mail®)	0	0
c. Total Paid Distribution (Sum of 15b (1), (2), (3), and (4))		296	293
d. Free or Nominal Rate Distribution (By Mail and Outside the Mail)	(1) Free or Nominal Rate Outside-County Copies Included on PS Form 3541	23	13
	(2) Free or Nominal Rate In-County Copies Included on PS Form 3541	0	0
	(3) Free or Nominal Rate Copies Mailed at Other Classes Through the USPS (e.g., First-Class Mail)	0	0
	(4) Free or Nominal Rate Distribution Outside the Mail (Carriers or other means)	0	0
e. Total Free or Nominal Rate Distribution (Sum of 15d (1), (2), (3) and (4))		23	13
f. Total Distribution (Sum of 15c and 15e)		319	306
g. Copies not Distributed (See Instructions to Publishers #4 (page #3))		0	0
h. Total (Sum of 15f and g)		319	306
i. Percent Paid (15c divided by 15f times 100)		92.79%	95.75%

* If you are claiming electronic copies, go to line 16 on page 3. If you are not claiming electronic copies, skip to line 17 on page 3.

16. Electronic Copy Circulation		Average No. Copies Each Issue During Preceding 12 Months	No. Copies of Single Issue Published Nearest to Filing Date
a. Paid Electronic Copies	►		
b. Total Paid Print Copies (Line 15c) + Paid Electronic Copies (Line 16a)	►		
c. Total Print Distribution (Line 15f) + Paid Electronic Copies (Line 16a)	►		
d. Percent Paid (Both Print & Electronic Copies) (16b divided by 16c × 100)	►		

☒ I certify that 50% of all my distributed copies (electronic and print) are paid above a nominal price.

17. Publication of Statement of Ownership
☒ If the publication is a general publication, publication of this statement is required. Will be printed
in the **DECEMBER 2021** issue of this publication.   ☐ Publication not required.

18. Signature and Title of Editor, Publisher, Business Manager, or Owner		Date
Malathi Samayan - Distribution Controller	*Malathi Samayan*	9/18/2021

I certify that all information furnished on this form is true and complete. I understand that anyone who furnishes false or misleading information on this form or who omits material or information requested on the form may be subject to criminal sanctions (including fines and imprisonment) and/or civil sanctions (including civil penalties).

PS Form **3526**, July 2014 (Page 3 of 4)   PRIVACY NOTICE: See our privacy policy on www.usps.com

Moving?

Make sure your subscription moves with you!

To notify us of your new address, find your **Clinics Account Number** (located on your mailing label above your name), and contact customer service at:

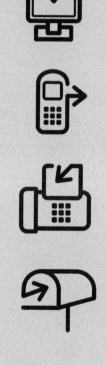

Email: journalscustomerservice-usa@elsevier.com

800-654-2452 (subscribers in the U.S. & Canada)
314-447-8871 (subscribers outside of the U.S. & Canada)

Fax number: 314-447-8029

Elsevier Health Sciences Division
Subscription Customer Service
3251 Riverport Lane
Maryland Heights, MO 63043

*To ensure uninterrupted delivery of your subscription, please notify us at least 4 weeks in advance of move.

ELSEVIER

Printed and bound by CPI Group (UK) Ltd, Croydon, CR0 4YY

03/10/2024

01040370-0009